Ultrasound in Veterinary Medicine

NIPA GENX ELECTRONIC RESOURCES & SOLUTIONS P. LTD.
New Delhi-110 034

About the Editor

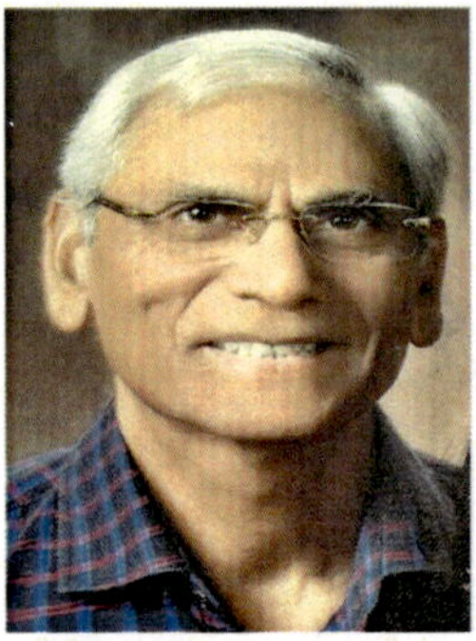

Prof. (Dr.) J.P. Varshney M.V.Sc.; Ph.D. (Veterinary Medicine) has been a best teacher, researcher and clinician of repute who has devoted his entire career to the cause of clinical medicine. Diagnosis of ailing animal has always been his passion. No matter to what extent he has to go in employing diagnostic modalities. He has a vast clinical experience of 55 years of diagnosing and treating the diseases of not only canine, feline, ruminant, equine but also of exotic pet and zoo animals. His inclination of integrating the findings of detail clinical examination, radiography, electrocardiography, echocardiography, ultrasonography and laboratory investigations in disease diagnosis has made him a distinguished clinical scientist of undisputable repute. He is still continuing his yeoman clinical services in alleviating the sufferings of the animals at Nandini Veterinary Hospital, Surat even after 14 years of retirement from Indian Veterinary Research Institute, Izatnagar as Principal Scientist. He is serving as a visiting faculty in veterinary colleges. He has been bestowed with Award of Merit-2001, Award of Honour-2002, Best Teacher Award 2003-2004 (IVRI, Izatnagar), PETCARE Award for Canine Excellence-2005 and Dr. C.M.Singh Memorial Lifetime Achievement Award-2020 besides other 30 awards. He has 390 publications in national/international scientific journals of repute, besides book chapter, bulletins, monographs at his credit. His books "Equine Parasitic Diseases and Their Management (ICAR-IVRI Izatnagar Publication, 2003),"Research Findings -Homeopathic Bio efficacy and Management of Animal Health (Sintex International limited, Kalol, 2007), "Electrocardiography in Veterinary Medicine" (Springer Nature, Singapore, 2020) and "Handbook of Exotic Pet Medicine" (Brillion Publishing, New Delhi, 2021) are the testimony of his clinical acumen ship in the field of clinical veterinary medicine.

About the Contributors

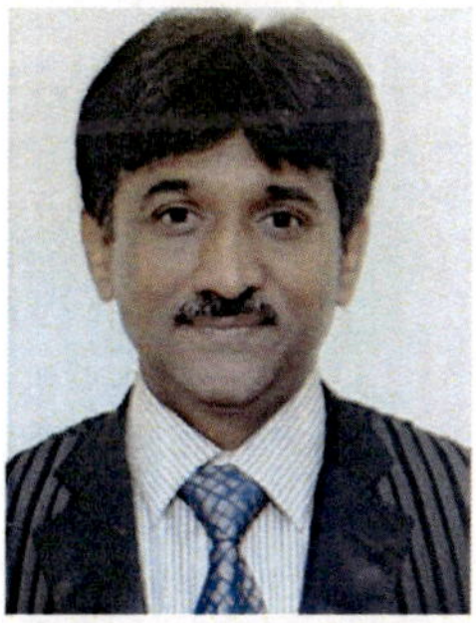

Dr. P.S. Chaudhary, M.V.Sc. (Veterinary surgery and Radiology), a chief surgeon at Nandini Veterinary Hospital, Surat, has a vast experience of imaging techniques and surgical interventions on various species of animals since 2000. He is known among his peer group for his minimum cut surgeries and diagnostic skill using radiography and ultrasound. His clinical publications and presentations have bagged him many awards.

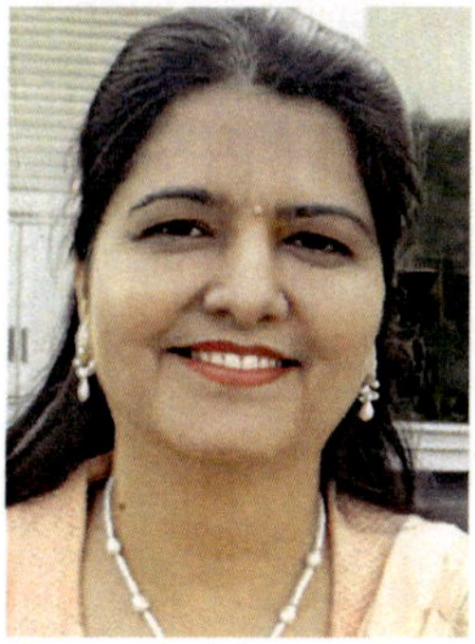

Prof. (Dr.) Neetu Saini M.V.Sc; Ph.D, Associate Professor (Veterinary Medicine). Guru Angad Dev Veterinary and Animal Sciences University, Ludhiana, Punjab, has a rich experience of 17 years in the field of veterinary cardiology. Her doctoral work on canine echocardiography has made her a distinguished veterinary cardiologist and bagged her Young Scientist Award besides many other awards. She is very reputed amongst students as an excellent teacher, trainer and clinician.

Ultrasound in Veterinary Medicine Fundamentals and Applications

Editor

J.P. Varshney

B.V.Sc. and A.H., M.V.Sc.(Medicine); Ph.D. (Vet. Med.)
Formerly Principal Scientist
Department of Veterinary Medicine
ICAR-Indian Veterinary Research Institute, Izatnagar, Uttar Pradesh
Presently Senior Consultant (Veterinary Medicine) Nandini Veterinary Hospital
Ghod-Dod Road, Surat-395001, Gujarat

NIPA GENX ELECTRONIC RESOURCES & SOLUTIONS P. LTD.
New Delhi-110 034

NIPA GENX ELECTRONIC
RESOURCES & SOLUTIONS P. LTD.
101,103, Vikas Surya Plaza, CU Block
L.S.C.Market, Pitam Pura, New Delhi-110 034
Ph : +91 11 27341616, 27341717, 27341718
E-mail:newindiapublishingagency@gmail.com
www: www.nipabooks.com

For customer assistance, please contact
Phone: + 91-11-27 34 17 17 Fax: + 91-11- 27 34 16 16
E-Mail: feedbacks@nipabooks.com

ISBN: 978-93-91383-04-6

Composed and Designed by NIPA.

Dedicated
To
My Parents & Teachers
Who
Nurtured, Steered, Inspired,
And
Made Me
What I am Today
And To
Those Who Lost
Their Life
During
Covid-19 Pandemic

Acknowledgements

I whole heartedly thank to my better-half Mrs. Jai Prabha Varshney and other family members (Dr.) Jai Pratibha Varshney (daughter) and Brigadier (Dr.) Atul Seth (son-in-law); Jai Prabhat Varshney (son) and Mrs. Ritu Gupta (daughter-in-law); Mrs. Jai Prabhanshi Varshney (daughter) and Ajit Varshney (son-in-law); and grandchildren (Agrima Seth, Vedaant Varshney, Devansh Varshney and Anvi Varshney) for their unconditional love, care, encouragement, support and being my strength through out and specially in the difficult and challenging time of Covid-19 pandemic without which this book would not have seen the light of the day.

I shall fail in my duty if I do not acknowledge the contribution of my learned colleagues Dr. P.S. Chaudhary, Chief Surgeon, Nandini Veterinary Hospital Surat; and Dr. Neetu Saini, Associate Professor (Veterinary Medicine) Department of Medicine, Guru Angad Dev Veterinary and Animal Science University, Ludhiana. I acknowledge both of them for contributing valuable material and sparing their valuable time.

I take this opportunity to thank Shri Nayan N. Bharatia Managing Trustee and all other members of the Board of Trustees, Nandini Veterinary Hospital, Surat, profusely for their all-time encouragement and support. Help rendered by all technical and supporting staff of the hospital is also duly acknowledged.

I also thank my all animal patients who provided me great opportunity to explore the applications of ultrasound in the disease diagnosis and management.

(J.P. Varshney)

Acknowledgements

It gives me an immense pleasure to thank my beloved father Late Shri Shankar Bhagwan Chaudhary and mother Smt. Saroj Shankar Chaudhary whose dream and efforts made me to become a veterinarian to serve the mute community. I whole heartedly thank my wife Mrs. Sharda Chaudhary for always providing her uncompromised support to build my professional career. Love, care and uncalled support of my daughter Ms. Prashansa Chaudhary and son Meet Chaudhary is highly appreciable.

Above all I am very much thankful to all pet owners who helped enthusiastically in scanning procedures for confirming diagnosis and sharing images in this book. I thank Shri. Nayan Bhartiya, Managing Trustee and Board of Trustees to provide an advanced ultrasound scanning machine at the hospital. Thanks are also due to all technical and supporting staff of the hospital.

(P.S. Chaudhary)

Preface

The success in the practice of any system of medicine (modern human medicine /veterinary medicine, traditional medicine, Ayurveda, or homeopathy etc.) rests on timely exact diagnosis and rational therapeutic approach. Clinical examination of the patient, laboratory investigations, electrocardiography, and imaging modalities (radiography, ultrasonography including echocardiography, magnetic resonance imaging, computerized tomography etc.), are the pillars of diagnosis. None of these diagnostic modality is perfect in isolation and has its own advantages and fall outs. Though, clinical examination of the patient is the basic and very important examination, it cannot ascertain the exact nature of the ailment and disease remains only speculative. Laboratory investigations provide valuable support to clinical suspicion and are the key for the exact etiological diagnosis of infectious diseases. These investigations can also reflect functions of the different organs but suffers from the lacunae of not touching many diseases. Electrocardiography is restricted to the evaluation of the heart rate, rhythm, conduction and to some extent chamber size. But diagnosis of valvular defects, ventricular wall defects, septal defects, type of cardiomyopathy, pericardial effusion and cardiac masses remains obscure. All the three diagnostic modalities (clinical examination, laboratory investigations and electrocardiography) do not visualize the architecture of the internal organs and fail to detect early lesions. The imaging modalities have a great promise in bridging these gaps. Though radiography is an important valuable and time tested imaging modality for many years, it suffers from the risk of radiation. This has led to the development of imaging modalities like ultrasound that is free from the risk of radiation.

Developments in veterinary medicine have followed the foot prints of human medicine. Fast developments in science and technology have opened new avenues. During last few decades developments in basic sciences have made the diagnosis of many diseases possible not only in human medicine but also in veterinary medicine. The technique of ultrasound/ultrasonography has revolutionized the diagnostic modalities. The application of ultrasound in veterinary medicine has extended diagnostic arsenal of veterinarians. As compared to other diagnostic techniques, ultrasonography is the latest diagnostic modality. It is a non-invasive, safe, radiation free and unique diagnostic modality as its results are instantaneously available. It has made the diagnosis of diseases of gall bladder possible which was otherwise impossible. Differentiation between fluid filled cysts, pus filled abscess or tumour has now become possible through the application of ultrasound. The technique was not so popular in veterinary practice in India during last century. But now veterinarians are inclined to use ultrasonography in their practice with an increased vigor because of improved portable ultrasound machines are easily available at their command and resource personnel are also available in almost all veterinary institutes. Exact interpretation of ultrasonographic findings is very crucial in the disease diagnosis otherwise misinterpretation may lead to chaotic results. Therefore proper professional training and continuous updating of knowledge is of paramount importance in order to interpret ultrasonographic findings correctly.

The book "Ultrasound in Veterinary Medicine: Fundamentals and Applications" is intended to provide standard scanning protocols for imaging different organs and structures of the body of different animal species, and adequate knowledge to facilitate correct diagnosis of diseases of different body organs as well to determine pregnancy status correctly. The book has been written in a simple and concise way along with illustrations so that the information may be used by the veterinarians to arrive at correct diagnosis in all clinical situations faced by them. The information on basic aspect of ultrasound; ultrasound machine; scanning procedure; land marks for imaging different body organs; image interpretation; ultrasound guided biopsy; ultrasound guided ovum collection; ophthalmic ultrasound; cardiac ultrasound; mammary ultrasound; sonographic features in diseases of different organ; pregnancy diagnosis; actual case studies with sonograms in different conditions; and ultrasound of ruminants, equines, leporine, reptiles (snake, turtle/tortoise), pet rodents and pet avian has been included in this book to increase the diagnostic horizon of the veterinarians. The other aspect of ultrasound i.e. therapeutic ultrasound has also been touched. Information on these important topics will not only be valuable to practicing veterinarians but also to academicians and blossoming veterinarians engaged in disease diagnosis and its rational treatment. It is a great pleasure and satisfaction to me to see a transition from restricted diagnostic modalities of yesterday to the present day repertoire of diagnostic techniques available at our command. The proper clinical use of the technique of ultrasonography has a great potential and future in disease diagnosis in veterinary medicine in coming years.

It is firmly and earnestly believed that veterinary students, researchers, academicians, specialist in veterinary medicine as well as practitioners will get adequate knowledge about ultrasonography and its application in veterinary medicine through this book and correct use of ultrasonography will be encouraged in the diagnosis of various medical, surgical and gynecological/obstetrical conditions of different species of animals.

Surat, Gujarat, India **J.P. Varshney**

Contents

Section 1. Basics

Section 2. Canine and Feline

Section 3. Other Animals

Section 4. Therapeutic Ultrasound

Section 5. Case Studies

List of Abbreviations

@	At the rate
AFAST	Abdominal Focussed Assessment with Sonography for Trauma
A:G ratio	Albumin : globulin ratio
A-Mode	Amplitude -Mode
ALT	Alanine aminotransferase
Ao	Aorta
AP	Alkaline Phosphatase
AST	Aspartate dehydrogenase
B-Mode	Bright-Mode
BPD	Biparietal diameter
BPH	Benign Prostate Hyperplasia
BSA	Body surface area
BUN	Blood urea nitrogen
°C	Celcius
CC	Cysto-colic
cm	Centimeter
cm2	Centimeter square
CFU	Colony Forming Unit
cmm	Cubic milli meter
CPU	Central Processing Unit
CEUs	Contrast Enhanced Ultrasound
CT	Computerized Tomography
CW- Doppler	Continuous Wave –Doppler
DH	Diaphragmatico-hepatic
DICOM	Digital Imaging and Communication in Medicine
dl	Deci-liter
DDFT	Deep Digital Flexor Tendon
E.canis	Ehrlichia canis
EDV	End diastolic volume
EDVI	End diastolic volume index
e.g.	Exampli gratia (for example)
EPSS	End- point to septal separation
ESV	End systolic volume
ESVI	End systolic volume index
FAST	Focussed Assessment with Sonography for Trauma
0 F	Fehrenheit
Fig	Figure
FS	Fractional shortening
g	Gram
GA	Gestation age
GSD	Gestational sac diameter

Hb	Haemoglobin
HD	Head diameter
Hg	Mercury
HR	Hepato-renal
HRU	Hepato-renal umbilical
Hz	Hertz
Hrs	Hours
ICC	Inner chorionic cavity diameter
ICL	Inferior Check Ligament
i.e.	That is
IM	Intramuscular
IU	International Unit
IV	Intravenous
IVCT	Isovolumetric contraction time
IVRT	Isovolumetric relaxation time
KHz	Kilohertz
Kg	Kilogram
<	Less than
L	Left
l	Liter
L1,L3,L5	Lumbar vertebra 1, Lumbar vertebra 3, Lumbar vertebra 5
LDH	Lactate dehydrogenase
LIPUS	Low intensity pulsed ultrasound
LVET	Left ventricular ejection time
LVFWd	Left ventricular free wall dimension in diastole
LVFWs	Left ventricular free wall dimension in systole
LVIDd	Left ventricular internal dimension in diastole
LVIDs	Left ventricular internal dimension in systole
>	More than
mcL	Microliter
mEq	Milli equivalent
mcg	Microgram
M Dec T	Mitral valve deceleration time
mg	Milligram.
MGS	Mean Grey Scale
MHz	Megahertz
M-Mode	Motion –Mode
mm	Millimeter
MPI	Myocardial performance index
MRI	Magnetic resonance imaging
MV A Vel	Mitral valve peak A velocity
MV E Vel	Mitral valve peak E velocity
µg	Microgram
µL	Microliter
m	Meter
mm	Millimeter
ng	Nano gram
OPD	Outdoor patient department
OPU	Oocyte pickup

%	Percent
PCV	Packed cell volume
pg	Pico gram
pH	Potential of hydrogen
PZT	Lead zirconate titanate
PV Vel	Pulmonary valve peak velocity
PW-Doppler	Pulse Wave -Doppler
R	Right
RBC	Red blood cells
SDFT	Superficial Digital Flexor Tendon
Sec /s	second
SR	Spleno-renal
TFAST	Thoracic Focused Assessment with Sonography in Trauma
TGC	Time gain compensation
TV A Vel	Tricuspid valve peak A velocity
TV E Vel	Tricuspid valve peak E velocity
USG-TV-OPU	Ultrasound guided trans vaginal ovum pick up
μs	Micro second
Vcf	Velocity of circumferential fiber
Viz	videlicet or namely
W	Watt

List of Figures

Section 1: Basics

1

Basics of Ultrasound

J.P. Varshney and P.S. Chaudhary

During recent years ultrasonography has become an indispensable diagnostic modality in human and veterinary medicine because of its non-invasive nature, providing visualization of internal organs, and quick results. Birth of ultrasound took place in 1794 when an Italian biologist Lazzaro Spallanzani discovered that bats used sound waves for navigation. Since then continuous developments and advancements in the technology have made the sonography a dependable and an easily accessible diagnostic modality. This chapter describes and discusses about various basic aspects of ultrasound viz. History, developments, basics, safety considerations, uses and limitations, terminology, and emerging innovations.

What is an Ultrasonography

- It is a non-invasive, radiation free and safe imaging technique to scan internal structures of the body.
- Ultrasound imaging involves three important components i.e. ultrasound machine, patient/animal and expert operator (sonographer).
- Basics of ultrasound are little complex but its clinical use is simple.
- The structures are imaged by recording echoes of ultrasonic waves.
- The ultrasound transducer sends a narrow beam of high frequency sound wave into the soft tissues to be imagined. The sound waves interact with the tissue interfaces. Some of the sound waves are transmitted into deeper tissues while some of the sound waves are reflected back to transducer as echoes.
- The reflected sound waves (echoes)are analyzed by the computer and are converted into an image that is displayed on the monitor creating a two dimensional image of the area viewed.

Ultrasound and Its Production

- Ultrasound is a high frequency sound above the 20 kHz (20,000 cycles / second).
- Sound with frequencies between 20 Hz to 20 kHz is audible to human ears.
- Medical diagnostic ultrasound is usually produced at MHz (millions cycle/second).
- Ultrasound at such high frequency is produced by piezoelectric crystals. These crystals transfer electrical energy into mechanical sound waves and reconvert sound waves into electrical energy. In this way on electrical stimulation piezo crystals perform the work of a transmitter as well as receiver.
- Ultrasound frequencies between 2 to 20 MHz are commonly used for the purpose of diagnosis of diseases in diagnostic ultrasound.

Piezoelectric Effect

- It is a phenomenon exhibited by generation of an electric charge in response to an application of mechanical force (squeeze or stretch) on certain materials.
- Mechanical deformation as a result of an application of electric field to such material is also known as piezoelectric effect.
- Quartz crystals, ceramics, and lead zirconatetitanate can demonstrate piezoelectric properties.
- Researches are being continued to develop lead free piezoelectric materials.
- Individual piezoelectric material produces small amount of energy, but when stacked into layers in the transducer enable the transducer to convert the electric energy into mechanical oscillations. These oscillations are then converted to electric energy.

Production of Ultrasound Wave

- Production of ultrasound waves is based on “pulse-echo-principle”.
- Piezo crystals placed in transducer are the source of ultrasound waves.
- These crystals have ability to transform electric current into ultrasound and vice versa. After generating and sending ultrasound wave, piezo crystals return to listening mode and wait for returning ultrasound echoes.

- Ultrasound monitor converts the echoes into image. The cycle of pulse generation and echo is repeated many million times per second and is called pulse-echo-principle.

Properties of Ultrasound

- Ultrasound waves have frequency,intensity, wave length and can pass through medium at certain speed/ velocity. The distance travelled in one cycle is termed as wave length Fig.1A.

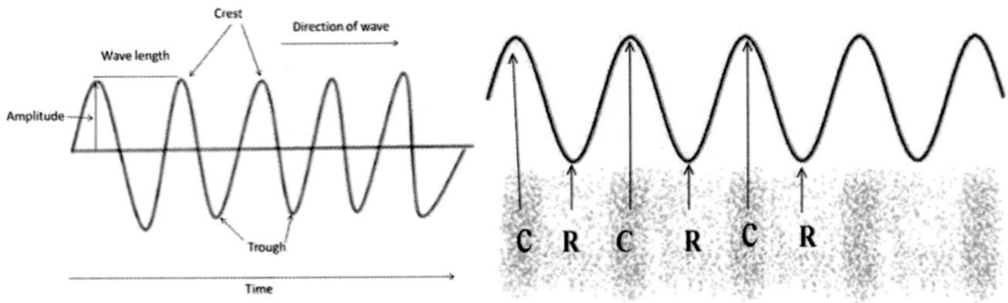

(A) (B)

Fig.1: Showing characteristics of sound wave. Frequency and wave length **(A)** are inversely related as the wave length increases, the frequency decreases. Each wave **(B)** has a cycle of compression (C) and rarefaction (R).

- Sound is a mechanical energy. When it travels through a medium/ material, it produces movement of the particles within the material/ medium. Sound waves are longitudinal waves. The direction of the movement of the particles within the wave is the same as of the sound wave. Each sound wave has a cycle of compression and rarefaction (Fig.1B).
- Number of cycles per second is termed as frequency .It is measured in MHz and depends on thickness and damping of piezo crystals.
- Intensity of the ultrasound has impact on resolution and penetration. Measurement of intensity is done in watts/cm^2.
- The speed of sound /ultrasound is the distance travelled in one second. Ultrasound velocity within soft tissues varies slightly. But it varies greatly between soft and hard tissues.

Attenuation or Weakening

When an ultrasound beam travels through tissues, it is attenuated or weakened. Attenuation or weakening do happens to returning echoes also. The attenuation is directly proportional to the frequency of the beam. The attenuation is due to absorption, reflection, refraction and scattering phenomenon.

- When an ultrasound wave enters the body, changes may occur in its loudness or intensity.It is used to construct the visual image.
- When ultrasound wave travels through tissues, its energy to some extent is absorbed by the tissues and is converted into heat. It is very small amount.Higher frequencies are absorbed at greater rate but gives better axial resolution. Frequencies between 6 to 12 MHz give adequate resolution for imaging.
- A part of ultrasound wave is reflected and other is transmitted when ultrasound wave encounters boundaries between different medium.

Reflection occurs when the ultrasound wave is deflected towards transducer. The major factors affecting the amount of reflection are angle of incidence, acoustic impedance mismatch, width of the tissue boundary and angle of tissue boundary.

- Scattering takes place when ultrasound wave strikes a rough surface or pass through heterogeneous media.
- Refraction occurs when ultrasound signal is deflected from a straight path and angle of deflection is away from the transducer. Ultrasound waves are only refracted at a different medium interface of different acoustic impedance. Double image artifacts in ultrasound can be caused by refraction.

Resolution

- Resolution is the distinguish echoes in terms of space, time or strength. Good resolution is important for the production of high quality images.
- There are three types of resolution namely spatial, contrast and temporal.
- Spatial resolution is the ability of ultrasound system to detect and display structures that are close together. Spatial resolution is of two types viz. axial (or longitudinal) and lateral
- Axial resolution is the minimum distance that can be differentiated between two reflectors located parallel to the direction of ultrasound beam. Axial resolution is related to frequencies and is better when frequency is higher.
- Lateral resolution is related with the width of the crystal and distance of the reflector from it. It is the minimum distance that can be distinguished between the two reflectors located perpendicular to the direction of ultrasound beam.
- Contrast resolution is the ability of ultrasound system to demonstrate differentiation between tissues having different characteristics. Differentiation of liver and spleen is the example of contrast resolution.

- Temporal resolution is the ability of ultrasound system to accurately show changes in the underlying anatomy over time. It has an important place in echocardiography.
- Image brightness depends on the loudness of echoes.
- Details of the image depends on frequency of stimulation, frequency of crystal, width of the crystal and depth from which echo is coming.
- Higher frequencies are associated with better resolution but less penetration. On the other hand lower frequencies are associated with less resolution but more penetration.

Ultrasound Modes

- There are three types of ultrasound modes such as B- mode (bright mode), M- mode (motion mode) and Doppler mode (Fig.2).

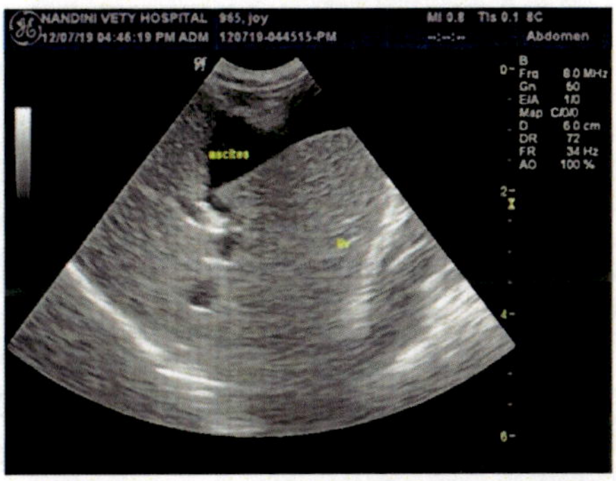

B-Mode

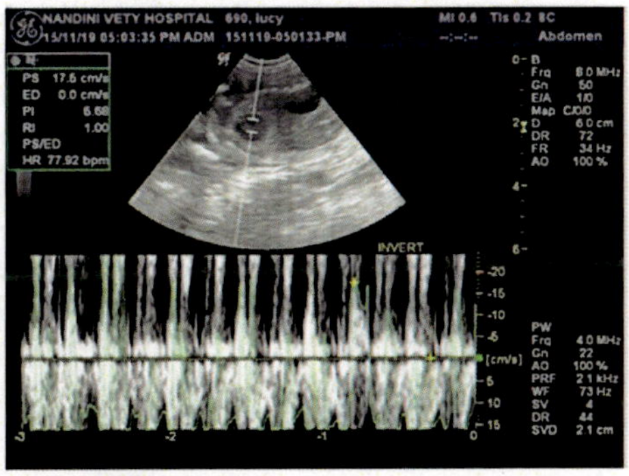

M-Mode

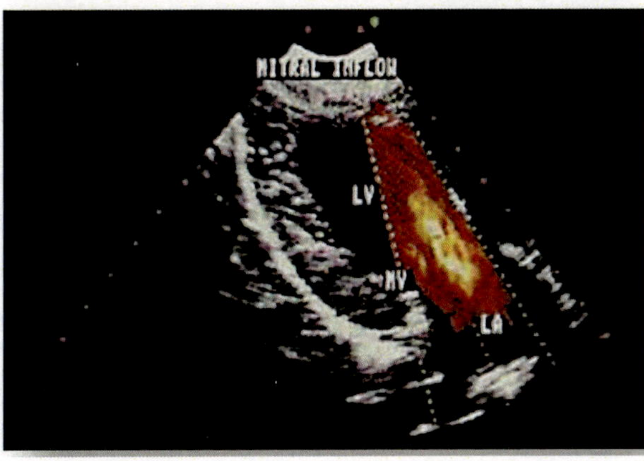

Colour Doppler

Fig. 2: Showing different modes of ultrasonography.

- The bright mode provides structural information in two dimensional images in different shades of grey i.e. different degree of brightness (Fig.2).
- While motion mode (M-mode) captures the returning echoes in one line of B mode image and displays them over a time axis (Fig 2). Generally both modes are displayed together on the monitor.
- In Doppler mode, the phenomenon of "Doppler shift" (frequency change from sent to returning echo) is used. The shift in frequency is generated in sound waves reaching the moving particles and correlates with velocity and direction of the moving particles. Doppler mode (Fig.2) is used to examine the blood flow and tissues in motion. Colour Doppler is used to examine blood flow velocity and its direction; and motion of the tissues in a selected two dimensional area. Power Doppler is used to examine vascular emergencies such as testicular or ovarian torsion. It focuses on returning frequency shift and can detect even very low flow. Spectral Doppler is used to examine foetal heart tones or patent vessels in pregnancy in humans.

Artefacts

- Artefacts are defined as alteration (s) in the image which does not represent an actual image of the area examined. They may be produced by technical imaging errors or may be produced as a result of complex interaction of the ultrasound with biological tissues. In simple term artefacts represent a false portrayal of image anatomy or image degradation related to false assumption, malfunctioning or maladjustment of the instrument.
- There are two categories of artefacts.
- Category 1 artefacts are produced by the faulty use of machine, machine setting, scanning procedure or incomplete / faulty preparation of the patient. Artefacts arising due to faulty scanning procedure and patient preparation are also termed as manipulation artefacts. It is advisable to prepare patient by fasting for 12-24 hrs., giving anti-flatulent and ample drinking water to make their urinary bladder full. The site should be prepared by shaving and cleaning the area and liberal application of acoustic gel. For good quality images ultrasound machine should be properly set with respect to power, gain and TGC. These artefacts can easily be corrected.
- Category 2 artefacts arise owing to sound wave characteristics and tissue interfaces. This category of artefact includes reverberation, comet tail, mirror image, acoustic imaging, acoustic enhancement, side lobe, side thickness artifacts and refraction.

- Artefacts are also grouped as attenuation artefacts, propagation artefact and miscellaneous artefact.
- There are three types of attenuation artefacts viz. shadowing, edge shadowing and posterior enhancement. Shadowing artefact (Fig. 3) is caused by partial or total reflection or absorption of sound energy. Such artefacts are seen while imaging cholelith, renal liths or bones. Edge shadowing artifacts are seen while imaging cystic structures. Thin acoustic edge shadow is seen behind edge of cystic structures. Posterior enhancement artifacts are seen because neighbouring signals are passed through more attenuated structures. Therefore returning echoes are weak.

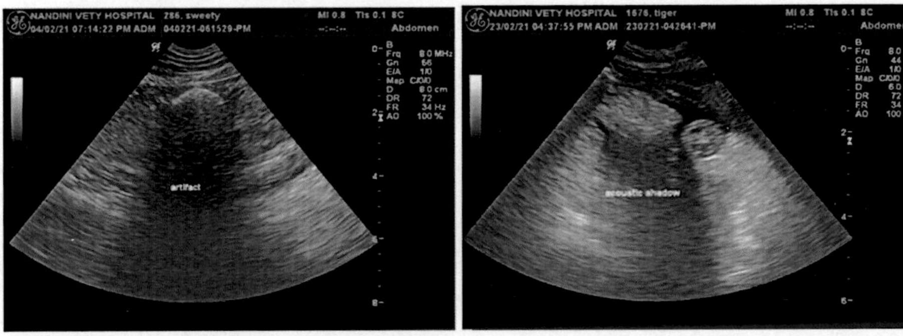

Fig. 3: Sonograms showing acoustic shadowing

- Reverberation, comet tail and mirror image artifacts fall under the category of propagation artifacts. Reverberation artefacts (Fig. 4) are series of equally spaced lines and occur when sound waves strike two highly reflective layers. Comet tail artefacts (Fig. 5) are similar to reverberation artefacts and are produced by the front and back of very reflective particles like air bubble. Mirror image artefacts (Fig. 6) are produced when there is a highly reflective interface near the structure being imaged. Diaphragm is a mirroring reflector.

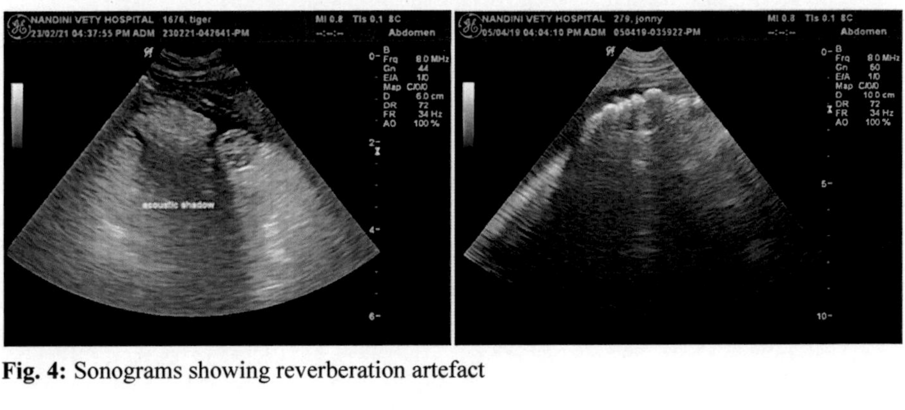

Fig. 4: Sonograms showing reverberation artefact

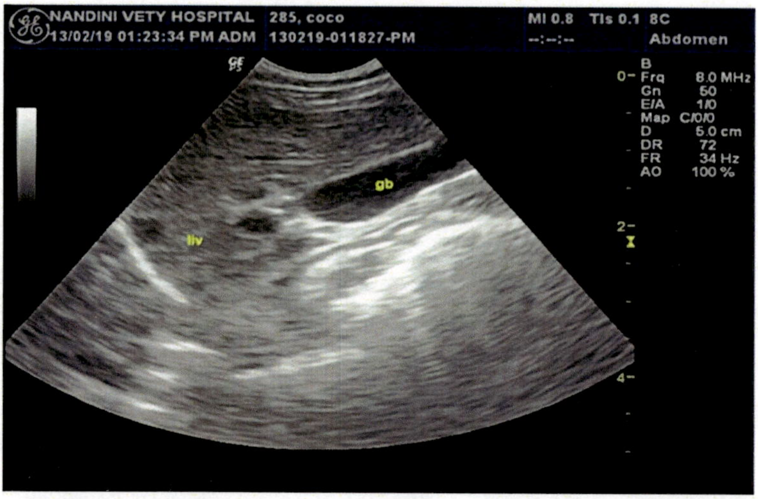

Fig. 5: Sonogram showing comet tail artefact

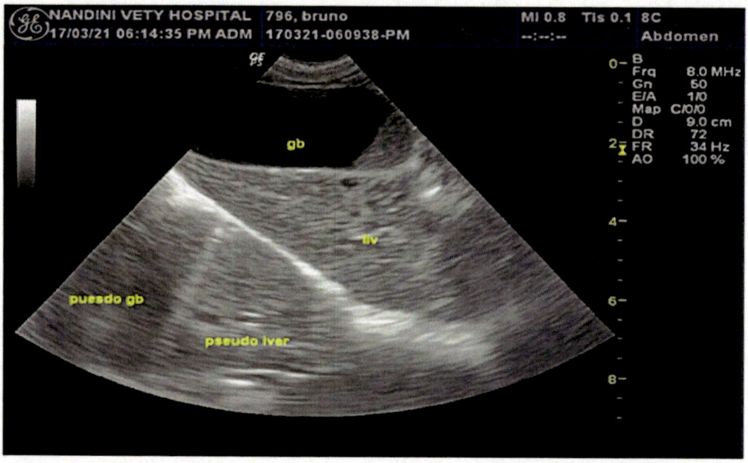

Fig. 6: Sonogram showing mirror image (liver and gall bladder) artefact

- The category of miscellaneous artefacts consists of ring down artefact and side lobe artefacts. The former one artefact is caused by resonance from collected gas bubbles and is similar to comet tail. While later one is caused by low energy side lobes of main ultrasound beam and are seen in hypoechoic or echo free structures as bright rounded lines. Ultrasound energy in side lobes is mostly dissipated in tissue without generating significant reflections. But when side lobes face strong reflectors such as calcification and pericardium, significant reflections (detectable by transducer) may be generated.

- Refraction artefacts occur due to bending of ultrasound beam from its original direction when the ultrasound beam passes through a boundary between tissues having different sound speeds (different acoustic impediments). Refraction artefacts lead to improper positioning and brightness of echoes displayed in sonograms. Refraction occurs between the spleen and adjacent fat or liver and adjacent fat and creates duplication of the organ. Refraction artefacts are easily recognised because they create implausible image findings such as duplication of ventricles or atria. Fat, pericardium and pleura behave as lens causing refraction. Refraction artefacts can be corrected by switching the image window, or adjusting the angle of the probe.
- Range ambiguity artefact is visualized as a group of echoic lines within fluid filled structure.

Transducers or Probes

- Transducers or probes consist of piezoelectric crystals, damping material and matching layer.
- Different types of transducers (Fig .7) such as large convex, micro convex, sector, and linear are available. Large convex probe produces sector shaped image with large convex top and are used for transabdominal sonography. Micro convex probe produces sector shaped image with small curved top and are used in transthoracic or transabdominal sonography. Sector transducer is used for transthoracic sonography and their image is pie shaped with angulated top. Linear probes produce rectangular image and are used in sonography of vascular and superficial soft tissues.

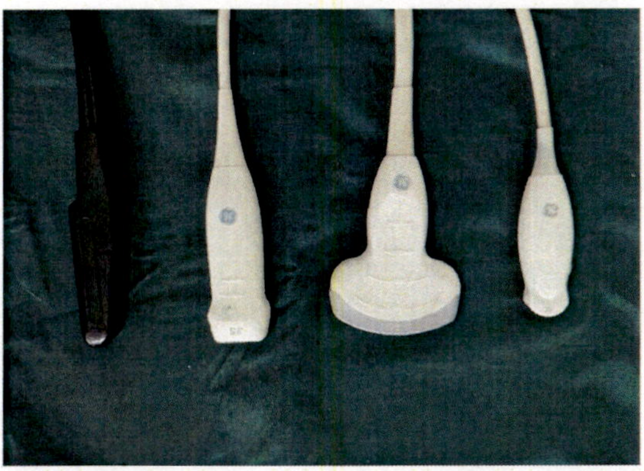

Fig. 7: Showing different types of transducers. From left to right linear transducer 5 MHz with large foot print, linear transducer 3 MHz with small foot print, curvilinear transducer 4 MHz, curvilinear transducer 8MHz

- Ultrasound transducers are made of transducer head, connecting wire or cable and a connector.
- The transducer has a foot print region (Fig. 8) where ultrasound wave leaves and returns to the transducer. It needs to remain in contact with the body to transmit and receive ultrasound waves.
- Each transducer also has a transducer or probe marker (Fig. 8) located next to the head of the transducer in order to assist identify its orientation. The probe marker can be a notch, a dot or light on the probe's head.

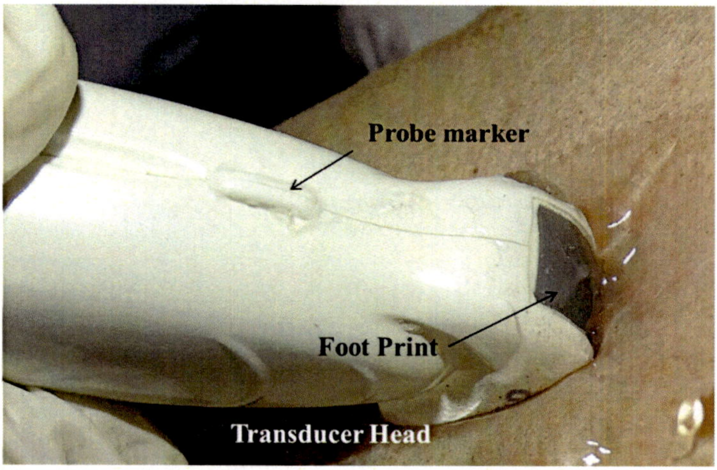

Fig. 8: Transducer Head showing probe marker and foot print region.

Components of Ultrasound Transducer

- Ultrasound transducer has five main components (Fig. 9) i.e. crystals with piezoelectric properties, positive and ground electrodes on the faces of the element, damping block, matching layer and housing.
- Crystal/ceramic element with piezoelectric properties-Usually lead zirconatetitanate (PZT) is used for this purpose. It may consist of a single element or multiple elements. Element thickness is determined by what resonance frequency is desired.
- Positive and ground electrodes on the faces of the element allows for electrical connection. Positive electrode is in the back of the element and ground electrode is on the front of the element
- Damping (backing) block is adhered to the back of the crystal (behind the positive electrode). It absorbs ultrasound energy directed backward and attenuates stray ultrasound signals from the housing. It dampens the resonant vibrations in the element.

- Matching layer interfaces between the transducer element and the tissue. It allows close to 100% transmission of the ultrasound from the element into the tissues by minimizing reflection due to traversing different mediums (acoustic impedance). It may consist of one or multiple layers. Each layer is one-quarter wavelength thick.
- Housing includes a plastic case, metal shield and acoustic insulator. It provides electrical insulation and protection of the element.
- Ultrasound transducers typically consist of 128-512 piezoelectric elements arranged in linear or curvilinear arrays. Each element is equal to or less than a ½ wavelength wide and transducer length is generally 5 to 15 cm. Each element is individually insulated.

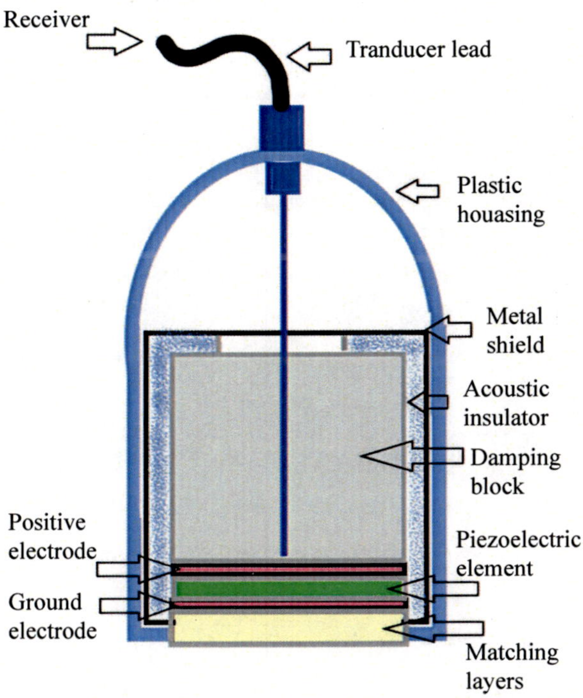

Fig. 9: Diagrammatic representation of anatomy of the transducer

Image Produced by Linear and curvilinear Transducers

- Curvilinear transducers produce pie shaped image (Fig.10).
- Linear transducers produce square or rectangular shaped image (Fig.10).

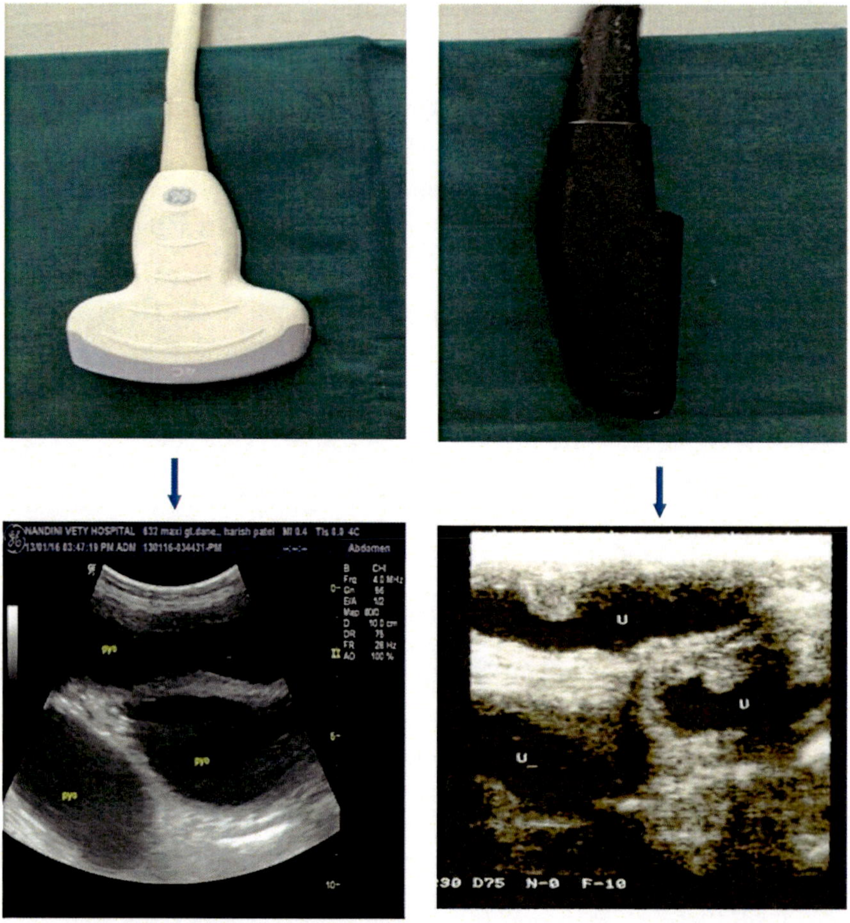

Pie shaped Image

Rectangular Image

Fig.10. Pie shaped image is produced by curvilinear transducer (A) and rectangular image is produced by linear transducer (B).

Anatomic Planes or Position of Probes

- Scanning anatomic planes are used to establish the direction of the entering ultrasound beam and the anatomic potion of the organ being seen from that particular direction.
- Three planes viz. transverse or axial or cross section, sagittal or longitudinal, oblique and frontal or coronal are used to detail relationship between adjacent structures/organs.
- Scanning planes provides two dimensional ultrasound images.

- Body structures are usually viewed longitudinally or sagittal and axially or transverse.
- Sagittal or Longitudinal Scanning Plane- Ultrasound beam enters the body from anterior or posterior direction and anatomical portion is visualized from anterior, posterior, superior or inferior directions.
- Transverse Scanning Plane- Ultrasound beam enters the body from either an anterior, posterior or lateral direction. When the beam is entering from anterior or posterior direction, the anatomical portion is visualized from anterior, posterior, right lateral and left lateral direction. When the beam is entering from right or left lateral direction, anatomic portion is visualized from lateral (right or left), medial, anterior or posterior direction.
- Frontal or coronal Scanning Plane-Ultrasound beam enters the body from either a right or left lateral direction and anatomical portion is visualized from lateral (left or right), medial, superior or inferior direction.

General Interpretation of Echogenicity

- Echogenicity is a qualitative assessment of the reflected energy within a tissue or at interface. It is displayed as brightness of the echo as compared to scanning back ground.
- The degree of echogenicity is classified as increased echogenicity (hyperechoic), normal echogenicity (isoechoic), decreased echogenicity (hypoechoic), or no echogenicity (anechoic) (Fig.11).

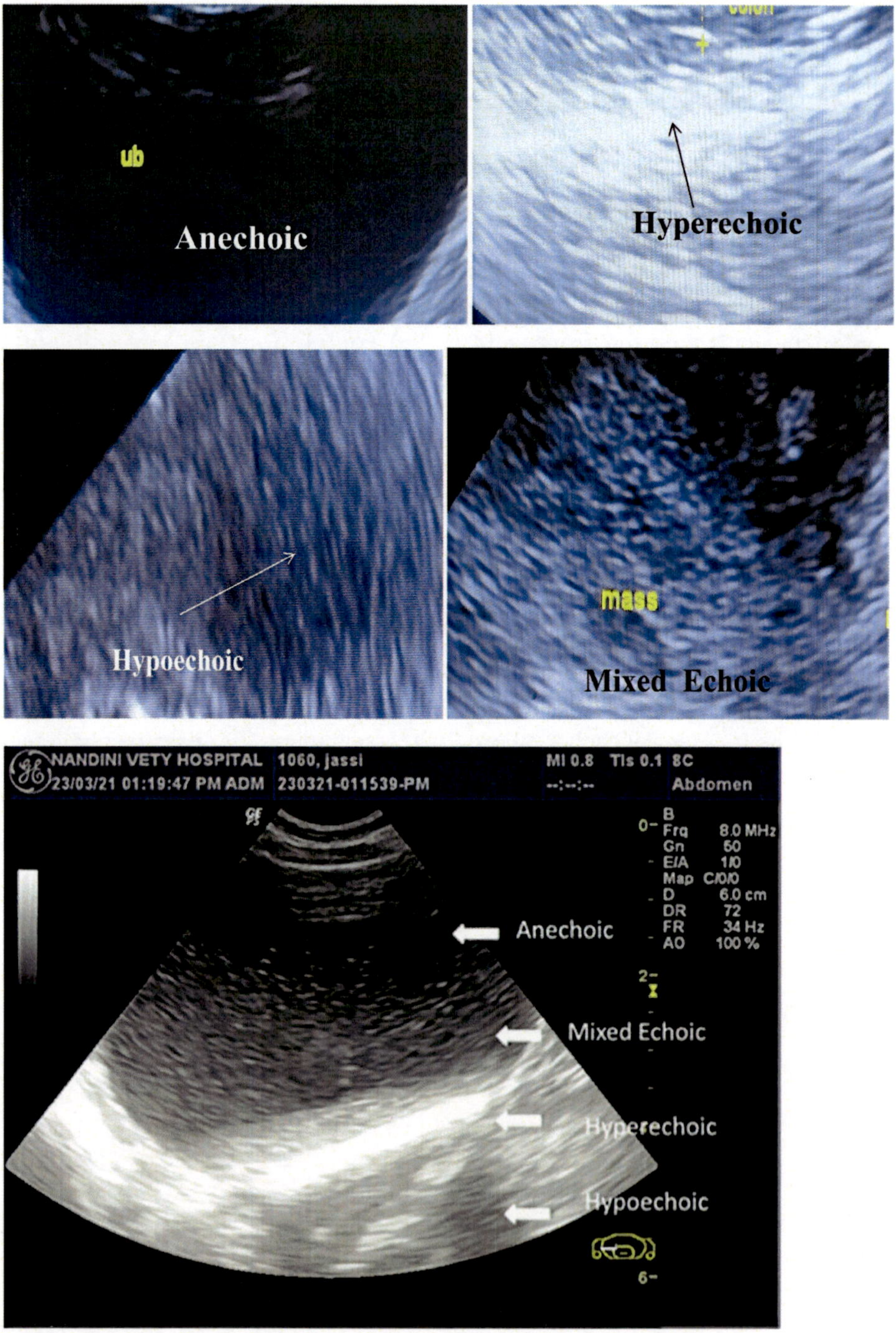

Fig. 11: Showing different degrees of echogenicity

- In pathological conditions various combinations of echo amplitudes are observed.
- Far enhancement and shadowing are artefact phenomenon generally observed in imaging ultrasonography.
- Far enhancement phenomenon is observed when sound calibrated for soft tissues travels through fluid resulting into increased echogenicity.
- Shadowing artefact is seen when an ultrasound beam encounters bones or intestinal gas.

Relative Echogenicity

Echogenicity of different organs/conditions is different. Their relative echogenicity in increasing order is as follows:

- Fluid – It is anechogenic. So it looks black.
- Renal Medulla
- Renal Cortex
- Liver
- Spleen
- Prostate glands having benign hypertrophy
- Peritonitis-The mesentery looks hyperechoic.

Echo Texture

Echo texture is described as

- Uniform
- Mixed, mottled or multi-focal
- Heteroechoic
- Target type (Hyper and hypoechoic concentric rings alternating).

Ultrasonographic Appearance of Different Tissues

Different body tissues have different echogenic appearance. Details are given below.

Tissues	Ultrasonographic Appearance
Vein	Anechoic compressible
Artery	Anechoic pulsatile

Fat	Hypoechoic with irregular hyperechoic lines
Muscle	Hypoechoic but separated with hyperechoic septa
Tendon	Hyperechoic and fiber like
Ligament	Like tendon but more compact
Bones	Hyperechoic lines with hypoechoic shadow
Nerves	Starry night appearance: transverse plane

Image Terminology

The following terminology is usually used to describe the image.

- Anechoic or Echolucent – There is no returning sound waves and area looks darker.
- Hypo-echoic – There are few returning sound waves and area is darker than the surrounding tissues
- Hyper-echoic or Echogenic – Structures look brighter than the surrounding tissues.
- To point out areas on the screen, the screen is divided into nine zones (Fig.12) so that sonographer can describe the location of the area of interest as near, mid, far, left, centre and right.

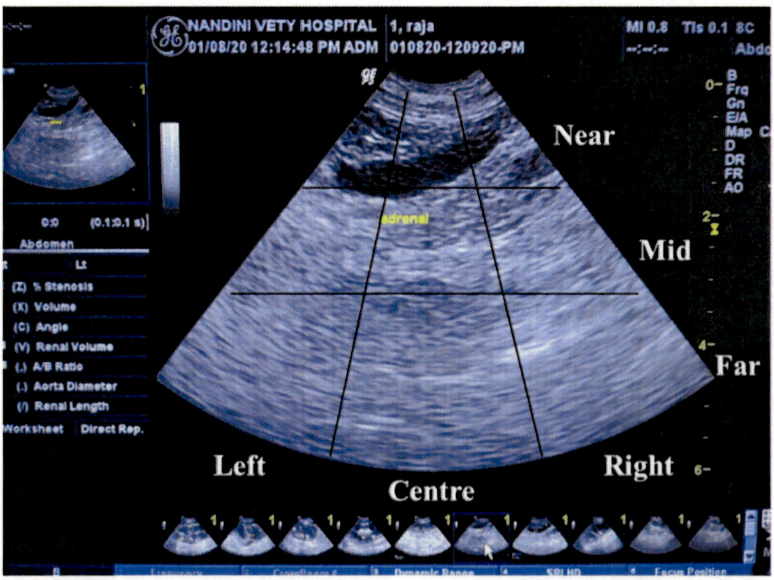

Fig. 12: Showing nine zones on the screen to point out an area of interest on the screen.

Other Terminology used in Ultrasound

Besides image terms, the following terms are also usually used in ultrasonography.

- **Period** - It is the time taken by the sound wave to complete one cycle and is measured in micro-second (μs).
- **Wave Length** - It is the length of the space covered by one cycle.

In other words it is distance travelled during the time period.

- **Frequency** - It is the number of complete cycles per unit of time and is measured in hertz (MHz). Frequency and wave length of sound wave is inversely related i.e. as the frequency increases, the wave length decreases.
- **Acoustic Velocity** - It is the speed at which sound wave travels through a medium. For soft tissues the velocity is similar. In living soft tissues average speed of ultrasound wave is 1540 m/sec.
- **Acoustic Impedance** - It is the degree of impediment shown by a sound wave when it is transmitted through a medium. In other words it is the resistance offered by the material to the propagation of an ultrasound wave. It is expressed as Z(Acoustic impedance)

$Z= pV$ (Kg/m^2 s). Where p is density of material and V is velocity of ultrasonic wave in the material.

- **Acoustic Pressure** - It denotes the amplitude of alternating stresses on a material by a propagating ultrasonic wave. It is expressed as P (Acoustic pressure)

  $P= Za$ (Z=Acoustic Impedance, a = amplitude of particle vibration).
- **Attenuation Coefficient**- It is a parameter used to estimate the decrement of sound wave amplitude in certain medium. Attenuation coefficient increases with increasing frequency i.e. when frequency is increased, sound wave penetration is decreased.
- **Types of Ultrasonic Waves**- There are three types of ultrasonic waves such as Longitudinal (particles vibrate along the direction of travel of the wave), shear or transverse, and surface or Rayleigh wave. Longitudinal waves can propagate in solid, liquid and gases), Shear or Transverse waves (particles vibrate at right angle or transverse to the propagation direction) and Surface or Rayleigh wave (produced in a semi – infinite material. Particles vibrate following an elliptical orbit).

Interaction of Ultrasound Waves with Tissues

When an ultrasound beam travels through tissues, it is attenuated. This also happens to returning echoes. The attenuation is directly proportional to the frequency of the beam. The attenuation is due to absorption, reflection and scattering phenomenon.

- When ultrasound wave travels through tissues, its energy to some extent is absorbed by the tissues and is converted into heat. It is very small amount.
- A part of ultrasound wave is reflected and other is transmitted when ultrasound wave encounters boundaries between different medium.
- Scattering takes place when ultrasound wave strikes a rough surface or pass through heterogeneous media.
- Higher frequencies are absorbed at greater rate but gives better axial resolution. Frequencies between 6 to 12 MHz give adequate resolution for imaging.

Speed of Sound Wave in Different Medium

The velocity of sound wave varies in different medium. Its velocity in air, water, tissues and bones is mentioned below.

- The velocity of sound wave in air is 330 m/s.
- The velocity of sound wave in water is 1480 m/s.
- The velocity of sound wave in tissues is 1540 m/s.
- The velocity of sound wave in bones is 4080 m/s.

Acoustic Impedance

- Acoustic impedance is the ability of living tissues to impede transmission of sound.
- The ability of different tissues to impede transmission of sound is different as follows as reported in the literature:
- In air acoustic impedance is 0.0004 x 10^5Rayls.
- In fat acoustic impedance is 1.38 x 10^5Rayls.
- In water acoustic impedance is 1.48 x 10^5Rayls.
- In blood acoustic impedance is 1.61 x 10^5Rayls.
- In kidney acoustic impedance is 1.62 x 10^5Rayls.

- In soft tissues acoustic impedance is 1.63 x 10^5Rayls.
- In liver acoustic impedance is 1.65 x 10^5Rayls
- In muscle acoustic impedance is 1.67 x 10^5Rayls
- In bone acoustic impedance is 7.8 x 10^5Rayls

Doppler Ultrasonography

- It is non-invasive technique used to estimate the blood flow in the blood vessels.
- It works by measuring sound waves that are reflected from the moving objects (such as red blood cells), known as Doppler Effect.
- This effect is employed in Doppler ultrasonography to generate the imaging of the movement of the tissues and fluid and their relative velocity to the transducer.
- It works by measuring sound waves that are reflected from the moving objects.
- There are different types of Doppler ultrasound such as colour Doppler, power Doppler, spectral Doppler, duplex Doppler and continuous wave Doppler.
- Colour Doppler uses a computer to change sound waves in to different colours. Colours show speed and direction of blood flow in real time.
- Power Doppler is a new type of colour Doppler that provides more details of blood flow without showing the direction.
- Spectral Doppler gives blood flow information on a graph. It is useful in detecting the extent of blood vessel blockage.
- Duplex Doppler converts the image of blood vessels and organs into a graph.
- Continuous Wave Doppler sends and receives sound waves continuously and provides more accurate measurement of blood flowing at faster speed.

Advantages of Ultrasound

- Ultrasound is of great assistance in the early diagnosis of health problems.
- Ultrasound facilitates visualization of even those internal abnormalities that may remain obscure by other imaging modality such as x-ray.

- Ultrasound may lead to more successful treatment outcomes as treatment can be started early with an early diagnosis of the condition.
- Images of ultrasound scanning can be electronically shared with the experts for consultation.
- It is non-invasive, painless and virtually risk free imaging modality.
- Ultrasound is a quick technique with immediate observable results.
- There is no risk of radiation with ultrasound.
- Diagnosis of wide range of benign and malignant diseases and medical problems is possible by ultrasonography.
- It can be used to detect congenital problems also in young pets.
- Ultrasonography is the integral part of cancer diagnosis

Safety Considerations of Ultrasound Wave

- Diagnostic ultrasound is considered as a safe procedure to patient and operator. Till date there is no confirmed report of any significant adverse biological effect of real time B- mode diagnostic ultrasound.
- It can be performed in any location without the need of any specific safety precautions
- Some amount of energy is absorbed by the tissue on exposure to ultrasound. Amount of absorption of energy depends on the composition of tissue and the frequency of ultrasound beam.
- Bones absorbs more ultrasound energy as compared to soft tissues.
- Absorption in tissues rises with increasing frequency.
- Absorption of energy within tissues leads to rise in temperature.
- The rise in temperature during ultrasonographic scanning is also limited by the use of scanned beams, with any point in tissue being interrogated for only a very short time.
- Significantly elevated temperature is only likely to be found when stationary beams are used (M-mode, spectral Doppler and colour flow imaging techniques).
- It is debatable that temperature rise above normal core level can be teratogenic.
- It is being considered by the majority of workers that temperature elevation of 1.0 -1.5 ^{0}C is not of much concern.

- There is a considerable debate on non-thermal effect of ultrasound as to whether diagnostic ultrasound exposure is able to induce cavitation effects in the absence of exogenous bubbles (such as those that are used as ultrasound contrast agents). The acoustic cavitation is commonly cited as potent side effect of the ultrasound but lacks sufficient confirmation.
- Bruising has been reported as another problem of ultrasound. But it is usually not at the current diagnostic level.
- In experimental studies using diagnostic exposure, lung haemorrhage has been observed by some workers, but the effects have not been reported in the foetus.
- Pulse Doppler transmits higher acoustic outputs in a stationary beam, and can produce increase in temperature leading to biological consequences.
- Safety margin is small in sonographic and pulsed Doppler examinations of the prenatal animals. Therefore, the acoustic output of the equipment, the exposure time, and the sensitivity of target tissues should always be considered.
- It is better to limit the exposure with pulsed or continuous wave Doppler ultrasound.
- The benefits of diagnostic ultrasound clearly outweigh the potential risk.

Landmarks in the Development of Ultrasound

- There is continuous evolution in ultrasound machines leading to improvised facility in the diagnosis of diseases.
- Today's ultrasound has more than 225 years journey.
- Birth of ultrasound took place in 1794 when Italian biologist Lazzaro Spallanzani discovered that bats used sound waves for navigation. The technique is now called as echolocation where locations are identified through sound waves reflected from the object in the environment. On the same principle present day ultrasound technique works.
- In 1877 piezo electricity was discovered by Pierre Currie and Jacques Currie. Probes emit and receive sound by way of piezoelectric effect.
- Paul Langevin invented first transducer in 1915.
- In 1915, navy used ultrasound to detect submarines.
- During 1920 to 1940, sonography was used as physical therapy.
- Karl Dussik in 1942 used sonography for the first time in the medical diagnoses.

- In 1948, George D. Ludwig developed A –mode ultrasound equipment and detected gall stones.
- During 1949-1951, Douglas Howry and Joseph Holmes contributed in the development of B –mode ultrasound equipment.
- First echocardiogram was taken by Inge Edler and C. Hellmuth Hertz in 1953.
- Ian Donald incorporated ultrasonography into obstetrics and gynaecology in 1958.
- In 1966, Pulse Doppler Ultrasound was designed by a team consisting of Don Baker, Dennis Watkins and John.
- In 1980s Kazunori Baba developed 3-D ultrasound technology.
- In 1994 B-mode ultrasound was used to block brachial plexus by Steven Kapral and his colleagues.
- Presently (after 2000) compact and handheld devices have also been developed. The i-phone now is having telesonography applications.
- Ultrasound was used for the first time as a diagnostic aid in veterinary medicine for the diagnosis of pregnancy in sheep (Lindahl, 1966).

Advances in Ultrasound Technology

Ever increasing concerns of people about radiation dose and appropriate use of imaging technology has attracted the attention of researchers to continuously develop and improve the diagnostic imaging modalities for better image of internal organs of the patients. Developments in ultrasound technology have made clinical application of diagnostic sonography more attractive and remunerative. It is expected that future ultrasound technology will be more cost effective without compromising high quality imaging, automated, mobile, definitive, and intuitive for users

Emerging Innovations in Ultrasound

- Advanced applications in 3-D imaging.
- Newer applications of ultrasound contrast. Contrast enhanced ultrasound (CEUS) are being used to scan digestive tract and heart. The technology is very effective at tumour detection. With some more advancements CEUS may replace the need for CT or MRI scans to test for cancer and other medical problems.
- Shear wave elastography.

- Developments of wireless transducers.
- App based ultrasound technology.
- Fusion with CT /MRI.
- Laparoscopic ultrasound.
- Engineering advances such as miniaturisation of electronics are leading to the development of hand held ultrasound scanners.
- With the development of hand held scanners without compromising the image quality, it appears that the ultrasound will become an easy diagnostic modality in the hands of primary health care and emergency physicians and veterinarians to enable quick assessment of patients/ ailing animals.
- Developments of LinkedIn parallel Digital Signal Processors promise to deliver similar speed with markedly greater flexibility than application specific integrated circuits.
- Development of Real –time volumetric scanning can reduce the need for operator skill, making ultrasound more reproducible and productive. This technique can help to create images with more depth and details than traditional ultrasound. The technique can be used to identify tumours, evaluate cardiac function and more making the diagnosis much easier.
- Advanced computing platforms might even make automatic feature recognition possible, as lesions and tissues are outlined, measured, and compared to databases containing normal and abnormal ranges.
- Introduction of touch enabled ultrasound systems will enhance mobility by sacrificing cumbersome key boards.
- Emergence of using a customer android or an apple device as an ultrasound scanner is the other innovation in pipe line.
- Integration of artificial intelligence with ultrasound is intended to automise time consuming tasks, quantification and picking out the ideal image slice from a 3-D dataset.
- Development of sono-elastography facilitates measuring tissue stiffness. This type of imaging will be helpful to better identify conditions such as liver fibrosis, prostate cancer, lumps in breast, and teat/udder fibrosis.

References

Lindahl, I.L. (1966). Detection of pregnancy in sheep by means of ultrasound.Nature212:642-643.

Suggested Further Readings

Kealy, J.K. and McAllister, H. (2005). Radiology and Ultrasonography of the Dog and Cat. 5th edn. Elsevier Saunders, St. Louis..

Mannion, P. (2006). Diagnostic Ultrasound in Small Animal Practice. Blackwell Science Ltd., Oxford, U.K.

Nyland, T.G., Mattoon, J.S., Herrgesell, E.J. and Wisner, E.R. (2002). Physical Principles, instrumentation, and safety of diagnostic ultrasound. In: Small Animal Diagnostic Ultrasound.

Nyland, T.G. and Mattoon, J.S. (eds), 2nd edn. WB Saunders, Philadelphia.

2

Ultrasonography and Ultrasound Machine

J.P. Varshney and P.S. Chaudhary

Ultrasonography or sonography is a diagnostic medical procedure that uses echoes of ultrasound pulses to produce images, of the objects or of the areas of different densities in the body, on the screen. This diagnostic procedure is performed through ultrasound machine. Sonogram is a visual image produced from ultrasonography. This chapter provides information about ultrasound machine, its different components, operating part of the machine, preparation of the animal for sonography, positioning of animals, scanning approaches and procedure, use and application of ultrasound, precautions and limitations of ultrasound

Ultrasound Machine

For successful sonography, adequate medical knowledge, the technical dexterity and know-how to navigate various knobs of the ultrasound machine is mandatory.

- Ultrasound machine (Fig.13) has different components such as monitor key board, processor (central processing unit-CPU), data storage transducer and printer.

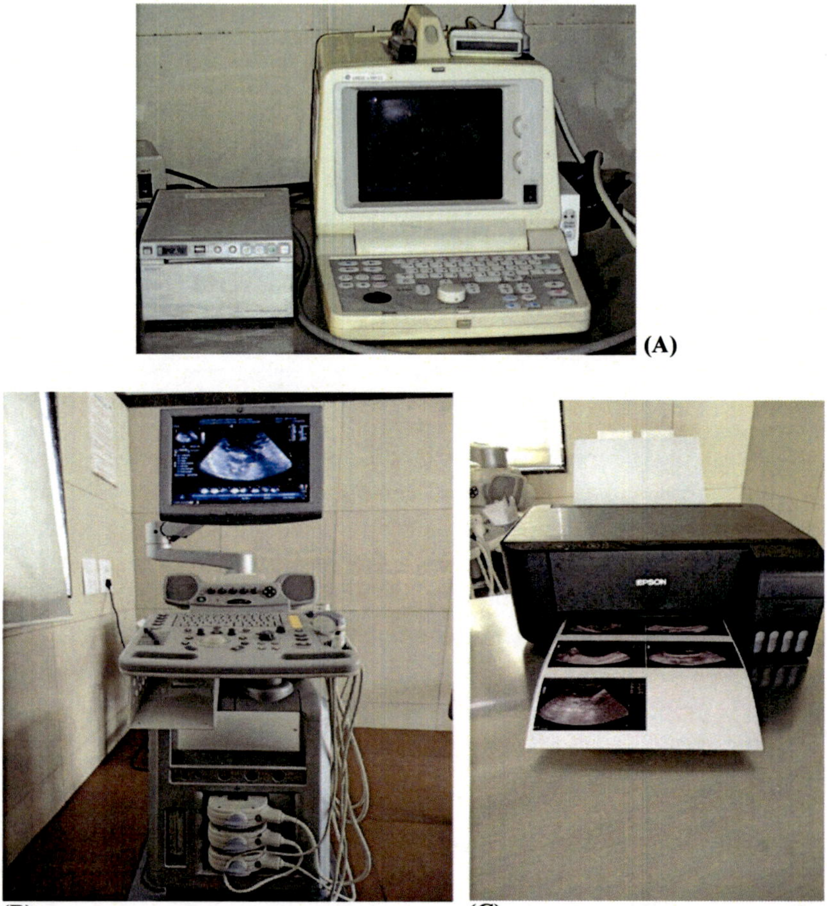

(A)

(B) (C)

Fig. 13: Different Ultrasound machines. Simple ultrasound machine **(A)**. Advance ultrasound machine with facility of M- mode and colour Doppler **(B)**. Printer of advanced ultrasound machine **(C)**.

- CPU(central processing unit) is the brain of the ultrasound machine. It is basically a computer having microprocessor, memory, amplifiers and power supplies for the microprocessor and transducer. The CPU sends electrical currents to the transducer to emit sound waves, and receives the returning echoes. The CPU does calculations involved in processing the data. After processing raw data, the CPU forms the image on the monitor. The CPU can also store the processed data and/or image on the disk.

- Transducer, another very vital component of the ultrasound machine, has dual function of emitting sound waves at a definite frequency as well as capturing the returning echoes (returning frequency depends on the tissue through which the ultrasound waves traverse). The returning wave is digitized as echoes or dots on the screen.
- Images are acquired in real time and in any imaging plane. Ultrasound may be conventional real time or Doppler. Ultrasound machines available today are complex and quite advance in electronics and post processing capabilities.
- The main function of ultrasound machine is to change the returning echoes (received by the transducer) into visible dots forming the anatomic image on the ultrasound screen. The brightness of each dot relates to the strength of echo and agreyscale image is produced.
- Linear and curved transducers are generally used. A linear transducer produces linear scan and a curved transducer produces an arc-shaped image. The most important part in diagnostic ultrasound is probe or transducer. Axial resolution is improved and image looks enlarged when high frequency transducer is used. With low frequency transducers axial resolution is less but penetration is more.

Transducers or Probes

- Ultrasound transducers or probes (Fig.14) are made of transducer head, connecting wire, and a connector. Details are given in chapter 1.
- Head of the transducer has a foot print region from where sound waves are emitted and received. A marker is also located next to the head in order to assist identification of orientation.
- Type of transducer or probe depends on the arrangements of piezo crystals and firing sequence.
- There are many types of the probes viz. linear array, annular array, and sector. The piezo crystals are arranged in a straight line in linear array and in concentric ring in annular array probes. Sector probe has only one or two crystals which are in motion when stimulated.
- Linear array probes are further categorized as phased linear array and steered linear array depending upon the number and arrangement of crystals.
- Overlapping the crystals in linear array probe creates phased linear array transducer.

- Steered linear array probe is created by altering the direction of electric stimulus.
- Probes or transducers are also classified according to their usage as endovaginal probes (designed to scan genital structures from within the vagina),trans rectal probes (designed for pregnancy examination in large animals in veterinary practice and also for human prostate examination),
- Probes are also categorized according to ultrasound frequency produced as 2.5 MHz, to 50 MHz.
- Transducer is, therefore, selected as per species of animal to be examined, and area to be scanned as selection of transducer or probe is important for generating good sonographic images.

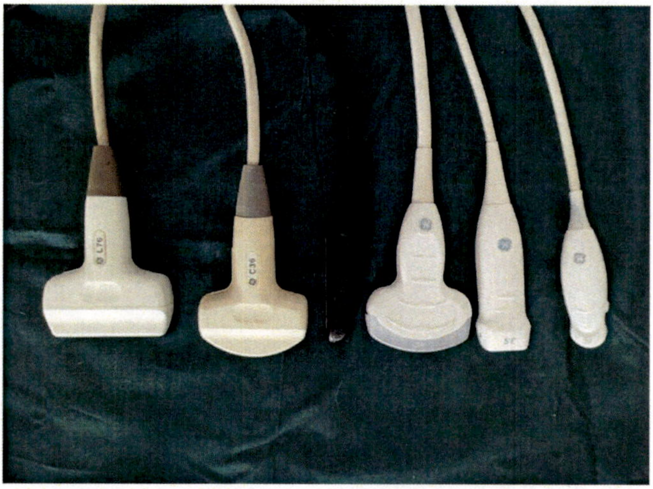

Fig. 14: Transducers of different MHZ and foot prints

Control panel of ultrasound machines (Fig.15).

Ultrasound equipment has a wide variety of features and options. The features are operated either from the console of the equipment or touch screen monitor or a combination of both.

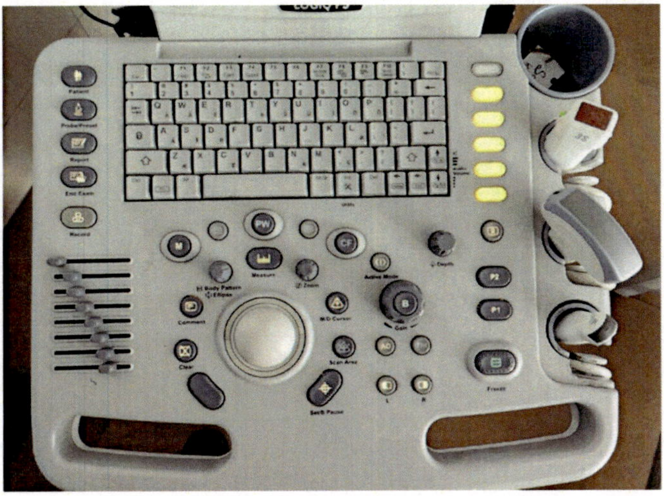

Fig. 15: Control panel of Ultrasound machine

- Power on and off switch - This is sued to switch the machine on and off.
- Alpha Numeric Key- It is used to write numbers.
- Patient Key- It is used to write the details of the patient.
- Select/ Change probes/Probe selection-This is for selecting the specific probe.
- Set- This is pressed to select from activated menu. Press to fix measurement point.
- Present Menu- Scroll ball is used to navigate the menu. Selection is made such as abdomen/vascular/procedures etc.
- Scroll/ Track Ball- It is used to move the cursor within image or navigation through menu. It has multi-function and can be used in conjunction with calliper placement, screen annotation or moving the zoom or Doppler boxes to the desired location.
- Frequency Adjustment- This is used to increase resolution at the cost of penetration.
- Focal zone Adjustment- It is used to adjust the depth at which the image has highest resolution.
- Gain Knob - It functions as amplifier and is used to change the strength of returning echoes. It adjusts the overall brightness of the image. The overall brightness of the image can be increased or decreased.

- Time Gain Compensation – It is to change strength of returning echoes in a certain depth. Gain is adjusted in specific area of the image. It allows adjustment of brightness at a specific depth of the image (Fig.16).

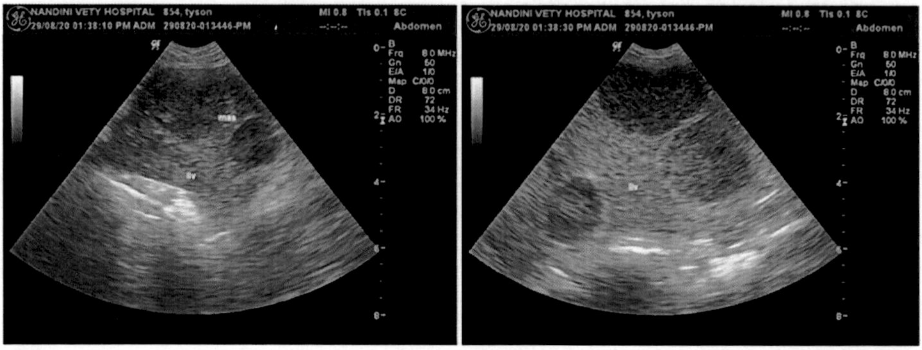

(A) **(B)**

Fig. 16: Overall gain and power affects overall brightness on the screen. Sonogram at **(A)** displays adequate overall brightness due to adequate overall gain, whereas sonogram at **(B)** displays increased overall brightness due to higher overall gain.

- Sector Width – It is the angle of sector image. For high resolution it is better to use a small angle.
- Frame Rate – Rate at which images are updated on the screen is called frame rate. The type of the examination affects the frame rate.
- Dynamic range(compression) - It is used to adjust the number of grey shades displayed.
- Depth Adjustment – It is to change the depth of the ultrasound beam. The depth of the field of the view on the monitor screen can be decreased or increased. Area of interest should be maximised on the monitor and depth of the field of view should be decreased.
- 2-D knob- It stands for 2-D mode of scanning or traditional B-mode imaging.
- The M-Mode knob – It activates the M-Mode function. The M-Mode display corresponds to the anatomic components that the M-Mode cursor intersects. It is used primarily to document motion, such as cardiac activity of the foetus in early gestation.
- Colour Flow knob – It activates colour flow or colour Doppler. Colour flow or colour Doppler detects blood flow in the insonated tissue and assigns colour to the blood flow based upon the direction of blood flow.

Red colour indicates blood moving towards the transducer (up) and blue colour indicates blood moving away from the transducer (down)

- Persistence –It affects the duration of the stay of the image on the screen before it is updated. For better and smooth image, persistence should be as low as possible.
- Split Frame – Some Ultrasound machines have facility to display 2 or more images on the screen for side by side comparison.
- Freeze key -It is used to freeze the current image measurements can be taken when the image is frozen.
- Print / Save –It is used to print a frozen image and/or save an image to a hard drive.
- Measurement / Cursor - After activating the first measurement button – a marker appears on the screen. Scroll button is used to place it over the desired area. By pushing 'set' or 'mark' - the first cursor is placed there and second cursor appears. Scroll ball and set are used.
- Additional measurements can be obtained by pushing the cursor button again. Some machines will have extra measurement buttons.
- Change Mode –It is used to change the mode of the ultrasound machine as M- mode button to M-mode, Doppler button to Doppler mode, colour Doppler to colour, etc.
- Focus – It is used to change or add focal zones to the image.
- Change Paper – 'Open' button on printer is used to open and insert new roll. Printer is closed manually. Then printing can be started.

Gain Controls

- Gain speaks about the amplification of electrical signals generated by returning echoes.
- Brightness of the image depends on intensity of the echo.
- Gain control is used to adjust amplitude to create image with good contrast.
- Near field echoes are brighter than that of far field. Adjustment of near field gain control may lead to better image
- Gain control should be done before image is frozen.

Other Controls

- Depth of field – It is used to change the size of the image to visualize the structure that might be out of field.
- Reject – It is another gain control option to reject near field echoes of high intensity.
- Orientation – It is used to document plane in which probe is oriented (Transverse, sagittal).
- Pulse Doppler cursor
- Biopsy Cursor
- Format
- Pointers
- Polarity
- Left-right Invert
- Annotation.

Patient Preparation

- A fast for 8 to 12 hours prior to abdominal ultrasonography is desirable to reduce gas in the abdomen.
- For the examination of urinary bladder and prostate glands, drinking a lot of water prior to sonography is advisable so that urinary bladder is full. The full bladder makes the visualization of these organs better.
- The site is prepared by shaving and cleaning the area in dogs (Fig.17 A) and cats (Fig.18).
- For transrectal sonography, rectum should be cleaned off faecal material.
- Acoustic gel is applied on the area to ensure good contact (Fig.17B).

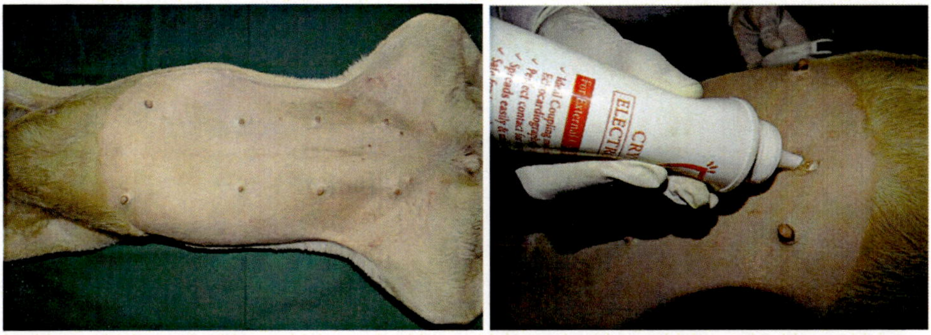

(A) **(B)**

Fig.17. Preparation of the site for ultrasonographic examination in dog by shaving **(A)** and application of acoustic gel **(B)**.

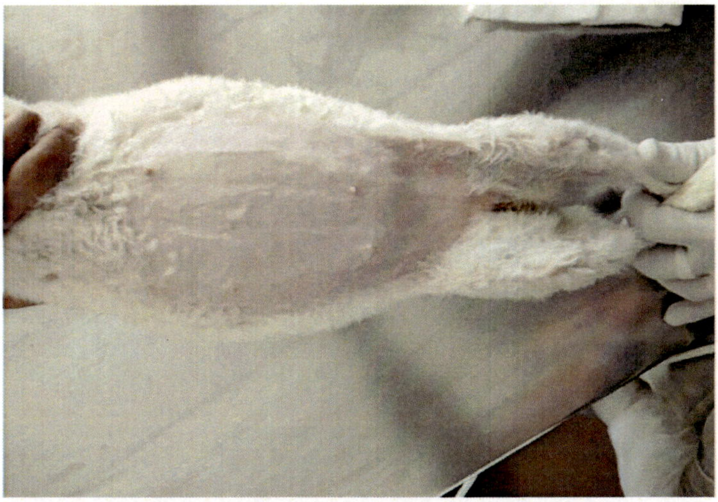

Fig. 18: Preparation of site for ultrasonographic examination in cat by shaving and applying acoustic gel

Positioning of Dogs and Cats for Ultrasonographic Examination.

- For ultrasonographic examination dogs and cats are placed in dorsal (Fig.19A), right lateral (Fig.19B), left lateral recumbency (Fig.19C) or in standing position depending upon the organ to be visualized.
- Scanning in done in at least two planes i.e. transverse and sagittal or longitudinal plane.
- For echocardiography a table with a central window is appropriate.

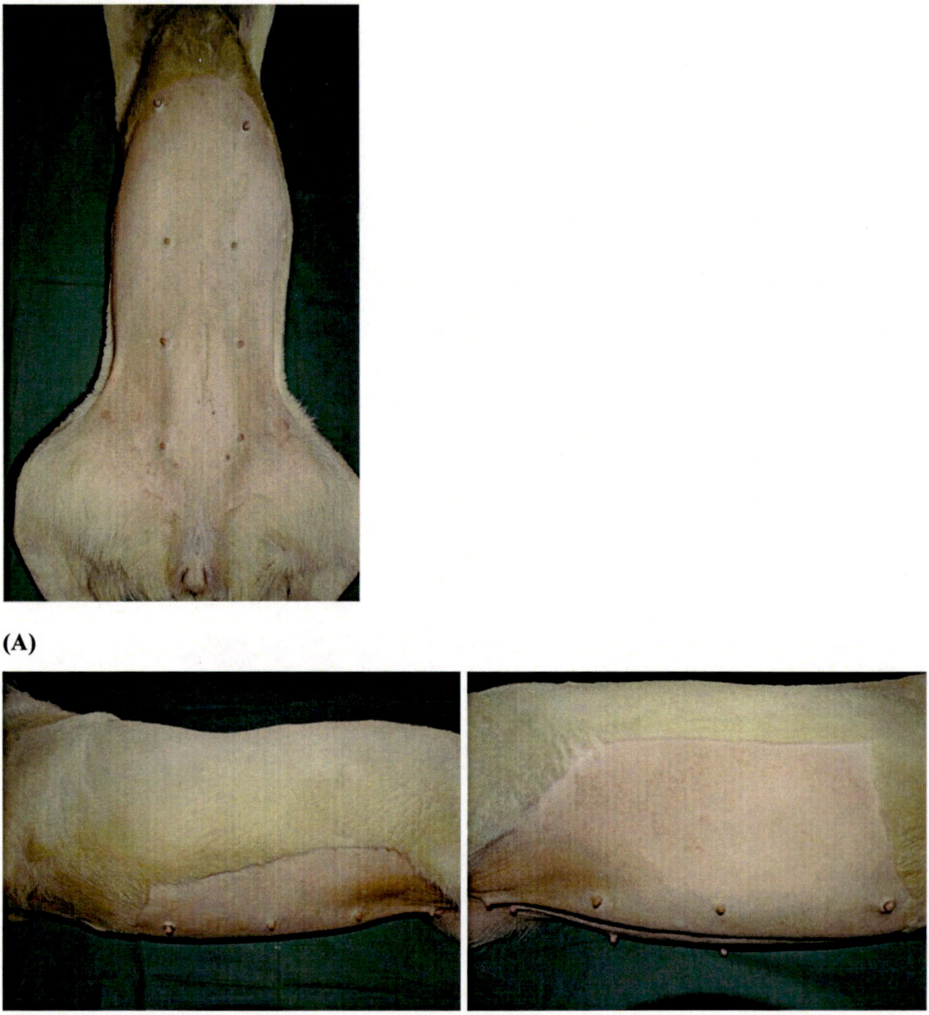

(A)

(B) (C)

Fig. 19: Positioning of dogs for ultrasonographic examination. Dorsal recumbency **(A)**, right lateral recumbency **(B)** and Left lateral recumbency **(C)**.

Things to be Set Prior to Actual Ultrasonographic Examination

- Selection of transducer, setting of gain in the machine and preparation of the patient determine the quality of sonographic image.
- The strength of ultrasound beam decreases with increasing depth in tissue. To compensate this loss of signal, gain setting is done in the machine.

- Select the transducer based upon thickness of the area to be scanned. If the depth of the tissues to be scanned is more, lower frequency transducer is selected.
- Using high frequency transducer at high gain setting may lead to incorrect interpretation.
- It is important to enter details of the animal (being examined) into the ultrasound equipment to be able to save ultrasound images on the hard drive. Minimum information includes, name of the animal, its species, sex and age; owners name, date of examination.

Information to be Detailed About the Organ Being Scanned

- Size of the organ
- Shape of the organ
- Position of the organ
- Contours or margins of the organ
- Relative echogenicity
- Echo texture of the organ

How to Drive Transducer

- Transducer is held like a pen. So that it can be rotated by 90 degrees by rolling between fingers and thumb without applying much pressure.
- The transducer should not be griped tightly.
- The transducer should not be pushed into the abdomen.
- There are three types of transducer's motion viz. distance motion, non-distance angle motion, and non-distance rotational motion.
- In distance motion transducer moves across physical distance. It moves cranial, caudal, left or right sided direction.
- In non-distance angle motion, the transducer remains at one position but angled in different directions.
- In non-distance rotational motion, the transducer stays in its position but rotated in clockwise or anti clock wise direction.
- A combination of these motions is used to finalize the image of the organ.

- Always keep the organ to be viewed in near field and perpendicular to the probe.

Imaging Approaches

- Transabdominal: For imaging abdominal wall, abdominal organs such as liver, gall bladder, spleen, stomach, intestines, pancreas, kidneys, urinary bladder, prostates, urethra, uterus.
- Transthoracic: For imaging heart, major vessels, lungs, diaphragm.
- Transurethral and Transvaginal: For imaging mucosal surface of urethra, bladder, vagina, cervix (special sector or radical endoluminal transducers).
- Transrectal: This approach is used in large ruminants and equines for pregnancy diagnosis and evaluating reproductive and urinary tract.
- Miscellaneous: It is used for scanning tendons, ligaments, teat, udder, eyes.

Trans abdominal Approach

- Place the dog/cat in lateral or dorsal recumbency.
- All organs are to be visualized in two planes. The location for placing transducer for visualizing different organs in transabdominal approach is shown in Fig.20.
- Examination is started by scanning liver first. The transducer is placed just caudal to xiphoid process.
- The stomach is scanned by sliding the transducer caudally.
- The transducer is slide further caudally and to the left to scan spleen.
- The transducer is moved with a medial and slightly caudal distance motion to visualize left kidney.
- Then transducer is angled medially to visualize abdominal aorta in long axis.
- Left adrenal gland is located. Celiac and cranial mesenteric arteries are cranial and left renal artery is caudal to adrenal.
- Caudal to left kidney, left ovary can be located in the near field.
- Transducer is moved further caudally to a central and caudal abdominal position to locate urinary bladder.

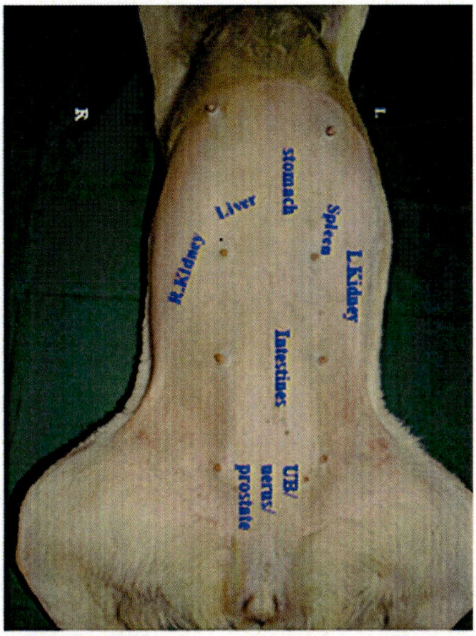

Fig. 20: Showing locations for placing transducer for visualizing different organs in transabdominal approach.

Transthoracic Approach

- Transthoracic approach is used to scan heart, major vessels, lungs and diaphragm. It is common in dogs and cats with heart disease.

Transurethral or Transvaginal Approach

- Transurethral approach is used in humans to image prostates, urethra and bladder
- Transvaginal approach is used in human females to image vagina, cervix or uterus.

Transrectal Approach

- Rectal transducer is used for trans-rectal sonography. It is commonly used in large animals (cows, buffaloes, horses) to detect pregnancy.

Miscellaneous Scanning Approaches

- Tendons, udder, teats, eyes are also examined using ultrasonography.
- Superficial structures poses problem as image is obscured due to near field reverberations. Using standoff pad is beneficial in solving this problem. A homemade fluid filled plastic bag can be used as a standoff pad. Using water bath for scanning teats, limbs or morbid samples give better resolution.

Purpose of Scanning Different Organs

- Liver: Liver is scanned for size, congestion, vessels, abscess, cyst, tumour, echotexture (hypoechoic, hyperechoic), and portosystemic shunts.
- Gall bladder: It is scanned for detecting cholecystitis, sludge, mucocele, bile duct obstruction, calculi and mass.
- Spleen: It is scanned for size, infarction,splenic vessels, mass, hypertrophy, and congestion.
- Esophagus: It is scanned for detecting mega esophagus, diverticulum, and foreign bodies.
- Stomach: It is scanned for detecting foreign bodies, ulcers, dilatation, and volvulus.
- Intestines: Intestines are scanned for foreign bodies, intussusceptions, obstruction, mucosal pattern, emptying time, intestinal wall thickness etc.
- Pancreas: It is scanned for pancreatitis, and tumours
- Kidney : It is scanned for tumours, nephroliths, hydronephrosis, nephritis
- Urinary bladder: It is scanned for cystitis, cystoliths, bladder volume, tumour, cysts etc.
- Prostate: It is scanned for its size, inflammation, hyperplasia, tumour, abscess etc.
- Female Reproductive organs: Female reproductive tract is generally scanned for ovarian follicular dynamics, pregnancy detection, foetal well being, foetal sexing, ovum pick up technology and detecting diseases of uterus and ovary.

Documenting an Ultrasound Examination

- A report is required at the end of the ultrasound examination. It is important to know that image documentation is an essential component of the ultrasound examination and its report. Images can be produced in paper format or stored digitally on the ultrasound equipment. Several ultrasound systems have knobs for images, which can be formatted to allow for printing on a thermal printer and for saving a digital copy in a DICOM format on the equipment hard drive.
- A permanent copy of the ultrasound report, including ultrasound images should be kept and stored in accordance with national regulations.

- Record of each sonogram should be kept for future reference and follow up.
- All findings of the case should be noted down during sonography or immediately after sonography is over.
- A format of the ultrasound report is given below. It can be modified as per requirement of the hospital.

Format of Ultrasound Report

Name and Address of the Hospital:

OPD No.: Date:

Name of the Patient:

Species of the Patient: Breed:

Age: Sex: Body weight:

Owner's name and address:

Mobile Number of the Owner:

Brief History of Illness:

Clinical diagnosis:

Details of Previous Ultrasound Examination if any:

Referred by Dr.

Specification of the area to be visualized (Entire abdomen/cranial abdomen/ mid abdomen/caudal abdomen or pelvic region/ urinary system /any specificorgan/ pregnancy/echocardiography/thoracic/ophthalmic/tendon,ligament/or subcutaneous tissues/ etc.)

Date of Sonographic Examination

Sonographic Examination Number

Sonographic Findings:

Interpretation:

Signature

Name and Qualification of the
Sonographer/Veterinarian

Note: Please correlate the findings clinically

Common Errors During Ultrasonography

- Ultrasonography is considered as safe, non-invasive, sensitive diagnostic modality of great clinical utility. As no diagnostic imaging technique is 100% accurate in diagnosing many diseases, some errors in interpretation of the image may occur with any imaging modality (Daneman and Navaro, 2009).
- Errors in diagnostic imaging have been categorized as errors due to perception, errors due to cognition, equipment-related errors, inevitable errors or multifactorial errors (Kassier and Kopelman 1989; Taylor et al., 2011).
- The expertise of the person performing and interpreting the imaging has a great bearing on the results of the imaging examination.
- Perceptual errors relate to failure of recognizing the abnormal finding present on the image.
- Cognitive errors are owing to over interpretation or misinterpretation of the findings on the image.
- Equipment-related errors are due to equipment failure and /or inadequate training. Inevitable errors occur due to masking or absence of expected abnormal imaging findings.
- More than one type of the error falls under the category of multifactorial errors. Such types of errors occur not only in radiography but also in ultrasonography.

Uses of Ultrasonography

A. Ultrasound is used as a diagnostic modality.

B. Ultrasound is also used for therapeutic purpose.

C. Ultrasound is also being used in medical biotechnology

A. Application of Diagnostic Ultrasound

- It is safest non-invasive imaging modality
- Two dimensional ultrasonography is used to assess body organs and cavities.
- It is also complementary to radiography.
- It reveals more specific information than radiography.

- It is of great value in the differential diagnosis of abscess, cysts, tumours and haematomas.
- It is being used to detect growth in stomach, intestines, liver, spleen, kidney, prostate, ovaries, and uterus.
- It is of great value in identification of architecture (size, shape and location) of a mass or organ.
- It facilitates identification of focal pathological area within parenchymal organs.
- Real time ultrasonography facilitates aspiration or needle biopsy.
- In small animals alterations in the structure of liver, gall bladder, spleen, kidneys, urinary bladder, spleen and prostate can be detected easily.
- Ultrasonography is used to detect portosystemic shunts in liver.
- It is used to detect liths/crystals in kidneys, urinary bladder and urethra.
- Ultrasonography has also been employed in evaluation of abdominal blood vessels.
- In females ultrasonography is being used to evaluate uterine anatomy, involution and pathology.
- Detection of pregnancy, embryonic mortality, monitoring foetal development and identifying foetal sex is another very important application of ultrasonography in animals.
- M- mode or two dimensional echocardiography facilitates assessing cardiac size, thickness of ventricle wall, valves, septa, great vessels and cardiac contractility.
- Echocardiography has made the evaluation of heart an easy task and the technique is useful in assessing pericardial effusions or masses (intra cardiac or pericardial).
- Ultrasonography has facilitated taking of ultrasound guided needle biopsy of internal organs with minimum invasion.
- Diagnosing ascites and haemoabdomen has become an easy task by employing ultrasonography.
- Ultrasonography has facilitated evaluation of soft tissues (muscles, tendons, ligaments). Some important information can be derived from ultrasonographic examination of muscles, tendon, joints, orbit and brain (Qiu *et al.,* 2015).

- Evaluation of adrenal glands and abdominal lymph glands has also become an easy task by the application of ultrasonography.
- Ultrasound guided nerve block is a new application of ultrasonography and intends to revolutionize the field of regional anaesthesia.
- It is the best technique to distinguish solids from fluid filled cavities.
- Transabdominal ultrasound has been used in evaluation of location, diameter of lesion, intestinal wall and motility, and intraluminal contents of the intestines in the goats with John's disease (Thrawat *et al.,* 2012).
- It has also been used in evaluation of animals with peritoneal or pleural fluids.
- Information about mediastinal masses can also be obtained.
- Pulmonary lesions are usually not accessible unless involved lung is against the thoracic wall or surrounded by soft tissue.
- Ultrasonography is not very useful in examining axial, appendicular skeleton, or skull.

B. Application of Therapeutic Ultrasound

- Hastening healing in animals.
- Repair of tendon and ligament injuries in animals
- Application of Ultrasound in human Medicine
    - High intensity ultrasound (10 W/cm^2) has been used for purposeful destruction of tissues in humans.
    - It has been used successfully in the treatment of Meniere's disease in man.
    - Ultrasound irradiation (up to 25 W/cm^2) has been employed in the management of vertigo in humans.
    - It has also been used in the surgical management of cataract in humans.
    - It has also been tried in the management of Parkinson's disease, wart management, and treatment of laryngeal papillomatosis in humans.
    - Ultrasonic renal lithotripcor, a new development, is showing promise in breaking renal stones in humans. Extracorporeal shock wave lithotripsy is the common technique for treating stones in the

kidney and ureter in humans in United State. Lithotripsy is also being employed in breaking gall stones.

- Interest is being renewed in the use of ultrasonic hyperthermia in cancer management.
- Ultrasound is also being employed in the management of arthritis, bursitis, muscle spasms, traumatic soft tissue injuries and certain collagen diseases as a physical therapy.

C. Application of Ultrasound in Medical Biotechnology Research

- Recently ultrasound is being promoted as a new modality in molecular research and therapy such as apoptosis and autophagy induction sonoporation (small pore formation) and cell membrane repair in gene transfer research, changes in gene expression, and construction of gene promoter regions. Low intensity pulsed ultrasound (LIPUS) has shown promise in accelerating bone fracture healing.

Application of Colour Doppler

- To check heart function in association with electrocardiogram.
- To detect blockages in blood flow.
- To detect damage in blood vessel and in the structure of the heart.
- To detect narrowing of blood vessels.
- To monitor blood flow after surgery.

Veterinary Point of Care Ultrasound

- It is the ultrasound examination carried out by the attending veterinarian in emergency department.
- It is invaluable test performed at the point of care to confirm suspicious findings of physical examination and to identify underlying pathologies in unstable animals.
- It is focused ultrasound scan aimed at determining the presence or absence of specific pathologies such as effusions (pericardial or peritoneal), pneumothorax and interstitial alveolar disease.
- The common indications of veterinary point of care ultrasound examination are traumas (blunt or penetrating), acute collapse, cardiovascular emergencies, effusions, respiratory distress, pneumothorax, haemorrhages and post-operative complications.

- Its aim is to quickly direct further diagnostic procedures and/or initiate life saving interventions.

Limitations of Ultrasound

1. It is of little value in examining organs containing air such as lungs, or air sacs.
2. It is of no use in examining bones as ultrasound waves cannot pass through.
3. Because of bony cage, examination of brain and spinal cord is not feasible.

Precaution

- Although ultrasonography is very useful technique in defining and assessing disease process, expertise is very much essential in interpreting the obtained images.
- Casual reading of sonograms may defeat the purpose.
- Clinical specialist (cardiologists, radiologists, internists, surgeons, veterinary medicine specialist, or veterinary gynecologists) are the potential resource.

Advantages of Ultrasound in Veterinary Medicine

- It provides real time look at internal organs.
- It is non-invasive.
- It does not require medication, analgesia or anaesthesia.
- It is affordable technique.
- It can be repeated without any harm.
- There are no side effects of ultrasound examination.
- It allows visualization of internal organs with more precision.
- The ultrasound procedure is easy and distress free.
- It facilitates to get biopsy sample of the internal organs.
- Now a day's ultrasound is easily accessible.
- Ultrasound can help in detecting foreign objects like fabric, plastic, wood and others that are occasionally ingested by pets.

Limitations of Ultrasound in Veterinary Medicine

- Major limitation of ultrasound is its inability to travel through air. So lungs cannot be properly evaluated.
- In large animals, visualization of stomach and intestines is limited because of large amount of gas and ingesta.
- It is very much dependent on the skill and experience of the operator.
- Results of ultrasound may vary widely between individuals.

References

Daneman, A. and Navaro, O.M. (2009). Common pitfalls in paediatric abdominal imaging. Paediatric Radiol. 39, S369-S37.

Kassier, J.P. and Kopelman, R.I. (1989). Cognitive errors in diagnosis: Instantiation, classification, and consequences. Am. J. Med. 86: 433-441

Qiu, Y.M. (2015). Piezoelectric micro machined ultrasound transducer (PMUT) arrays for integrated sensing, actuation and imaging Sensors. 15:233-240.

Thrawat, M., Alsobiyal, E., Hasahud, M and Buczinski, S. (2012). Trasnabdominal ultrasonographic findings in goats with paratuberculosis. Can. Vet. J., 53: 1063–1070.

Taylor, G.A., Voss, S.D., Melvin, P.R. and Grahem, D.A. (2011). Diagnostic errors in paediatric radiology. Paediatric Radiol. 41: 327-334.

3

Doppler Ultrasound

J.P. Varshney and P.S. Chaudhary

Doppler ultrasound is a non-invasive diagnostic tool being employed in evaluating blood flow in major vessels, veins and arteries. Information regarding perfusion in an organ or an area can also be obtained through Doppler ultrasonography. Doppler ultrasound is an important part of echocardiographic examination in dogs and cats. Its more recent application is in the investigation of the tissue wall motion while evaluating the heart. B-mode ultrasound is used to examine cardiac structures. Doppler is used to measure normal or abnormal blood flow within the heart and through different valves. Doppler ultrasound is also used to examine the foetal heart. (Fig.21).

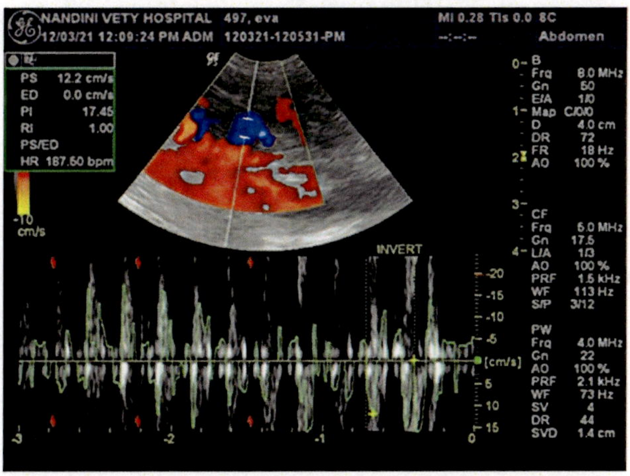

Fig. 21: Examination of foetal heart by Doppler ultrasound

Indications of Doppler Ultrasound

The main indications of Doppler ultrasound are in the diagnosis of following diseases:

- Congenital heart defect.
- Heart valvular defects.
- Arterial occlusion.
- Arterial stenosis.
- Deep vein thrombosis.
- Ventricular wall movement.
- Arteriovenous malformations.
- Venous insufficiencies.

Principle of Doppler Sonography

- Doppler principle is named after physicist and mathematician Christian Johann Doppler who discovered that the coloured appearance of moving stars was due to their motion relative to earth. This relative motion causes a red or blue shift in the frequency of light. The resultant shift in frequency of light from moving source is termed as Doppler Effect. This effect is also applicable to sound waves.
- In simple term the Doppler Effect is found in all types of waves where the source and the receiver are moving relative to each other.
- The change in frequency between emitted and returned sound waves is proportional to the velocity of moving reflector. This change in frequency is termed as the Doppler shift.
- Images of colour flow or Spectral Doppler are obtained from measuring the movement.

Application of Doppler Effect in Diagnostic Ultrasound

- Detecting presence or absence of blood flow.
- Detecting the direction of blood flow.
- Detecting the velocity at which blood is flowing.
- Blood flowing toward transducer produces positive Doppler shifted signal
- Blood flowing away from the transducer produces negative Doppler shifted signals.

Types of Doppler Instrumentation

- **Continuous wave Doppler (CW Doppler).** It is a simple instrument. It has hand held unit with an integrated speaker connected to a pencil probe transducer. It employs two piezo electric crystals in a single head. One crystal transmits a continuous sonic signal at a known frequency. The other crystal receives the returning echoes and records their frequency. There is continuous transmission and reception of ultrasound waves in this system. Direction of blood flow can be ascertained with CW Doppler but it is difficult to ascertain various depths of the source of signals. Doppler signals are obtained from all vessels in the path of the ultrasound beam. This type of Doppler is also used in adult cardiac scanners to investigate the high velocities in the aorta in humans.
- **Colour Doppler.** Velocity information determined from Doppler measurements is displayed as a feature of image itself. Velocities away from the transducer appear as shades of blue, towards transducer shades of red, and aliasing shades of green. Colour flow imaging can be used to identify vessels, to identify the presence and direction of the flow, and to highlight the gross circulation abnormality.
- **Power Doppler.** It is also referred to as energy Doppler, amplitude Doppler or Doppler angiography. It does not display velocity information. It simply displays the amplitude of returning Doppler shift echoes. Power Doppler is less dependent on angle of insonation.
- **Pulse Wave Doppler (PW).** The sensitive volume from which flow data are sampled, can be controlled. It can detect the depth at which a returning signal has originated. The detection of such mobile structures needs high pulse repetition frequency, an optimum transducer frequency for depth and use of correct insonation angle. It has one transducer. It sends pulse. Gate closes. After sometime gate opens. Gates remain open briefly. Gate closes. General Doppler and obstetric ultrasound scanners uses pulsed wave ultrasound. Pulse wave Doppler suffer from aliasing ambiguity i.e. the Doppler frequency is half the pulse repetition frequency. It is used to provide analysis of the flow at specific sites in the vessel being investigated.
- **Spectral Doppler.** It is a combination of B- mode and pulse wave Doppler. It is used in vascular flow imaging. The Doppler signal is of a complex nature in a given sampled volume of blood flow. Therefore, analysis of the entire spectrum helps in assessing the characteristics of vascular flow. Vascular flow is categorised into peak systolic and diastolic

velocities, systolic / diastolic ratio, resistive index, pulsatility index, acceleration time, and acceleration index and volume flow. Application of sets of these indices is paramount in detection of stenosis, its degree and related flow abnormalities.

- The Doppler ultrasound equipment has filters to cut out the big amplitude, low frequency Doppler signals resulting from tissue movements.

Size of the Doppler Signal

- As blood velocity increases, Doppler frequency also increases.
- Higher ultrasound frequency gives higher Doppler frequency. While in B mode ultrasound lower frequencies have better penetration.
- The choice of the frequency is a compromise between better penetration or better sensitivity to flow.
- More aligned Doppler ultrasound beam to flow direction increases the Doppler frequency.

Limitations of Doppler Ultrasound

- Fat, gas, faeces, motion (respiratory, peristaltic, cardiac or restlessness) interfere with image quality.
- Changes in blood flow pattern proximal or distal to stenosis of a vessel occurs only when degree of stenosis is significant.
- Multiple level stenosis result in obscure blood flow pattern
- Flow patterns are subject to individual variations.

Suggested Further Readings

Mannion, P. (2006). Diagnostic Ultrasound in Small Animal Practice. Blackwell Science Ltd. Oxford, U.K.

4

Ultrasound Guided Biopsy

J.P. Varshney and P.S. Chaudhary

Ultrasound is an excellent diagnostic modality for detecting visceral abnormalities. Detection of masses, nodules or effusions through sonography provides non-specific diagnosis. For specific/definite diagnosis tissue samples are necessary for histopathological examination. The techniques of ultrasound guided fine needle aspiration and core biopsy are of great help in establishing etiological diagnosis.

- Ultrasound is also used to take biopsy from organs like liver, gall bladder, adrenal glands, pancreas, kidney, spleen, prostate, abdominal mass, lymph nodes, ovaries, uterus, or thyroid.
- This technique is called ultrasound guided biopsy.
- Ultrasound is non-invasive technique, but ultrasound guided biopsy is a minimal invasive technique.
- It is an image guided procedure using ultrasound technology to assist specialist to perform needle biopsy.
- Percutaneous route is used to take biopsy of abdominal organs.
- It is always better to evaluate haemostatic parameters of the patient before taking ultrasound guided biopsy.
- The patient should be given either general anaethesia or a combination of heavy sedation and local anaesthesia before biopsy sampling procedure is performed in uncooperative dogs.
- The site is prepared by shaving, applying antiseptic (povidone –iodine or alcohol) and sterile acoustic gel.
- Sterile gel is also applied on the transducer. The transducer may be covered with a sterile sleeve if it is to be used per rectal. In case, transducer is used trans abdominally, no covering is needed.

- Target organ is imaged.
- Once a good view of the target organ is obtained, a small incision is made on the skin adjacent to the transducer to facilitate the insertion of sampling needle through abdominal wall via a clip on guide at an angle of 15 to 30 ^{0} to the transducer.
- A variety of needles (Fig.22) are available for taking biopsy sample. A large bore needle (gauge 14, tri cut biopsy needle) is recommended for taking tissue core sample for histopathological examination.

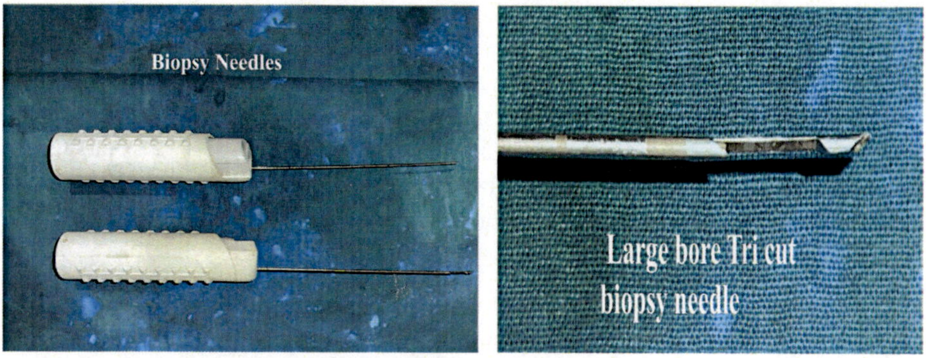

Fig. 22: Showing variety of needles for taking ultrasound guided tissue biopsy

- For taking aspirate for cytological examination, a fine biopsy needle of 18 to 22 gauges is suitable. The needle is pushed forward up to target region under the guidance of ultrasound (Fig.23) and fluid is withdrawn.

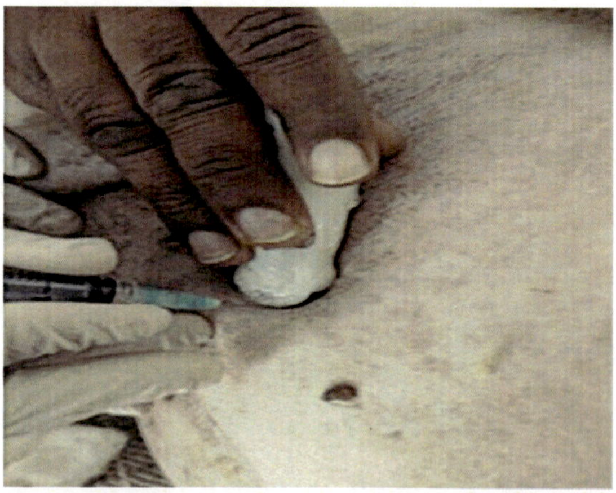

Fig. 23. Showing aspiration of fluid under the guidance of the ultrasound. A 22 gauge needle is pushed slowly into the abdominal cavity monitoring its passage on ultrasound monitor.

- An automatic biopsy device facilitates superior sample for histopathological examination.
- For small lesions (<3 cm), echogenic biopsy needle stylet enhances precision.
- Biopsy needle is pushed forward to the lesion site under the guidance of ultrasound.
- Needle is released from the biopsy guide and transducer is removed after needle is positioned. Sample is collected and needle is withdrawn.
- Percutaneous ultrasound-guided fine needle aspiration (FNA) and biopsy procedures are being routinely used in small animal practice to determine the nature of a lesion (inflammatory, infectious, or neoplastic).
- Abdominocentesis (Fig. 24), pleurocentesis, and pericardiocentesis can also be performed with the guidance of ultrasound.

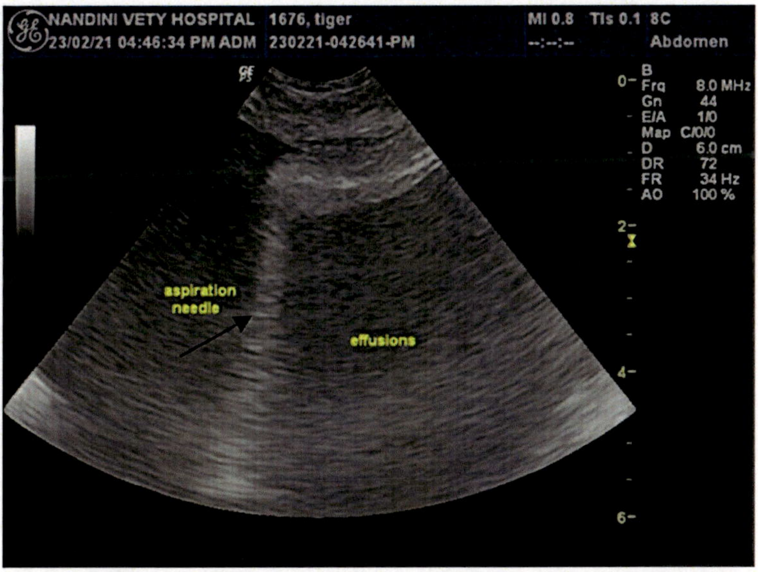

Fig. 24: Showing ultrasound guided abdominocentesis in a dog. Black arrow shows needle in the abdomen to aspirate peritoneal fluid for cytological, biochemical and microbial examination.

- Fluid samples obtained from these sites can be used for cytological, culture, and/or biochemical investigations.

Challenges of Ultrasound Guided Sampling

- It is not possible to take biopsy sample where gas or bones prevents access to the lesion.
- Structures and lesions located deep in pelvic canal may not be accessible by trans abdominal approach.

Advantages of Ultrasound Guided Biopsy

- It is a safe, minimally invasive, rapid technique.
- There is no radiation exposure.
- It allows precise, real-time observation of the sampling device and immediate post procedure monitoring.
- Low diagnostic yield regions, such as central tumour necrosis, and high-risk regions, such as blood vessels and the renal medulla can be avoided.
- The information obtained from ultrasound-guided biopsy sampling can help in surgical planning, chemotherapy options, radiation treatment and prognosis of the case.

Complications of Ultrasound Guided Biopsy Sampling

- The risk of complications of ultrasound guided biopsy is influenced by sonographer's training and experience; size of the needle; tissue being sampled; and location of the lesion.
- Penetration of other viscera may occur.
- Haemorrhage, accidental puncture of adjacent organs and infections are a few complications of the ultrasound guided biopsy. Occurrence of these complications is far less than those with blind biopsy technique.
- Haemorrhage is most common complication but it is minimal in most cases and self-limiting. It is more likely with neoplastic lesions.
- Pneumothorax can be a complication when aspirations and biopsies are done on the thoracic cavity. It is usually small and self-limiting.
- In rare cases seeding of neoplastic cells along the needle tract has been reported in certain cancers (transitional cell carcinoma, prostate cancer, feline pulmonary adenocarcinoma). Bladder and prostate sampling through urethral catheterization can eliminate the risk.
- Fatal shock reactions have been associated with the use of fully automatic biopsy needle in cats.

- Large gall bladder and excessive intestinal gas may limit visibility of the target organ.

Suggested Further Readings

Mannion, P. (2006). Diagnostic Ultrasound in Small Animal Practice. Blackwell Science Ltd., Oxford, U.K.

Section 2: Canine and Feline

5

Ultrasound of The Liver and Gall Bladder

J.P. Varshney and P.S. Chaudhary

Liver is situated in cranial abdomen. Scanning of abdomen is started with the examination of liver. Hepatic ultrasonography is a non-invasive diagnostic modality to evaluate liver parenchyma. Differentiation of focal disease from diffuse disease, cystic lesions from solid masses, and obstructive jaundice from non-obstructive jaundice is possible by hepatic ultrasonography.

Indications for Hepatic Ultrasonography

- Elevated or decreased values of liver enzymes.
- Ascites.
- Hepatic neoplasia.
- Detection of abdominal metastasis.
- Diagnosis of congenital/ acquired portocaval or portosystemic shunt.
- Blood flow abnormalities by Doppler ultrasound.
- Ultrasound guided percutaneous hepatic biopsy.
- Diagnosis of biliary diseases.

Procedure for Scanning

- Dogs and cats are placed in dorsal or lateral recumbency.
- Area is shaved and acoustic gel is applied just caudal to xiphoid process.
- After applying gel on skin of the animal, transducer is placed directly under sternum just caudal to xiphoid process. The sound beam is directed cranio-dorsally.

- Scanning of liver is started with the transducer in long axis plane.
- Diaphragm (Fig. 25) is used as a landmark for liver scanning.

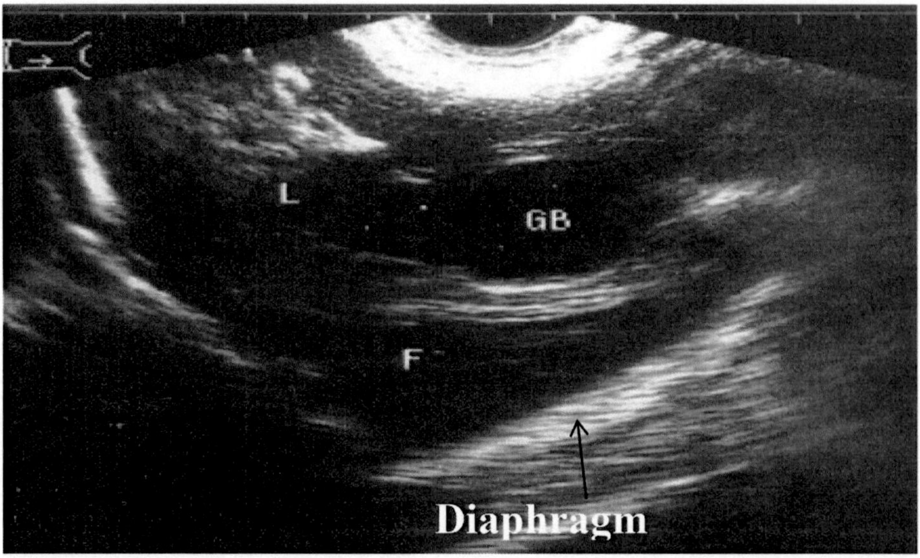

Fig. 25: Hepatic sonogram of a dog. Diaphragm serves as a land mark for identifying the liver.

- Probe is angled cranially to view mid-section of the liver.
- Angle the probe back to mid line and towards right to view gall bladder.
- Then rotate it 90 degree and angle the probe ventrally and dorsally to scan entire liver.
- Scanning of the liver can be done from right mid and left side. On the left laterally and caudally the liver touches the spleen; and on the right dorsally it touches the right kidney.
- Systematically portahepatis, liver size and interportal vasculature are screened keeping caudal vena cava as a land mark.
- Liver size of dogs of corresponding body weight can be calculated using a regression equation (Bhadwal *et al.*, 1999). The distance from skin surface to the midpoint of diaphragm is measured with the help of built in caliper to have an idea of sonographic liver size

Calculated liver size (Z) cm =4.14 + 0.19 x B.Wt (kg)

Calculated liver weight (g) =Ultrasonographic liver size x 127 – 348.68

Calculated liver weight (for calculated liver size of corresponding body weight) g = Z x 127 – 348.68.

Anatomical Considerations of Canine Liver

- Liver is composed of right lateral, right medial, and quadrate, left medial left lateral lobes; caudate process of caudate lobe and papillary process of caudate lobe. Gall bladder is encircled by left lobe (medial sub lobe) quadrate lobe and right lobe (medial sub lobe).
- In normal circumstances hepatic lobes distinction is not feasible during ultrasonography. Nevertheless, division between hepatic lobes becomes more apparent in dogs having significant ascites.
- Liver parenchyma has coarse echo texture in dogs (Fig.26) and cats (Fig.27).
- Portal vessels are predominant vessels throughout liver.
- The portahepatis is central area to the right of mid line where portal vein hepatic artery and bile duct enter and exit.
- Portal veins can be recognised by their hyperechoic wall due to fibro-fatty connective tissue.
- Hepatic veins are hypoechoic tubular structures. They taper towards periphery of the liver. Hepatic veins drain into caudal vena cava.
- Hepatic artery can be visualized using Doppler scanning.
- The blood vessels within liver parenchyma appear as anechoic channels in transverse and sagittal scans.
- Normally gall bladder wall is< 1 mm thick and is not sonographically visible.

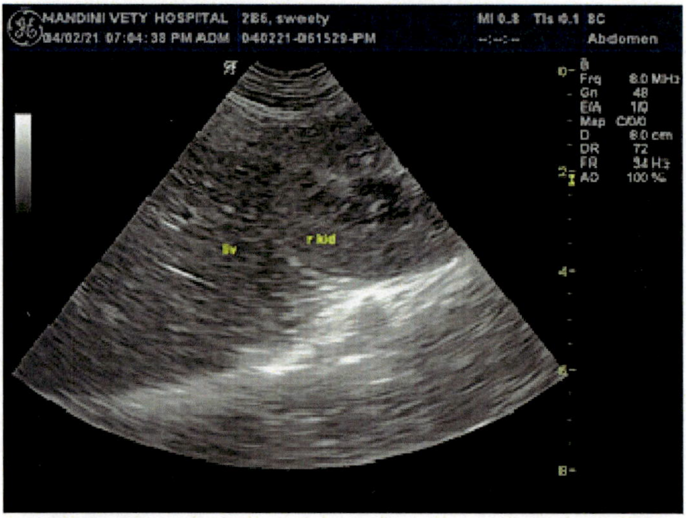

Fig. 26: Hepatic sonogram of a healthy dog showing coarse echo texture. Right kidney is also visible adjacent to liver

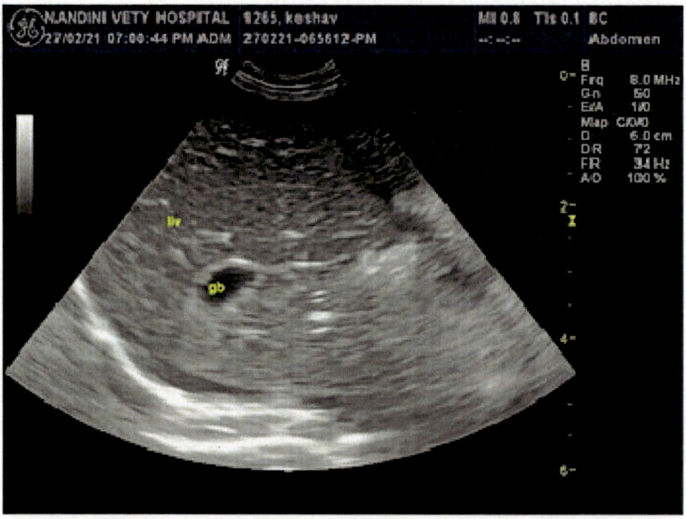

Fig. 27: Sonogram of a healthy cat showing coarse echo texture of the liver and a thin walled gall bladder with anechoic contents.

Ultrasonographic Features of the Liver

- Normal liver is comparatively hypoechoic with a coarse echo texture (Fig. 27 and 28) as compared to spleen; or equal to /slightly more echogenic than the cortex of right kidney; or hypo/isoechoic to falciform fat and has a uniform homogenous and medium level of speckled echogenicity interrupted by hepatic and portal veins. Adjustment of gain is very important as too much gain increases echogenicity and too little gain decreases echogenicity and thus may mislead interpretation.

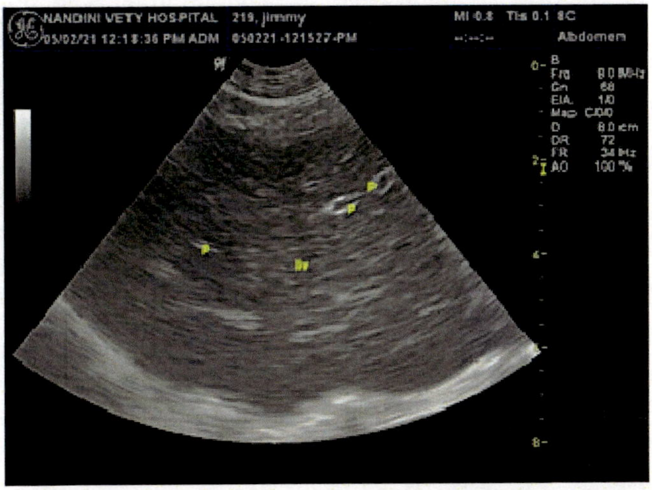

Fig. 28: Hepatic Sonogram of a healthy dog showing coarse echo texture of the liver and portal vein with hyperechoic wall (marked as P).

- The liver margins are sharp and smooth.
- The liver capsule is uniformly smooth.
- Diaphragm separates the liver from pleural cavity. In sonogram taken in dorsal recumbency, diaphragm is visualized as an echogenic, curvilinear continuous line ventral to liver parenchyma.
- Identification of lobes and sub lobes may not be sonographically clear. Broadly gall bladder and portal vein divide the liver into left and right lobes. The caudate lobe is just ventral and to the left of the gall bladder.
- The right gall bladder wall touches the right medial sub lobe of the liver.
- Caudate process of the caudate lobe and right lateral liver lobe is on the dorsal right of caudal vena cava and portal vein.
- The papillary process of the caudate lobe is in the left of portal vein.
- The left lateral hepatic sub lobe is just cranial to the gastric fundus.
- Being a large organ total liver cannot be visualized in a single scan.
- Assessment of liver size can be done by a single linear measurement from the skin surface to the midpoint of the diaphragm.

- Hepatomegaly is speculated when the distance between stomach and diaphragm increases, or ventral right kidney is displaced more caudally.
- Reduced distance between the stomach and the diaphragm or cranial displacement of right kidney is indicative of reduction in the size of the liver.
- Portal veins are in hepatic parenchyma and are identified by their hyperechoic outer wall (Fig.28).The intrahepatic portal veins are a continuation of portal vein.
- Hepatic veins are identified as hypoechoic tubular structures (Fig.29). Their walls are not hyperechoic.

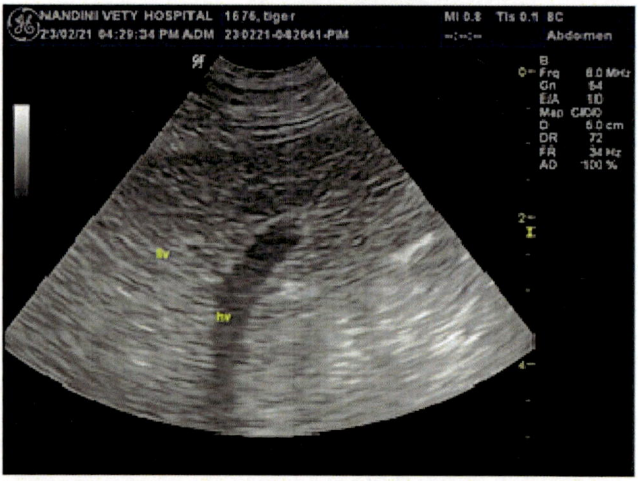

Fig. 29: Hepatic sonogram of a German Shepherd dog showing hyperechoic liver and distended hepatic vein (hv) as a tubular hypoechoic structure.

- In normal conditions cystic and bile ducts are not visualized in dogs. While these can be visualized in cats.
- Gall bladder is visualized as hypoechoic area with thin wall (Fig. 27 and 30).

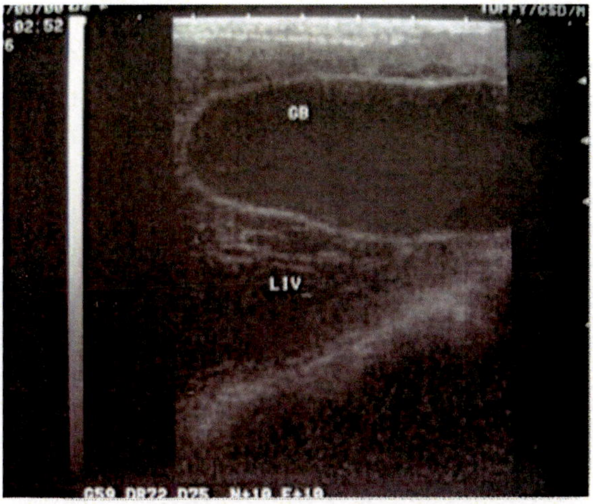

Fig. 30: Hepatic sonogram of a dog showing gall bladder as a thin walled stucture with hypoechoic contents

- Liver parenchyma is coarser than that of spleen at the same scanning plane.
- As compared to spleen, liver is slightly less echogenic (Fig.31).

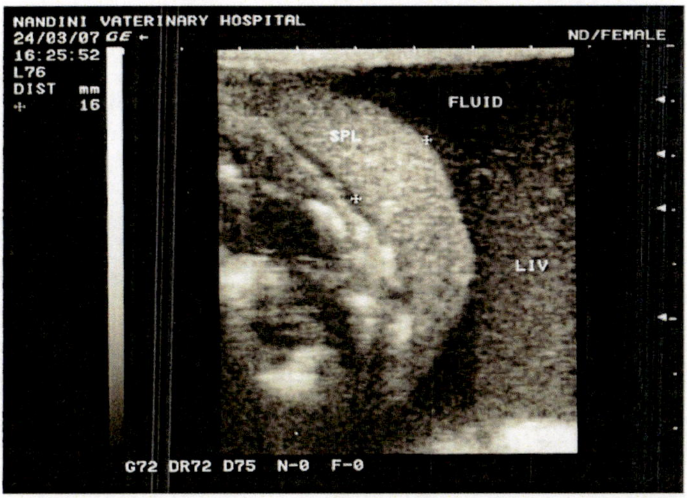

Fig. 31: Trans abdominal sonogram of a healthy dog showing liver and spleen. The spleen has increased echogenicity and fine grained texture as compared to liver

- As compared to cortex of right kidney, the liver is almost equal or slightly more echogenic at the same scanning depth and gain setting.

- Ultrasonographic identification of lobes and sub lobes of the liver is not always possible.
- Visualization of entire liver in a single scan cannot be done.
- For determining liver size multiple scan are needed.
- The size of the liver can be assessed by a single linear measurement from the skin surface to the midpoint of the diaphragm.
- Hepatomegaly is suggested by the increased distance between the stomach and diaphragm or caudal displacement and ventral covering of right kidney by the liver.

Point to be Noted During Liver Scanning

- Size of the liver (increased or decreased).
- Volume of liver.
- Generalised echogenicity of liver parenchyma.
- Presence of hepatic and portal veins.
- Presence of any abnormality.
- Whether abnormality is focal/multifocal or generalized.

Liver Echogenicity and Associated Conditions

- Generalized or diffuse hypoechoic liver (Fig.32) is suggestive of acute hepatitis, acute cholangio-hepatitis, amyloidosis, histocytic neoplasia, leukemia, lymphoma, or passive congestion.

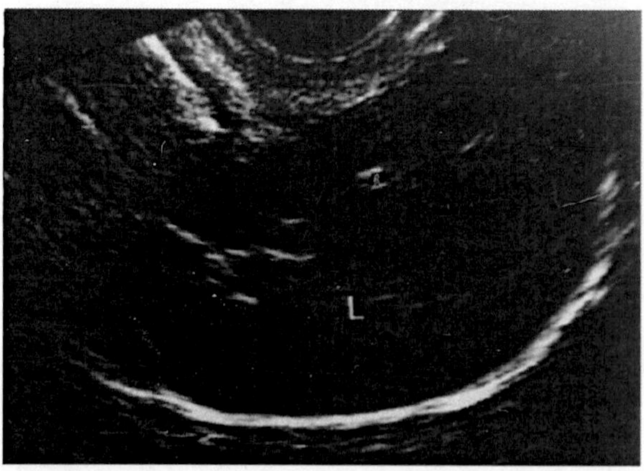

Fig. 32. Hepatic sonogram of a dog showing diffusely hypoechoic liver

- Generalized or diffuse hyperechoic liver (Fig.33 and 34) is suggestive of chronic hepatitis, cirrhosis, fibrosis, lipidosis, lymphoma, mast cell tumor, or steroid hepatopathy.

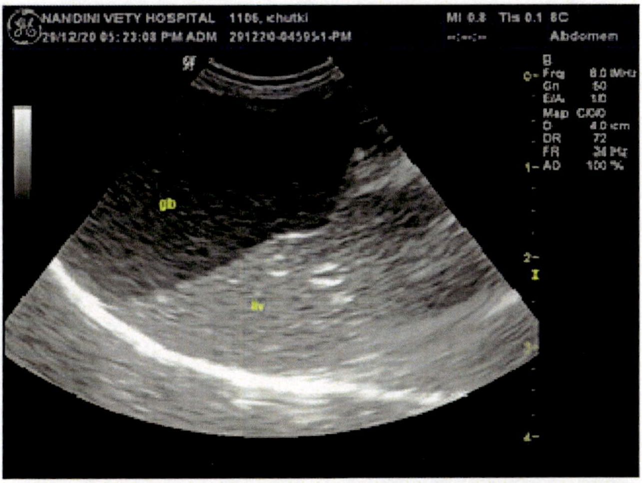

Fig. 33. Hepatic sonogram of dog showing diffusely hyperechoic liver

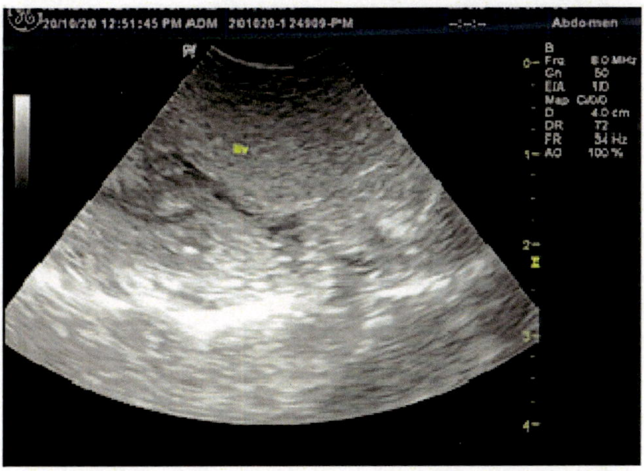

Fig. 34: Hepatic sonogram of an adult cat showing diffusely hyperechoic liver.

- Generalized or diffuse hetero echoic liver (mixed echogenicity) is suggestive of amyloidosis, hepatitis, hepatocellular carcinoma, lymphoma, metastasis, necrosis or steroid hepatopathy with hyperplasia.
- Hepatic tumours are focal or multifocal hyperechoic or mixed masses (Fig. 35, 36).

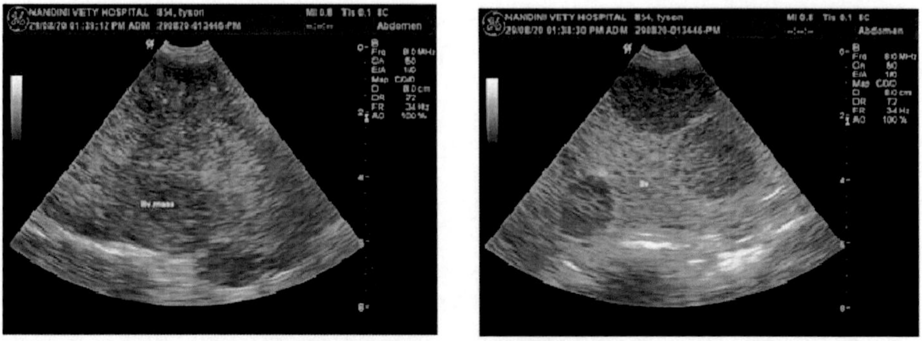

Fig. 35: Sagittal hepatic scan of dogs with anorexia, abdominal pain, vomiting showing masses of mixed echogenicity in liver suggesting hepatic tumour

- Solitary liver lesion with normal liver size in otherwise healthy subjects is suggestive of benign lesion.

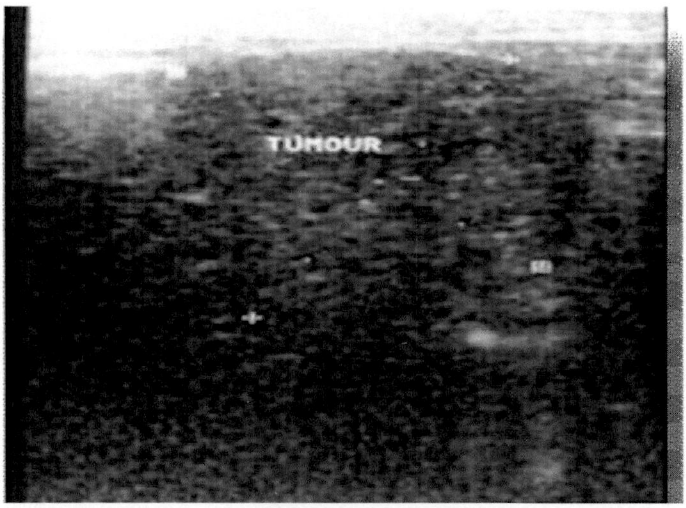

Fig. 36: Hepatic sonogram of a dog showing a focal mass with hetero- echogenicity suggestive of tumour

- Focal or multifocal anechoic lesions in liver are suggestive of cyst, abscess, haematoma, necrosis, biloma or cystic tumor.
- Cysts (Fig.37) have thin well defined walls, no internal echoes, sharp borders, peripheral reflective zones and strong acoustic enhancement.

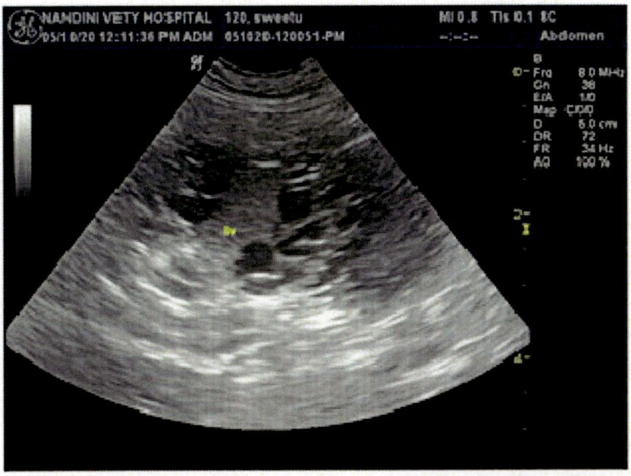

Fig. 37: Hepatic sonogram of a dog showing multiple thin walled anechoic structures with peripheral reflective zones suggesting hepatic cysts.

- Abscesses have centralized anechoic to hypoechoic region with an irregular poorly defined hyperechoic margin (Fig.38).

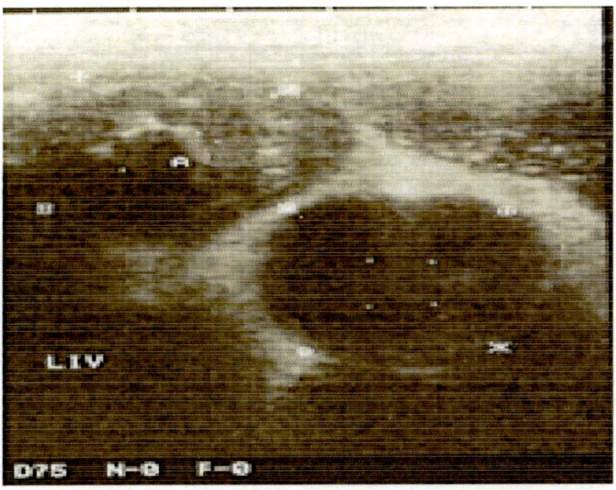

Fig. 38: Hepatic sonogram of a dog with persisting pyrexia (temperature 103- 104^{0}F) and anorexia showing hypoechoic regions with irregular poorly defined echogenic margins suggesting liver abscess.

- Haematomas are visualized as anechoic/hypoechoic structure (Fig.39). With clotting of the blood internal contents become echogenic.

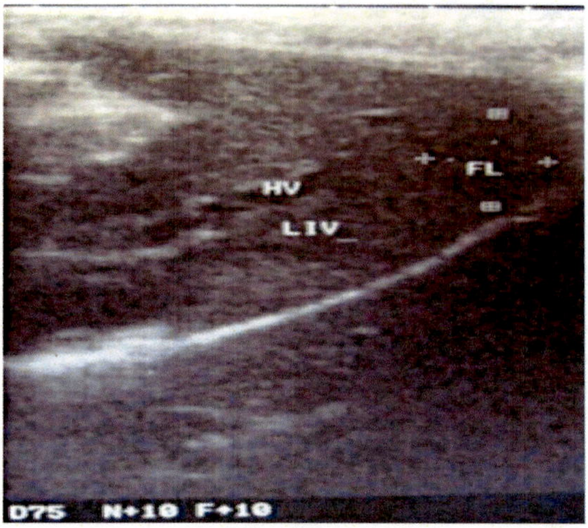

Fig. 39: Hepatic sonogram of a dog showing hypoechoic lesion in the liver suggestive of cyst, abscess, haematoma.

- Small hepatic nodules (<3 cm) can be anechoic, hyperechoic, hypoechoic (Fig.40), and /or heteroechoic. Nodules with hyperechoic centre and hypoechoic rims are often metastatic.

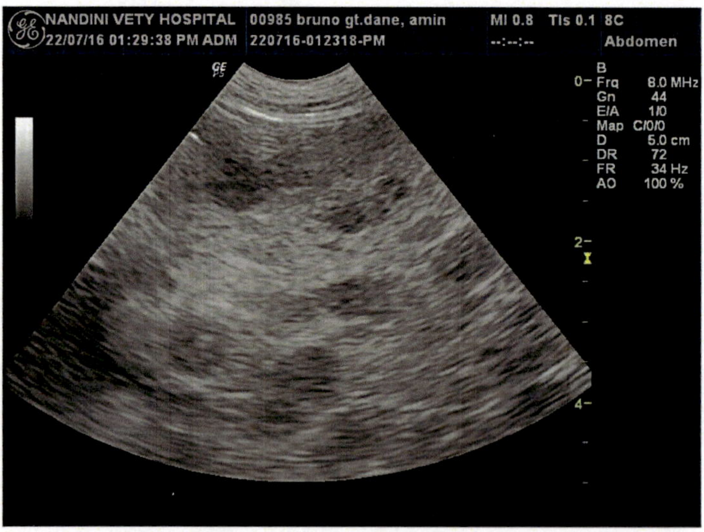

Fig. 40. Hepatic sonogram of a dog showing small multiple hypoechoic patches of variable size on liver lobe suggesting hepatic nodular hyperplasia.

- Focal or multifocal abnormalities can also be due to areas of mineralization (hyperechoic focus with distal shadowing) or intraparenchymal gas (hyperechoic focus with distal acoustic reverberation).

- Though, lymphoma, disseminated mastocytosis, acute hepatitis or cholangiohepatitis affect liver parenchyma diffusely, may not affect overall echogenicity. Therefore definite diagnoses of hepatic abnormalities necessitate cytological or histopathological examination of biopsied material.
- Shunts between intrahepatic vena cava and portal vein (Fig.41) or portal and hepatic vasculatures have been reported. Liver in such cases of intrahepatic portosystemic shunts shows patchy hyperechoic small bright areas with an overall reduction in scanning area. In portosystemic shunts liver becomes small with few detectable veins.

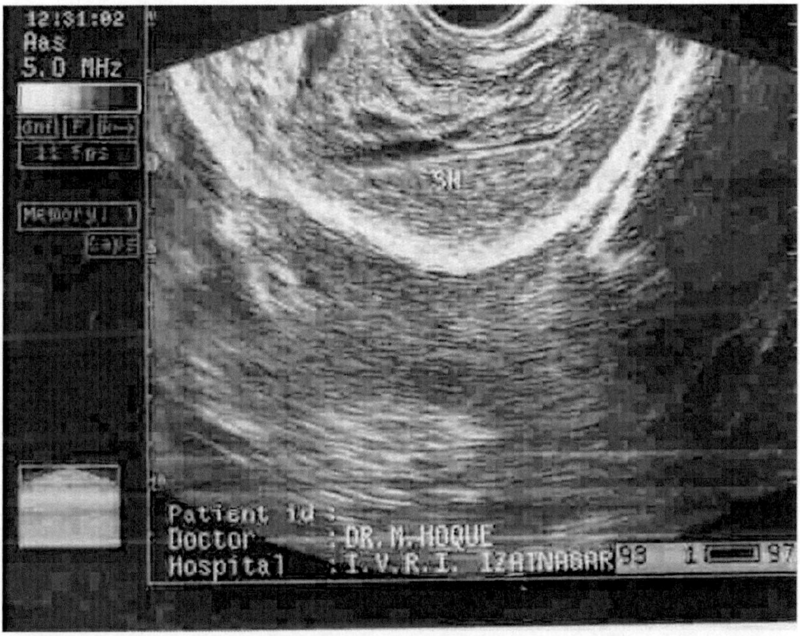

Fig.41: Hepatic sonogram of a dog showing shunt between intrahepatic vena cava and portal vein and patchy hyperechoic bright small areas with an overall reduction in scanning area suggesting intrahepatic portosystemic shunt (Varshney and Hoque, 2002).

- Cases of hepatic arteriovenous fistulas may be seen with dilated and tortuous vessels.
- Arteriovenous fistulas can be differentiated from conventional portiosystemic shunts by employing Doppler ultrasound.

Liver Size and Volume and Associated Conditions

- Liver size and volume is increased in amyloidosis, lipidosis, diffuse neoplasia (primary /secondary), or vacuolar hepatopathy/congestion.
- Liver size and volume decreases in cirrhosis, congenital portosystemic shunt, fibrosis, portal vein hypoplasia or microvascular dysplasia.
- Asymmetric enlargement is generally visualized when there is an abscess, cyst, granuloma, liver lobe torsion, or primary/secondary neoplasia in the liver.

Gall Bladder

The gall bladder is situated in the fossa between quadrate and right medial lobe of the liver and is usually visualized on the right of midline surrounded by hepatic parenchyma. In healthy dogs gall bladder wall, cystic and bile ducts are usually not visible. Ultrasonographic appearance of gall bladder of dogs is an anechoic round or oval shaped structure. In healthy dogs thickness of gall bladder wall is < 2-3 mm (Fig.42). On the other hand cystic and bile ducts are visible in cats. Gall bladder in some cats can be bilobed. In healthy cats thickness of gall bladder wall is approximately 1 mm (Fig.43).

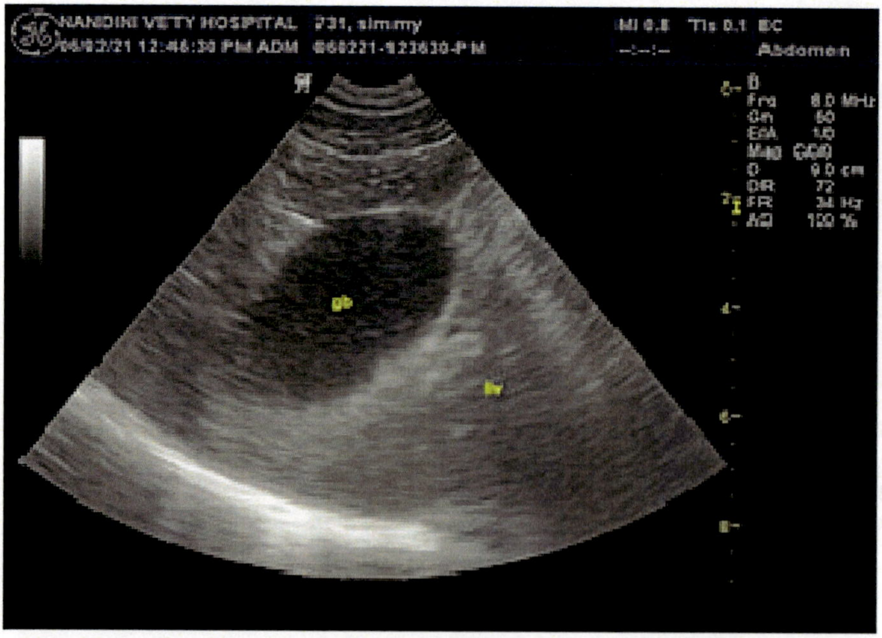

Fig.42. Hepatic sonogram of an adult healthy dog showing normal gall bladder as anechoic fluid filled oval shaped structure with thin hyperechoic wall (< 3 mm thick).

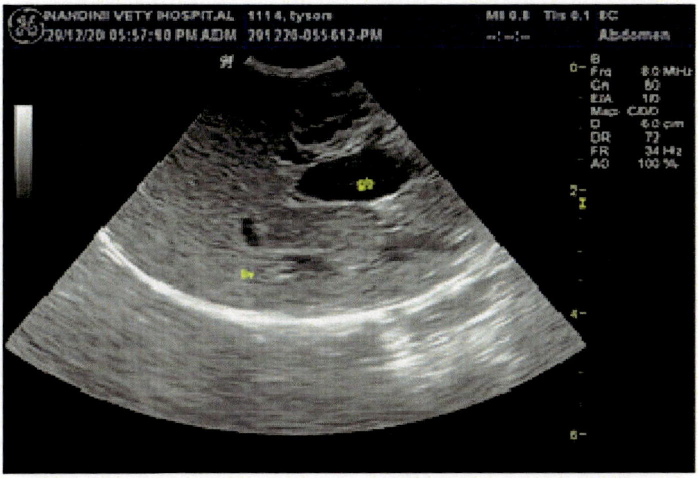

Fig. 43. Hepatic sonogram of a cat showing normal gall bladder as anechoic fluid filled oval shaped structure with thin hyperechoic wall.

- Gall bladder scanning in done in dorsal recumbency using a ventral subcostal and right sided intercostal approach.
- The gall bladder, common bile duct, portal vein, aorta and caudal vena cava can be scanned at 11th and 12th intercostal space. Gall bladder should be scanned in both longitudinal and transverse planes (Fig.44).

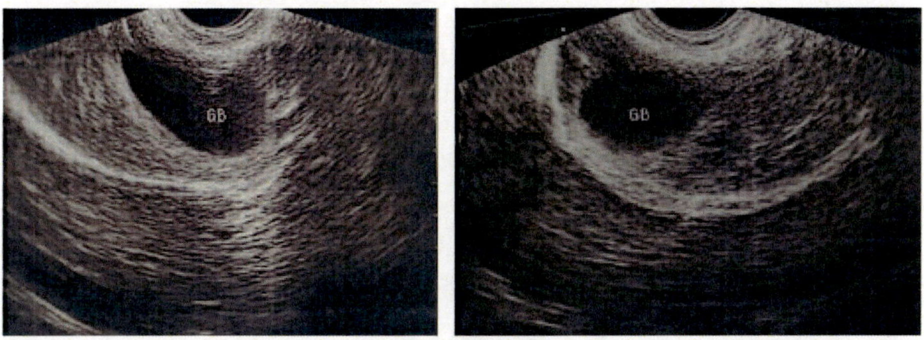

(A) **(B)**

Fig. 44: Hepatic sonograms of the dog showing gall bladder in longitudinal **(A)** and transverse **(B)** views. The gall bladder appears as round anechoic structure in transverse plane and elongated anechoic structure in longitudinal plane.

- The wall of gall bladder appears as thin echogenic line and is < 3 mm thick (Fig. 42 and 43).
- The volume of the gall bladder can be measured with the help of built-in-calipers.

- In anorectic or fasting animals, gall bladder appears full while it is contracted after feeding (Fig.45).

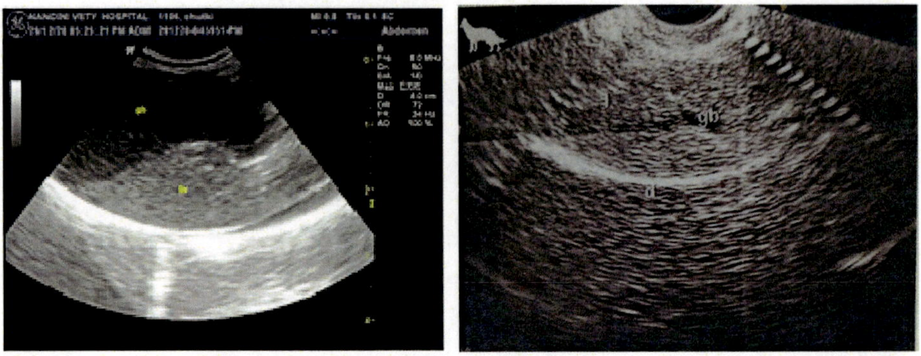

(A) (B)

Fig. 45: Hepatic sonograms of dogs showing gall bladder. Gall bladder is distended in anorectic dog **(A)** and contracted in dogs after meals **(B)**.

- Some echogenic material may be seen in gall bladder in dogs .It is termed as sludge (Fig. 46), generally seen in old dogs. Sludge, a well-defined mobile hyperechoic material, gravitated to the dependent portion of the gall bladder. Its etiology is nonspecific. It may be associated with inflammation. Sonographically sludge appears as a low amplitude echo pattern without acoustic shadowing in the dependent part of the gall bladder. Two different types of sludge pattern may be seen. In one type there is a clear line of interface between echogenic sludge and anechoic bile (Fig.46 B). In another type of sludge there is ill defined accumulation of echogenic bile (Fig. 46 C). It is considered as a precursor of cholelith in humans but clinical significance in dogs is not fully understood.

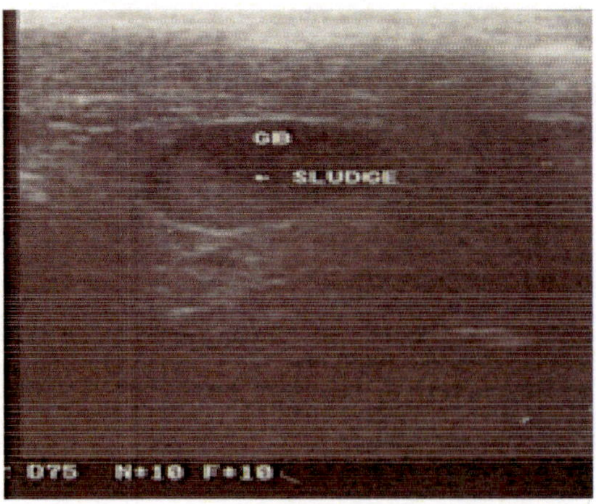

(A)

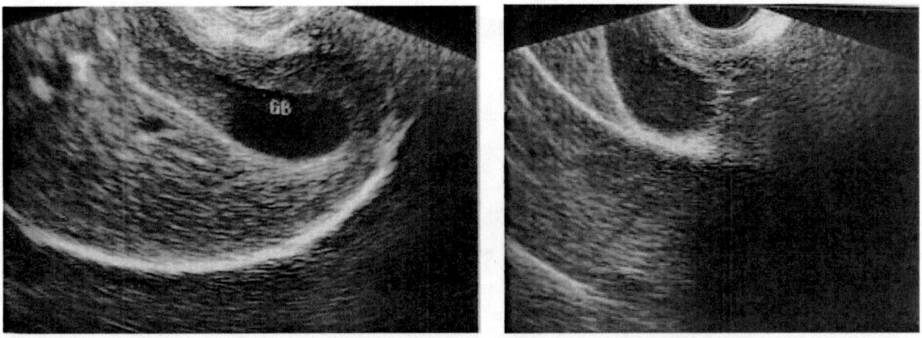

(B) **(C)**

Fig. 46: Hepatic sonogram of dogs showing some echogenic particles in the gall bladder suggesting sludge **(A,B and C)**. Sonogram B shows a clear line of interface between echogenic sludge and anechoic bile. While sonogram C shows ill-defined accumulation of sludge particles in the gall bladder.

- Mineralized and non-mineralized choleliths are other luminal abnormalities in gall bladder.
- In cats echogenic material in gall bladder with its thickened wall is suggestive of cholecystitis.
- Mucocele is abnormal collection of bile salt and mucus in the gall bladder and are suggestive of important hepatobilliary disease in canines. Many times mucocele has been observed in dogs with no clinical manifestations. Mucocele may lead to gall bladder wall necrosis, hepatobilliary obstruction and gall bladder rupture in extreme cases. Abnormal retention of bile salt, hypomotility of gall bladder, decreased contractility of gall bladder, excess secretion of mucus by biliary epithelium is some of the important factors ascribed to mucocele formation. Dogs with hyperadrenocorticism are at increased risk of mucocele (Mesich *et al.*, 2009). Ultrasonographic features of mucocele (Fig.47) include variations in mucus collection ,linear striations (stellate or kiwi like appearance), echogenic material in gall bladder, distended gall bladder with thickened wall .The striations are secondary to fracture lines between mucus collections. There is two types of mucocele pattern viz. finely striated (Fig. 47 B) and stellate type (Fig. 47 C). The gall bladder contents (echogenic mucocele) generally do not move with the changing position of the patient.

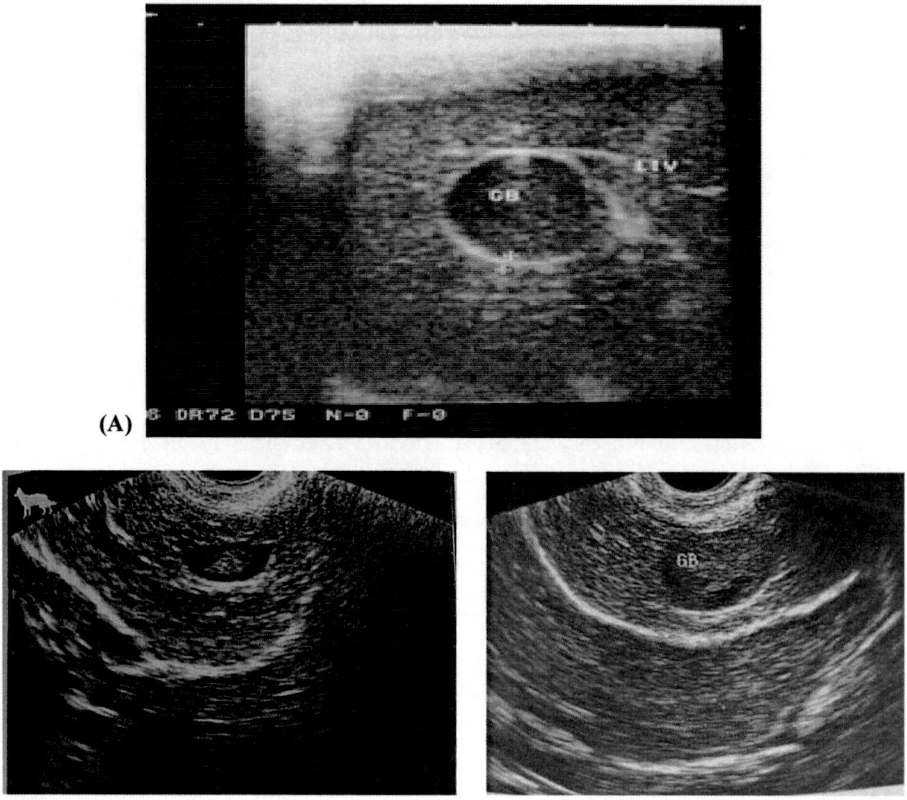

(A)

(B) (C)

Fig. 47. Hepatic sonograms of dogs showing abnormal collection of bile salts and mucus termed as mucocele **(A,B,C)**. Sonogram B shows linear striated pattern of mucocele. While sonogram C shows stellate pattern of mucocele and bile at the periphery is anechoic.

- Sometimes leakage of bile contents into peritoneal cavity is observed due to necrosis of gall bladder wall .Leakage of bile contents give an increased echogenicity to mesentery in contact with the gall bladder wall.

- Extra hepatic biliary obstructions are generally associated with pancreatitis, choleliths, biliary tumour and duodenal strictures at major duodenal papilla. Inflammation of tissues surrounding bile duct may leads to bile duct obstruction. In cats' cholecystitis/cholangiohepatitis, pancreatitis, and inflammatory bowel disease may occur concurrently. This condition in cats is called as triaditis.

- The thickness of gall bladder wall > 3 mm in dogs is suggestive of cholecystitis. Thickened gall bladder wall (Fig.48) may be due to cholecystitis/cholangiohepatitis, hepatitis, pancreatitis, cystic hyperplasia, gall bladder polyps or gall bladder wall edema (caused by hypoproteinaemia, right sided congestive heart failure, portal hypertension of biliary obstruction or neoplasia).

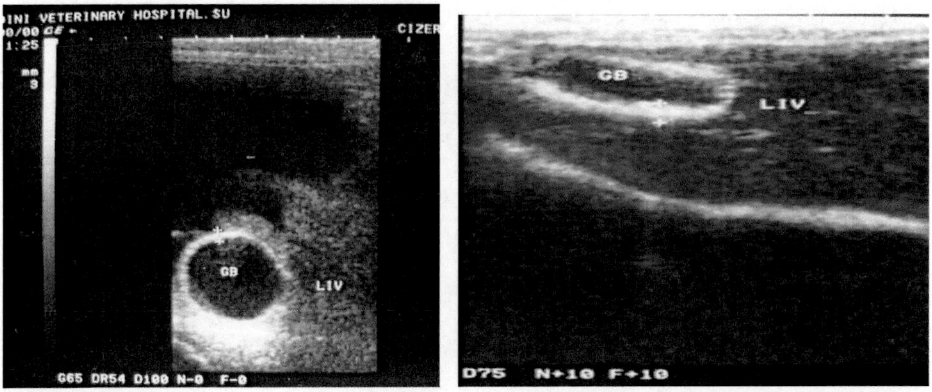

Fig. 48: Hepatic sonograms of dogs showing echogenic thickened gall bladder wall (>3 mm) suggesting cholecystitis.

- Sometimes gall bladder wall edema may cause bi -lobed appearance of gall bladder in dogs (Fig.49).

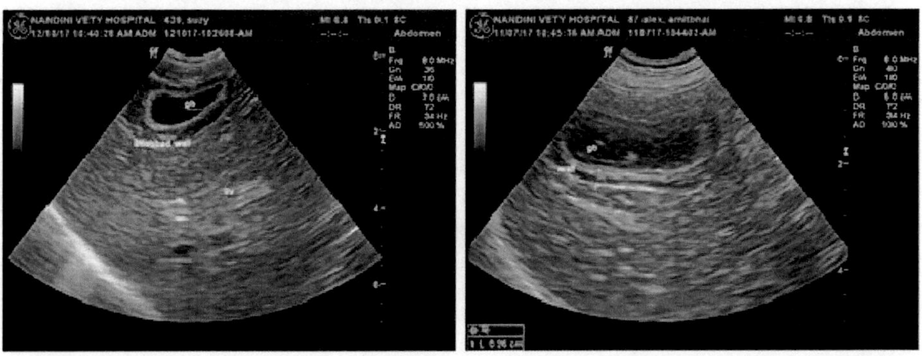

Fig. 49: Hepatic Sonogram of dogs showing edematous wall of the gall bladder giving an appearance of bilobed gall bladder

- Choleliths (Fig.50) are variable in size and appear as hyperechoic with acoustic shadowing. Choleliths may be secondary to biliary stasis, dietary factors, cholecystitis/cholangiohepatitis, or changed bile composition.

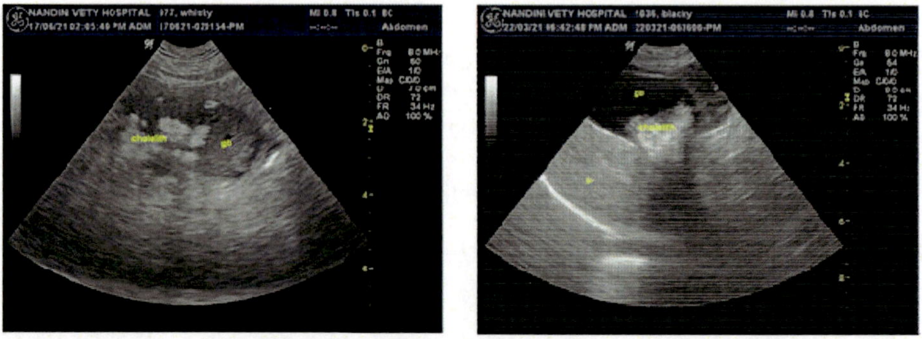

Fig. 50: Hepatic sonograms of dogs showing hyperechoic images of variable size with acoustic shadowing in the gall bladder suggesting cholelith.

- Sometimes echogenic material without acoustic shadowing is visualized in gall bladder (Fig.51).It is termed as inspissated bile.

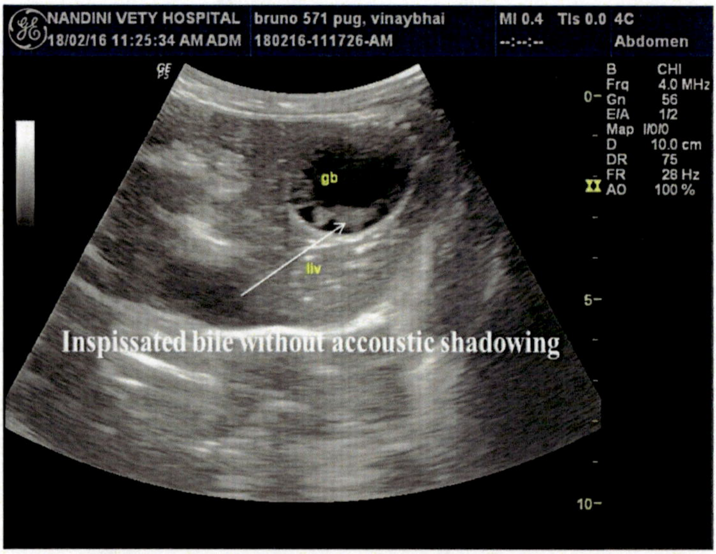

Fig. 51: Hepatic sonogram of a dog showing echogenic material without acoustic shadowing in the gall bladder suggestive of inspissated bile. The hyperechoic material is formed but with no acoustic shadowing suggesting that it is not mineralized.

Cholecystocentesis

- Bile samples can be obtained for cytological and cultural examinations employing ultrasound guided percutaneous cholecystocentesis.
- Cholecystocentesis can also be performed to drain gall bladder when there is extrabilliary obstruction.

General Abdomen

- Abdomen is visualized for the presence or absence of free abdominal fluid.
- Free abdominal fluid in the abdomen appears as anechoic areas (Fig. 52) separating various intra-abdominal structures.
- Normal abdominal lymph nodes are difficult to visualize.
- Enlarged lymph nodes appear as homogeneously hypoechoic.

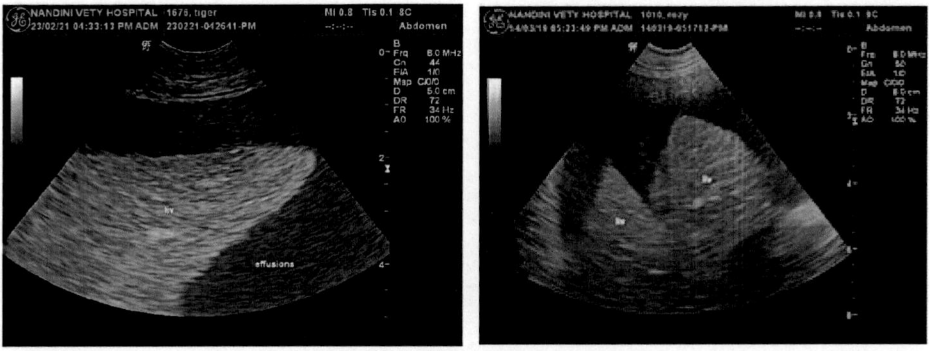

(A) **(B)**

Fig. 52: Abdominal sonogram of dogs with distended abdomen showing anechoic fluid accumulation in the abdomen suggesting ascites.

References

Bhadwal, M.S., Mirakhur, K.K. and Sharma, S.N. (1999). Ultrasonographic imaging of the normal canine liver and gall bladder. Indian J.Vet.Surg.20:10-14.

Mesich, M.L., Mayhew, P.D. and Pack, M. (2009). Gallbladder mucoceles and their association with endocrinopathies in dogs: A retrospective case-control study. J. Small Anim. Pract.50:630-635.

Varshney, J.P. and Hoque, M. (2002). Clinicopathological and ultrasonographic observations in canine hepatopathies. Indian J. Anim. Sci.72: 423-427.

Suggested Further Readings

Bandyopadhyay, S.,Varshney, J.P., Hoque, M., Sarkar, M. and Ghosh, M.K.(2007). Prevalence of cholecystic diseases in dogs : An ultrasonographic evaluation. Asian J. Anim. Vet. Advances 2:234-238.

Chaudhary, P.S.,Varshney, J.P. and Deshmukh,V.V. (2008). Application of ultrasonography, radiography and clinico-biochemical profile in the diagnosis of hepatic diseases and their clinical management. Intas Polivet 9:168-176.

Cuccivillo, A. and Lamb, C.R. (2002). Cellular features of sonographic target lesions of the liver and spleen in 21 dogs and cats. Vet. Radiol. Ultrasound 43:275-278.

Hoque, M. and Varshney, J.P. (2001). Sonographic evaluation of hepatobiliary system in dogs- An overview. J. Canine Dev. Res. 1:7-15.

Hoque, M. and Varshney, J.P. (2002). Ultrasonographic examination of hepatobiliary system in dogs: An analysis of 35 cases. Indian J.Vet.Med.21:76-81.

Tiwari, P., Varshney, J.P. and Hoque, M. (2002). Biliary obstruction in dogs: Diagnosis and Treatment. Indian J.Vet. Med. 21:115-116.

Tiwari, P., Varshney, J.P. and Hoque, M. (2005). Significance of biliary sludge in dogs with hepatobiliary diseases. Indian Vet.J. 82:533-534.

Tiwari, P., Varshney, J.P. and Hoque, M. (2003). Ultrasonographic survey of canine gall bladder diseases. Indian J. Anim.Sci.73:1126-1128.

Varshney, J.P. (2019). Liver cirrhosis in a Persian cat-A case report. J Canine Dev.Resch.15: 66-69.

Varshney, J.P. and Hoque, M. (2003). Ultrasonography of liver and spleen in canine babesiosis. Indian J. Anim.Sci.73:642.

Varshney, J.P., Hoque, M., Tiwari,P., Bandyopadhyay, S. and Saghar, S.S. (2004). Intrahepatic portosystemic shunt in dogs: Clinico-pathological observations. Indian J. Vet. Surg. 25: 107-109.

6

Ultrasound of The Spleen

J.P. Varshney and P.S. Chaudhary

Spleen is an elongated solid organ located on the left side along cranial and ventral abdominal wall. The size of spleen is variable in dogs. The spleen is larger in German Shepherds and Greyhounds. In cats the spleen is smaller and has fixed size. It is parallel to greater curvature of stomach within greater omentum. The position of spleen in dogs is variable as it is only attached by gastrosplenic ligament. The spleen of dogs is divisible into dorsal extremity (left cranio-dorsal), body (mid abdominal) and ventral extremity or tail (Fig. 53). While in cats spleen is smaller, superficial and is situated in left cranial abdomen.

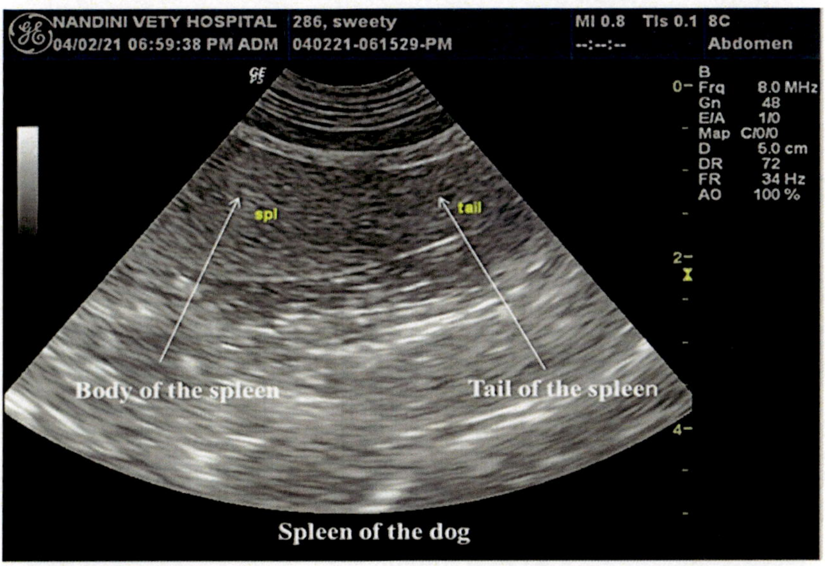

Fig. 53: Trans abdominal splenic sonogram of a dog showing body and tail portion of the spleen.

Landmarks for Identifying Spleen in dogs

- Stomach, left kidney and descending colon are landmarks to identify spleen (Fig. 54).

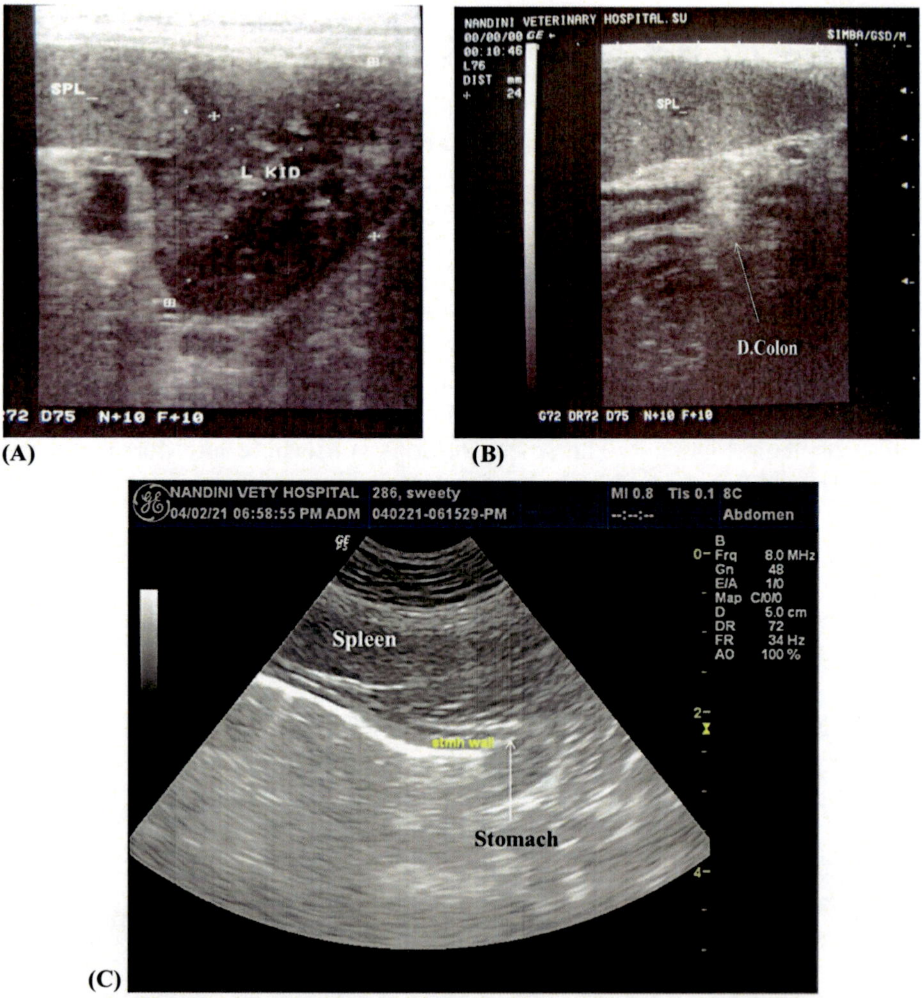

Fig. 54: Trans abdominal sonograms of dogs showing landmarks for the identification of spleen, Sonograms A, B and C are showing spleen adjacent to left kidney **(A)**, in the vicinity of colon **(B)** and adjacent to stomach **(C)**. Left kidney, colon and stomach are important landmark for identifying spleen.

- Spleen is caudal and lateral to stomach.
- Spleen is ventral, lateral (far field) and cranial to left kidney.
- Transverse colon is dorsal (far field), medial and caudal to the body of the spleen,

Scanning Technique

- Area to be scanned is prepared as described earlier.
- Acoustic gel is applied on the skin and transducer.
- Place the transducer on left cranial abdomen and slide it to left caudal abdomen until entire cranial border of spleen is evaluated. Then examine the body of the spleen in a distance motion back across the abdomen.
- Transducer is moved caudally along caudal border.
- Examine caudoventral extremity of spleen by moving transducer in a distance motion from left to right.

Ultrasonographic Features of Spleen

- In healthy dogs splenic parenchyma is slightly hyperechoic (Fig. 55) as compared to the liver.
- Splenic outer capsule is hyperechoic (Fig. 55).
- Spleen has homogenous echotexture (Fig. 55).
- Sometimes changes in size, shape, echogenicity and echotexture of spleen may be a normal response.
- Splenic vessel is visualized as hypoechoic tubular structure (Fig. 56).
- Splenic arteries can be visualized by Colour Doppler.
- A normal scan of spleen does not rule out disease.

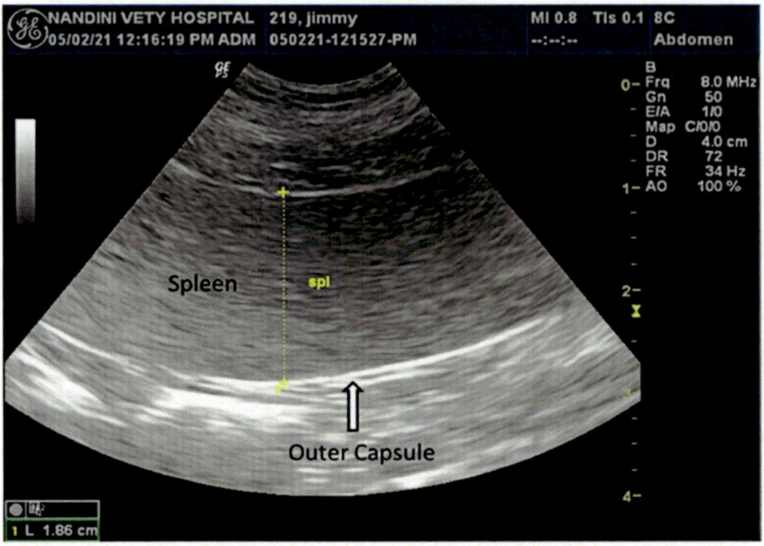

Fig. 55: Splenic sonogram of a healthy dog showing homogenously slight hyperechoic echotexture and hyperechoic outer capsule.

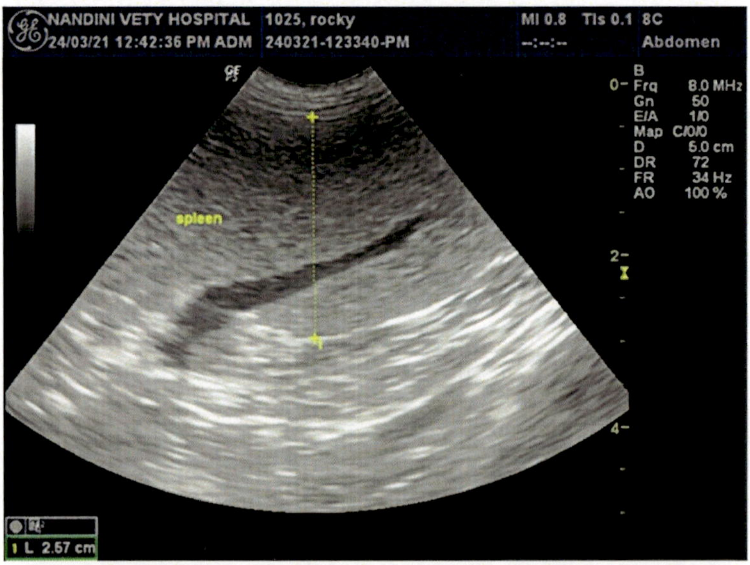

Fig. 56: Splenic sonogram of a dog showing splenic vessel as a hypoechoic tubular structure in the spleen.

- Spleen of the cats is small (neither long nor thick) and is seen in near field. Echogenicity of the feline spleen (Fig. 57) is somewhat similar to that of dogs.

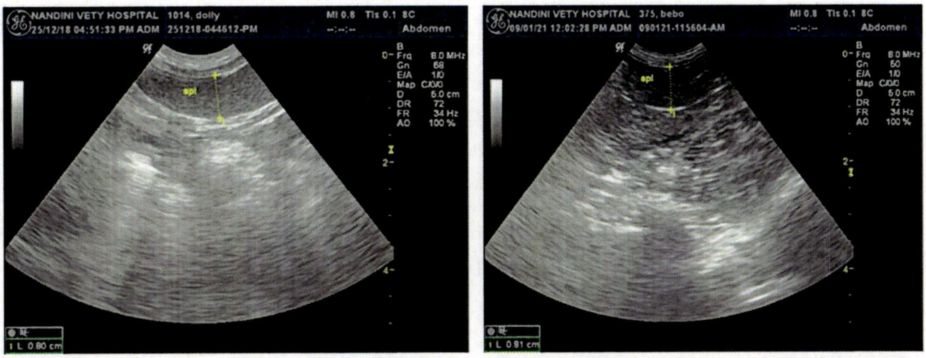

(A) (B)

Fig. 57: Splenic sonogram (long axis) of healthy cats showing homogenously slight hyperechoic echotexture with hyperechoic outer capsule similar to that of dogs.

Ultrasonographic Features of Splenic Diseases

- Broadly splenic diseases are grouped as focal or multifocal diseases: diseases with increased splenic size but no parenchymal change; diffuse nodular disease; and diseases with normal splenic ultrasound features.
- Nodular hyperplasia (Fig. 58) is characterized by hypoechoic to isoechoic nodules with sharp margins having no other parenchymal changes.

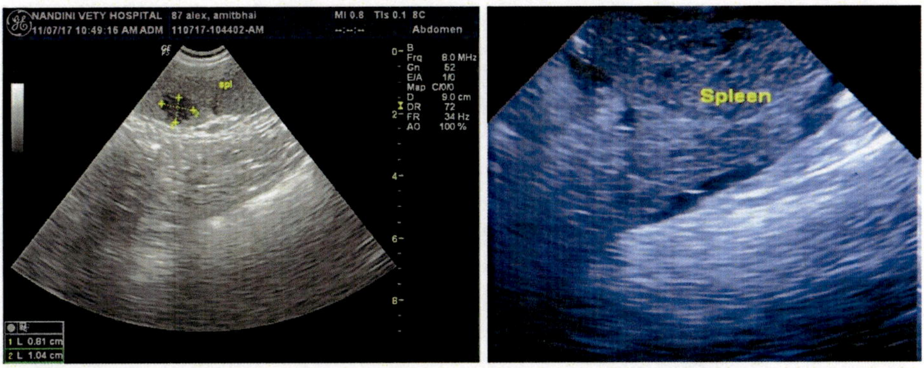

(A) (B)

Fig. 58: Splenic sonogram of dogs showing isoechoic and hypoechoic nodules with sharp margins suggesting nodular hyperplasia.

- Extramedullary haematopoiesis is also having sonographic features similar to nodular hyperplasia. Therefore requires cytological examination for differentiation.
- Myelolipomas are benign in nature and are irregularly shaped or rounded hyperechoic foci varying in size. It is difficult to distinguish them from

other poorly hyperechoic foci. Myelolipomas are more common in old aged dogs.

- Hyperechoic speckles with thin lines throughout the splenic parenchyma are suggestive of dystrophic mineralization.
- Splenic infarcts are hypoechoic poorly marginated foci (Fig. 59). Splenic infarcts are better evaluated on colour Doppler examination as they cause lack of blood supply.

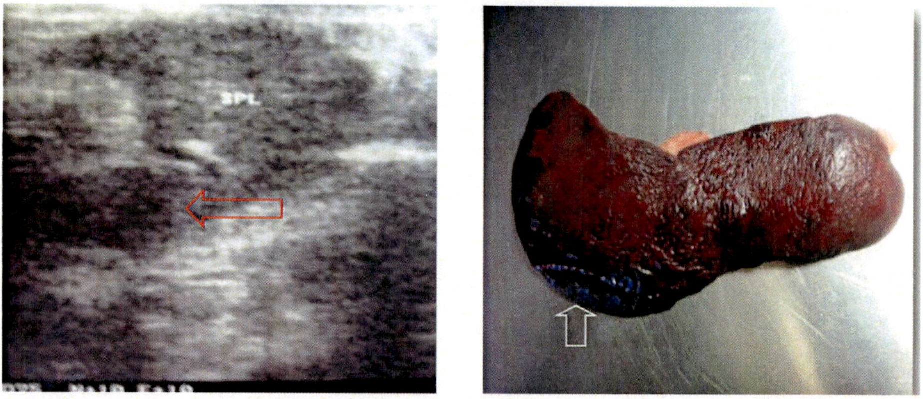

(A) **(B)**

Fig. 59: Splenic sonogram of a dog showing hypoechoic poorly marginated foci **(A)** suggestive of splenic infarct. Splenectomy confirmed area of infarct **(B)**.

- Though splenic abscesses are not common, they can be focal or multifocal. Sonographic appearance of abscesses varies from poorly marginated hypoechoic lesion to complex lesions with variable cystic components and echogenic debris (Ginel *et al.*, 2001). Hyperechoic foci with or without comet tail artefacts within lesion arouse suspicion of gas forming micro-organisms.
- Haematomas may occur in within splenic parenchyma, subcapsular region and /or near the spleen. Initially, haematomas in splenic parenchyma are hyperechoic and become anechoic to hypoechoic with large collection of unclotted blood (Hanson and Penninck, 1994). Therefore splenic haematomas may appear as anechoic, hypoechoic to hyperechoic areas in splenic parenchyma (Fig. 60) depending on the stage. Differentiation of haematoma from haemangiosarcoma may not be possible.

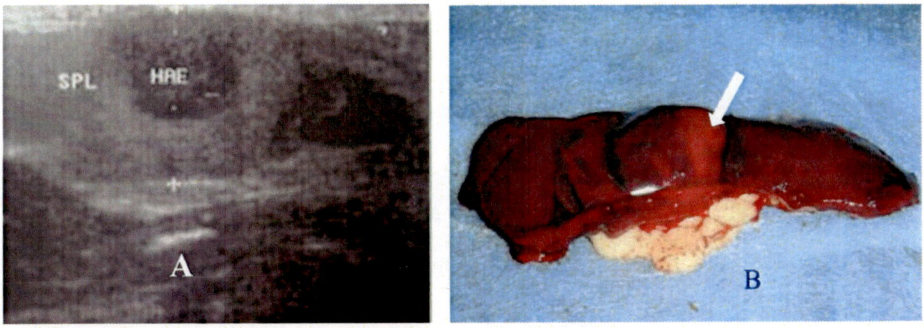

Fig. 60: Splenic sonogram of a dog showing anechoic, hypoechoic to hyperechoic areas in splenic parenchyma suggesting possible haematoma **(A)**. Splenectomised spleen showing area of haematoma **(B)**.

- Tumour in spleen may appear as a complex mass with hyperechoic, hypoechoic and anechoic echotexture (Fig.61). Haemangiosarcomas are common splenic neoplasia and have variable amounts of anechoic to hyperechoic areas throughout, occasionally with weak distal acoustic enhancement (Wrigley *et al.*, 1988).

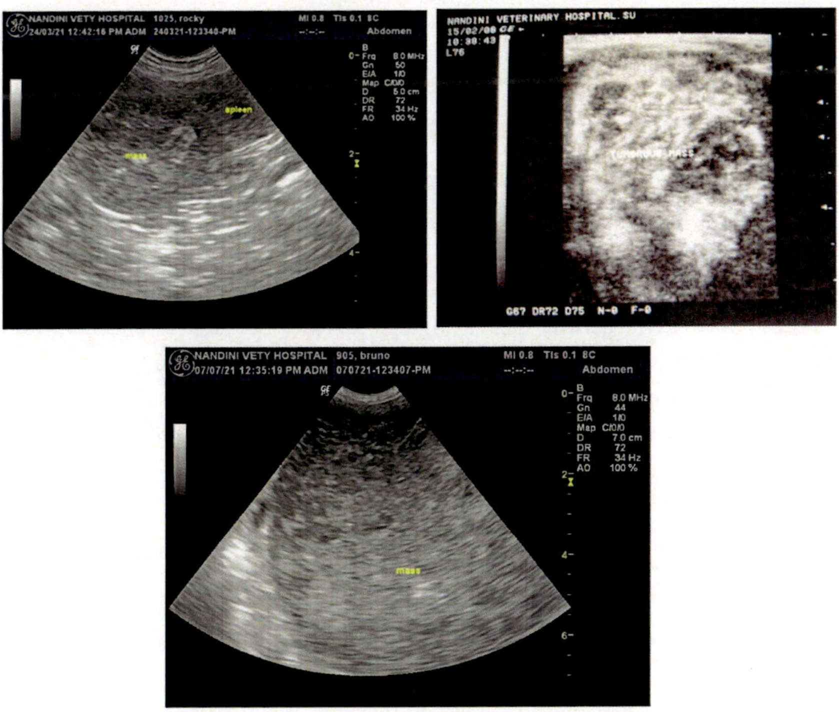

Fig. 61: Splenic sonograms of dogs showing a complex mass with hyperechoic, hypoechoic and anechoic areas suggesting tumour.

- Other neoplasia viz. malignant histiocytosis, malignant fibrous histiocytoma, and histiocytic sarcoma are described to have multiple well-defined, hypoechoic nodules causing distortion of the splenic margin (Ramirez *et al.* 2002).
- Mast cell tumours are characterized by diffuse hypoechogenicity of spleen or one /more hypoechoic nodules (Sato *et al.*, 2008).
- Multiple myeloma is characterized by small hyperechoic nodules (Fig. 62).

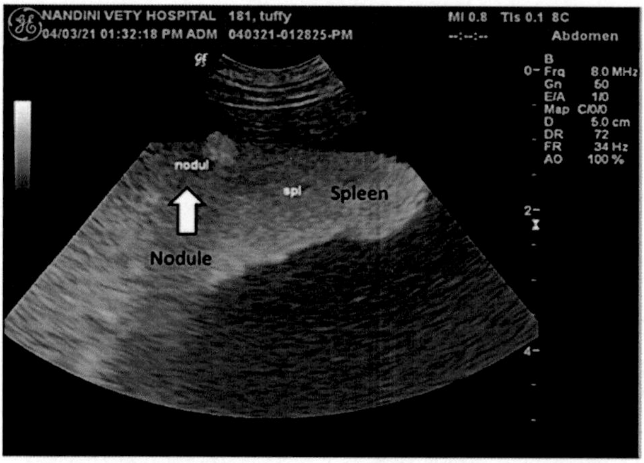

Fig. 62: Splenic sonogram of a dog showing hyperechoic nodule. Hyperechoic nodules are seen in splenic myeloma.

- Splenic torsion is more common in large breeds of dogs and is sonographically characterized by splenomegaly, coarse, diffuse, lacy hypoechoic to anechoic parenchymal pattern with interspersed linear echoes (Saunders *et al.*, 1988). Another pattern of splenic torsion is over all hypoechocity with hyperechoic spackles (Fig. 63) giving it a starry night appearance. Anechoic or slightly echoic fluid may also be seen near the spleen. Splenic torsion is not common in cats.

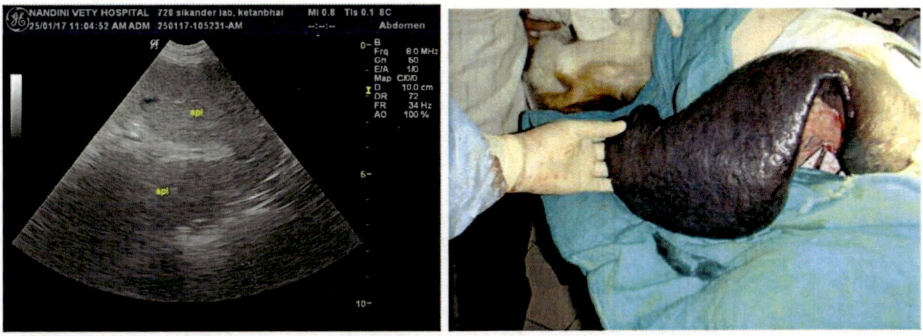

(A) **(B)**

Fig. 63: Splenic sonogram of a dog showing hypoechoicity with hyperechoic spackles **(A)** suggesting splenic torsion. Splenectomy confirmed torsion **(B)**.

- Chronic splenic torsion is characterized by hyperechoic foci with distal acoustic enhancement owing to gas secondary to gas producing bacteria (Gaschen *et al.,* 2003).
- Infectious splenitis is sonographically characterized by splenomegaly with hypoechogenicity (Fig. 64). In severe acute cases spleen is diffusely hypoechoic with mottled heterogeneous appearance (Ellison *et al.*, 1988).

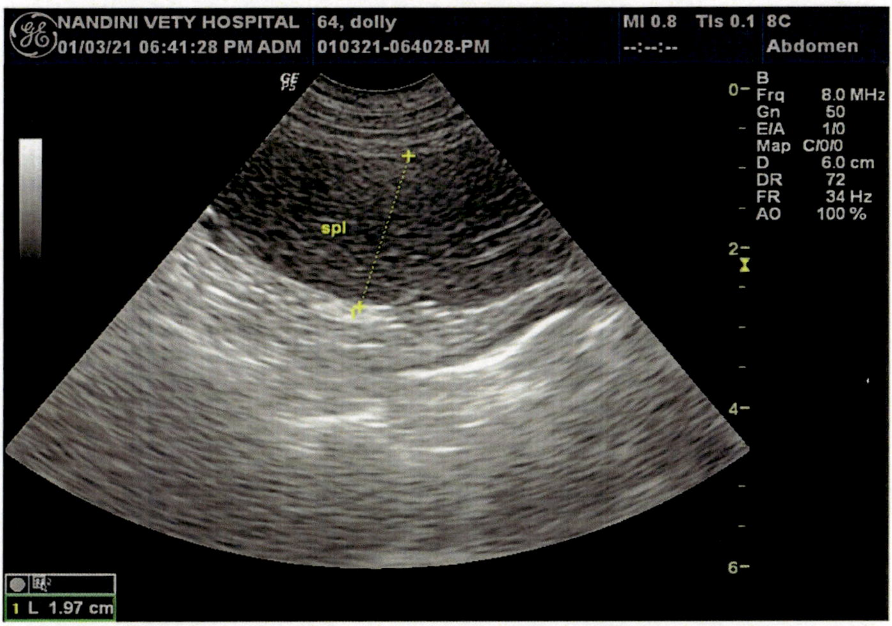

Fig. 64: Splenic sonogram of an eight year old dog showing hypoechoic and enlarged spleen suggesting splenitis.

- Extramedullary haematopoiesis and lymphoid hyperplasia are characterized by normal to reduced echogenicity of spleen.
- Different ultrasonographic patterns (Fig. 65) such as multiple, different sized hypoechoic nodules; diffuse hypo /hyper echogenicity with coarse echotexture; or multiple hypoechoic nodules (honeycomb pattern), moth-eaten appearance, spotted spleen, or leopard spots have been visualized in cases of splenic lymphoma in dogs.

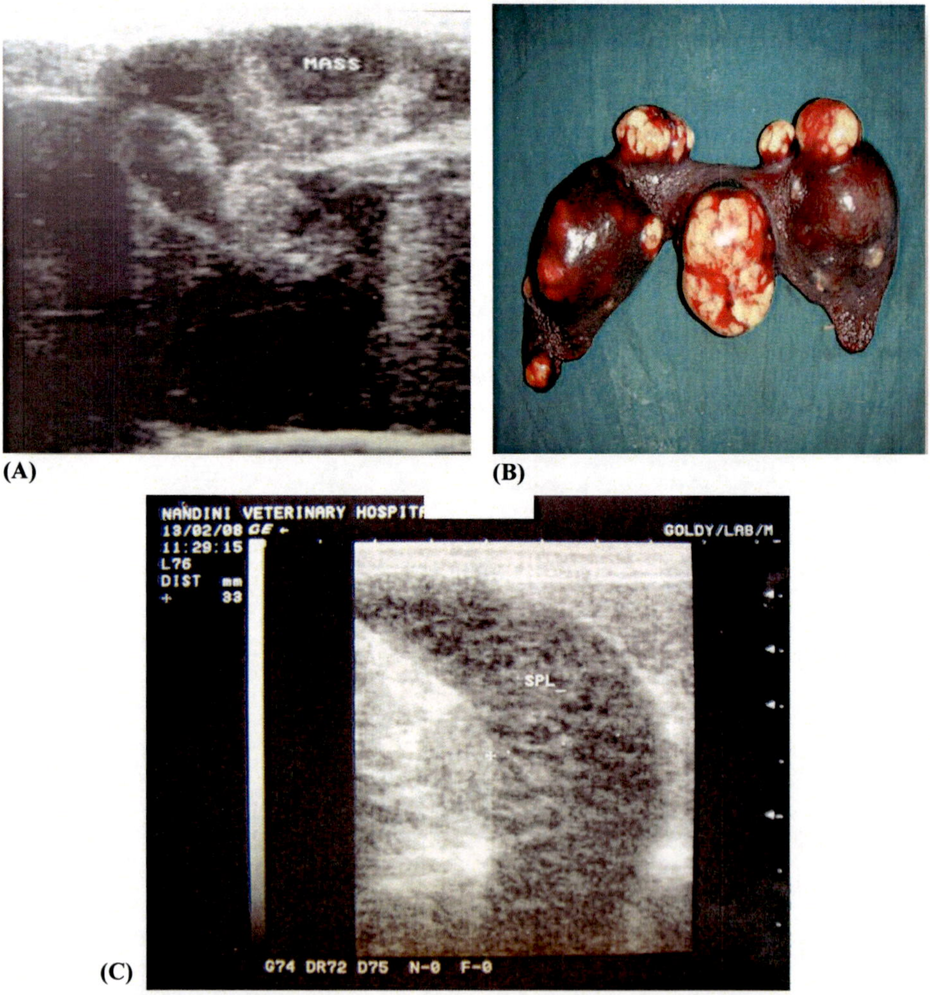

Fig. 65: Splenic sonogram of a dog showing variable hypoechoic to hyperechoic areas **(A)** suggesting mass/tumours. Splenectomy showed multiple growths of variable size **(B)**. Splenic sonogram of a male Labrador **(C)** showing mottled/Leopard spot parenchyma (multiple small oval shaped hypoechoic foci throughout splenic parenchyma) as has been reported in dogs with lymphoma.

References

Ellison, G.W., King, R.R. and Calderwood-Mays, M. (1988). Medical and surgical management of multiple organ infarctions secondary to bacterial endocarditis in dog. J.Am.Vet.Med. Assoc. 193:1289-1291

Gaschen, L., Kircher, P., Venzin, C., Hurter, K. and Lang, J. (2003). Imaging diagnosis: The abdominal air-vasculogram in a dog with splenic torsion and clostridial infection. Vet. Radiol. Ultrasound 44: 553–555.

Ginel, P.J., Lucena, R.and Arola, J.(2001). Diffuse splenomegaly caused by splenic abscessation in a dog. Vet. Rec. 149:327-329.

Hanson, J .A. and Penninck, D.G.(1994). Ultrasonographic evaluation of a traumatic splenic hematoma and literature review. Vet. Radiol. Ultrasound. 35:463-468.

Ramirez, S., Douglass, J.P. and Robertson, I.D. (2002). Ultrasonographic features of canine abdominal malignant histiocystosis. Vet. Radiol. Ultrasound 43:167-170.

Sato, A.F. and Solano, M.(2004). Ultrasonographic findings in abdominal mast cell disease: a retrospective study of 19 patients. Vet. Radiol. Ultrasound 45 :51-57.

Saunders, M.H., Neath, P.J. and Brockman, D.J. (1998). B-Mode and Doppler ultrasound imaging of the Spleen with canine splenic torsion: A retrospective evaluation. Vet. Radiol. Ultrasound 39: 349–353.

Wrigley, R.H., Park, R.D. and Konde, L.J. (1988). Ultrasonographic features of splenic hemangiosarcoma in dogs: 18 cases(1980-1986). J.Am.Vet.Med.Assoc. 192:1113-1117.

Suggested Further Readings

Varshney, J.P. and Hoque, M. (2003). Ultrasonography of liver and spleen in canine babesiosis. Indian J. Anim.Sci.73:642.

Varshney, J.P., Chaudhary, P.S. and Deshmukh, V.V. (2011). Splenomegaly and its successful treatment in an adult Labrador dog. Intas Polivet 12: 92-95.

7

Ultrasound of The Stomach

J.P. Varshney and P.S. Chaudhary

Ultrasonographic examination of gastrointestinal tract is not very much rewarding in dogs because of gas in the tract but it is crucial for a correct diagnosis. Imaging of stomach plays a significant role in the diagnosis of gastric diseases such as gastric dilatation, gastric foreign bodies, pyloric outflow obstruction, or gastric tumours.

Landmarks for Identifying Stomach

- The stomach in healthy dogs and cats is located caudal to the liver when transducer is placed at the level of xiphoid process and directed in sagittal plane. The transducer is slide from the liver position to the left and the stomach is visualized caudal to the liver.
- The sonographic appearance of the stomach in dogs is variable and depends on the size of the dog and food contents.
- The stomach is divisible into cardia, fundus, body and pyloric antrum leading into pyloric sphincter.
- Generally cardia is not identifiable.
- Fundus is located in left cranial abdomen.
- Gastric body is located right of midline if there is ingesta, gas and fluid.
- In cats the body of the stomach is located on the left of midline

Imaging Technique

- Dogs and cats are placed usually in dorsal recumbency. However, left or right lateral recumbency helps in displacing gas and fluid and may provide better visualization of the stomach.
- The site is prepared by shaving or clipping hairs and applying acoustic gel as detailed earlier.

- For gastrointestinal sonography fasting is always desirable as it prevents reverberation artefacts and beam attenuation (Feldman *et al.,* 2009).
- Curved array transducer of 8 to 10 MHz or linear transducer of 12 MHz is recommended for ultrasonography of gastrointestinal tract.
- Stomach should be visualized both in longitudinal and transverse axis.
- Sequential examination of stomach consists of examining fundus, body and pyloric antrum.
- When stomach is scanned in long axis plane relative to the patient, it provides transverse view of the stomach. The fundus is visualized in the left craniolateral quadrant. The body of the stomach can be visualized closer to midline as the transducer is taken to the right of the patient. The pyloric antrum can extend to the right side of the patient depending on the degree of distension.
- In cats pylorus and pyloroduodenal junction is close to midline.
- Pyloroduodenal junction in deep chested dogs can be visualized better by taking right dorsal intercostal approach.

Ultrasonographic Features of Stomach

- Reverberation artefacts (Fig.66) may sonographically be visualized as multiple equidistantly spaced linear reflections (Feldman *et al.*, 2009).

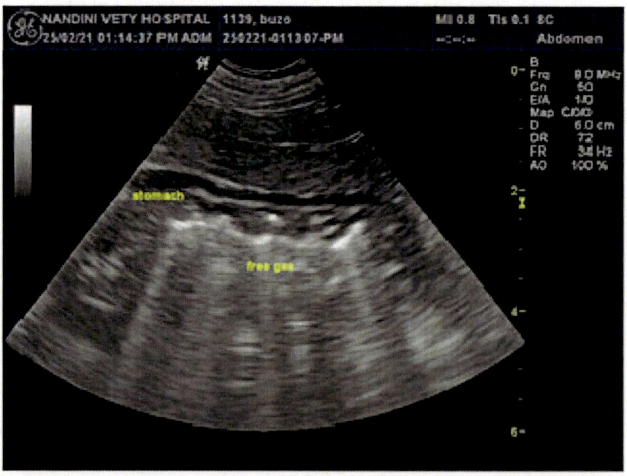

Fig. 66: Trans abdominal sonogram of a ten year old male Labrador showing wall of the stomach and reverberation artefacts. Stomach is showing characteristic pattern of alternating hyper and hypoechoic layers.

- Rugal folds and gastric fluid (Fig. 67) may be visualized when stomach is empty.

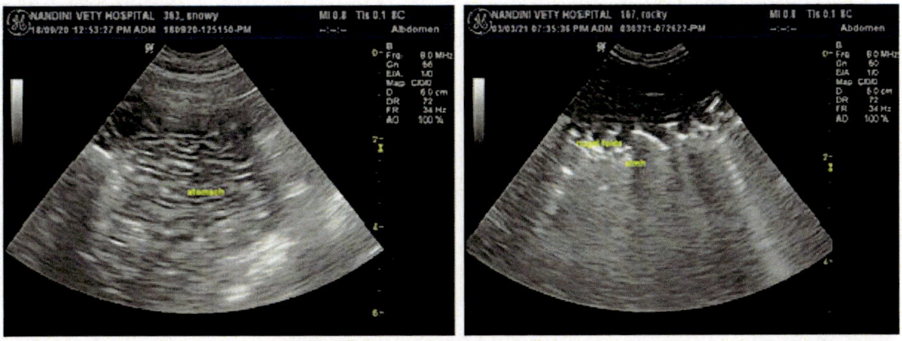

(A) **(B)**

Fig. 67: Gastric sonogram of healthy dogs taken empty stomach.Sonogram **(A)** showing normal hyperechoic gastric fluid between rugal folds giving stomach a stellate appearance. Reverberation artifacts are also visible in the right side sonogram **(B)**.

- Beam attenuation appears as reduction of ultrasound signal at depth in far field due to the attenuation of the ultrasound beam in the near field secondary to gastrointestinal contents (Feldman *et al.*, 2009).

- Wall of gastrointestinal tract has characteristic pattern of alternating hyper and hypoechoic layers. In all there are five layers (Fig.68). Luminal mucosal interface, submucosal and serosal layers are hyperechoic; and mucosal and muscularis layers are hypoechoic From lumen side gastro-intestinal layering are hyperechoic luminal mucosal interface, hypoechoic mucosa, hyperechoic submucosa, hypoechoic muscularis and hyperechoic serosa.

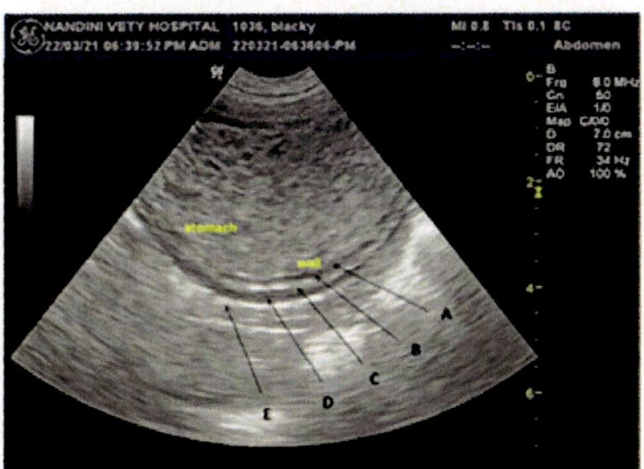

Fig. 68: Sonogram of the gastric wall of the healthy normal dog. The gastric wall has five layers of alternating hyperechoic and hypoechoic echoes. From inner side to outer side, the gastric wall layers are: hyperechoic mucosal surface **(A)**, hypoechoic mucosa **(B)**, hyperechoic submucosa **(C)**, hypoechoic muscularis propria **(D)**, and hyperechoic serosa **(E)**.

- The wall thickness of stomach of healthy dogs has been reported as 3-5 mm (Penninck *et al.*, 1989).
- Pyloric sphincter has hyperechoic mucosa while mucosa of pyloric antrum and duodenum is hypoechoic. Pylorodudinal junction is visualized as thickened of the muscularis between pylorus and proximal duodenum when probe is swept towards the right side.
- Empty feline stomach in transverse section has a wagon wheel appearance with a thick hyperechoic submucosal layer (Fig. 69) due to fat deposits.

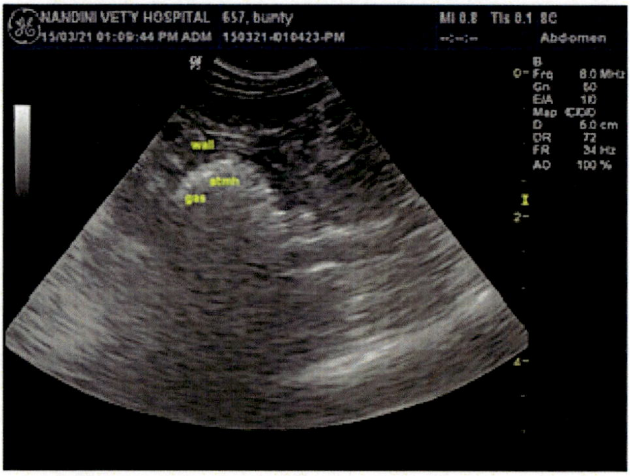

Fig. 69: Sonogram of a feline stomach showing wagon wheel appearance with thick hyperechoic submucosal layer.

- In cats inter-rugal and rugal fold thickness has been reported as 2 mm and 4 mm respectively (Newell *et al.*,1999).

Ultrasonographic Features of Stomach Abnormalities

- Stomach dilatation is characterized by thin stomach wall, no distinguished wall layering and less distinct rugal folds. Gastric contents may be hyper/ hypoechoic depending on composition.
- Dilatation of stomach due to gas may contain reverberation artifact within the far field of the image, making visualization of abnormalities of the dorsal aspect of the gastric wall or lumen, difficult.
- Congenital hypertrophic pyloric stenosis is characterized by circumferential thickening of pylorus, thickened gastric wall of more than 7 mm, and thickened muscularis layer of more than 4 mm (Penninck *et al.*, 1989).

- Foreign bodies (Fig.70) in the pyloric region may have irregular or geometric shape with strong acoustic shadowing. Foreign material in stomach has a hyperechoic interface with intense distal acoustic shadowing. Foreign bodies surrounded by fluid are readily seen.

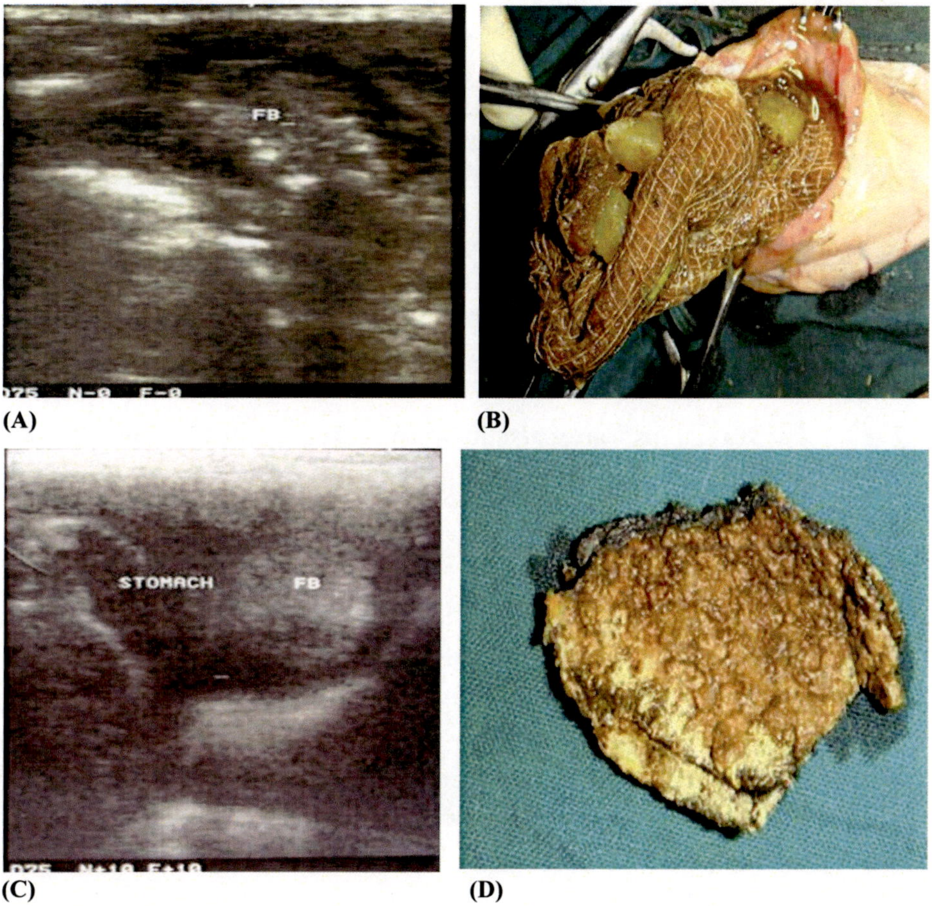

Fig. 70: Abdominal sonogram of a dogs showing irregular shaped material in stomach with acoustic shadowing **(A, C)** suggesting some foreign body.The dogs were operated and foreign bodies were retrieved from the stomach **(B, D)**.

- Chronic hypertrophic pyloric gastropathy in dogs is also characterized by muscular or mucosal hypertrophy; pyloric wall thicknesses (9 to 15.3 mm), and thickened (3 to 5.4 mm) muscular layer (Biller *et al.*, 1994).

- Gastritis is characterized by diffuse mild to moderate gastric wall thickening with distinguished wall layering.

- Neoplastic lesions or mass (Fig. 71) in stomach cause focal loss of wall layering along with varying degree of wall thickening (Larson and Biller, 2009).

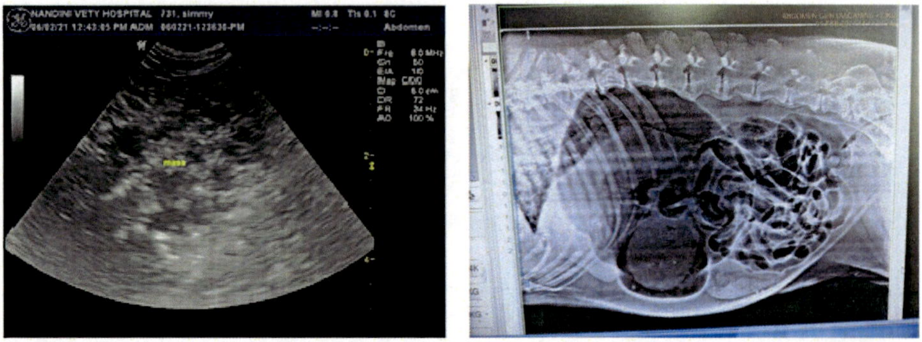

(A) **(B)**

Fig. 71: Abdominal sonogram of a dog showing hyperechoic mass with loss of gastric layring at some place **(A).** X-ray of the same dog **(B)** also revealed mass in stomach.

- Most carcinomas are seen in lesser curvature and pylorus of dogs. Gastric adenocarcinoma is characterized by pseudo layering pattern, asymmetrical transmural thickening, and changed wall layering with poor echogenic lining of mucosal and serosal wall layers (Beck *et al*., 2001).

- Leiomyosarcomas are characterized as small rounded masses protruding into gastric lumen at cardia, thickening of muscularis layer (Lamb and Grierson, 1999), and smooth luminal surface of the lesions.

- Lymphoma is common gastric tumor in cats and appears as focal mass / masses or diffuse infiltrative tumor characterized by wall thickening and /or loss of layering (Grooters *et al*.,1994).

- Adenomas in dogs and cats may appear as flat or polypoid (Gualtieri *et al.,*1999).

- Gastric leiomyomas in dogs form single or multiple, sessile, round polyps protruding into the lumen (Beck and Simpson, 1999) at gastric cardia or gastroesophageal junction (Culbertson *et al*., 1983). Definite diagnosis of tumors requires histopathology.

- Chronic hypertrophic gastritis is characterized by thickened gastric wall with intact layering pattern or thickened hypoechoic layer around pyloric lumen (Biller *et al*.,1994), or thickened rugal folds projecting into lumen (Vaughn *et al*., 2014).

- Eosinophilic sclerosing fibroplasia in cats is focal mass lesions or mural thickening at the pyloric antrum with a loss of wall layering pattern (Linton *et al.*, 2015).
- Uremic gastritis is characterized by thickened gastric wall (Fig. 72) and a hyperechoic line in mucosal or submucosal layer representing mineralization (Peters *et al.*, 2005).

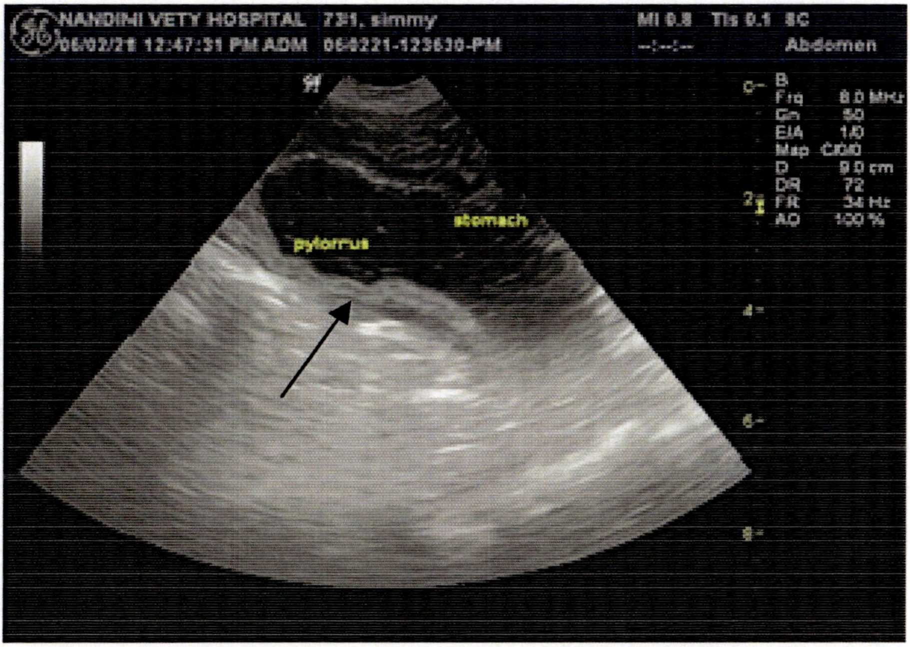

Fig. 72: Trans abdominal sonogram of the stomach of a Sieberian Huskie dog with vomiting showing thickened hyperechoic gastric wall of pylorus(black arrow) with loss of layering ; increased blood urea nitrogen (140 mg/dl) and serum creatinine (6.2 mg/dl) suggesting uremic gastropathy.

- Nonspecific gastritis is characterized by wall edema and wall thickening without a total loss of layering pattern. Many times normal visible ultrasound gastric pattern does not rule out gastritis.

References

Beck, J.A. and Simpson, D.S. (1999). Surgical treatment of gastric leiomyoma in a dog. Aust. Vet .J. 77:161-163.

Beck, C., O'Neill, T., Holloway, S.A. and Slocombe, R.F. (2001). The use of ultrasound in the investigation of gastric carcinoma in a dog. Aust. Vet. J.79:332-334.

Biller, D.S., Partington, B.P., Miyabayashi, T. and Leveille, R. (1994). Ultrasonographic appearance of chronic hypertrophic pyloric gastropathy in the dog. Vet. Radiol. Ultrasound 35:30-33.

Culbertson, R., Branam, J.E. and Rosenblatt, L.S. (1983). Esophageal/gastric leiomyoma in the laboratory Beagle. J.Am.Vet.med.Assoc. 183:1168-1171.

Feldman, M.K., Katyal, S. and Blackwood, M.S. (2009). Ultrasound artifacts. Radiographics 29:1179-1189

Grooters, A.M., Biller, D.S. and Ward, H. (1994). Ultrasonographic appearance of feline alimentary lymphoma. Vet. Radiol. Ultrasound 35: 468-472.

Gualtieri, M., Monzeglio, M.G. and Scanziani, E. (1999). Gastric neoplasia. Vet. Clin. North Am. Small Anim. Pract. 29:415-440.

Lamb, C.R. and Grierson, J. (1999). Ultrasonographic appearance of primary gastric neoplasia in 21 dogs. J. Small Anim. Pract. 40:211-215.

Larson, M.M. and Biller, D.S. (2009). Ultrasound of the gastrointestinal tract. Vet. Clin. North Am. Small Anim. Pract.39:747-759.

Linton, M., Nimmo, J.S. and Norris, J.M. (2015). Feline gastrointestinal eosinophilic sclerosing fibroplasia: 13 cases and review of an emerging clinical entity. J. Feline Med .Surg. 17:392-404.

Newell, S.M., Graham, J.P. and Roberts, G.D. (1999). Sonography of the normal feline gastrointestinal tract. Vet. Radiol. Ultrasound 40:40-43.

Penninck, D.G., Nyland, T.G., Fishe, P.E. and Kerr, L.Y. (1989). Ultrasonograph of the normal canine gastrointestinal tract. Vet. Radiol. Ultrasound 30:272-276

Peters, R.M., Goldstein, R.E., Erb, H.N. and Njaa, B.L. (2005). Histopathologic features of canine uremic gastropathy: a retrospective study. J. Vet. Intern. Med. 19:315-320.

Vaughn, D.P, Syrcle, J. and Cooley, J. (2014). Canine giant hypertrophic gastritis treated successfully with partial gastrectomy. J.Am.Anim.Hops. Assoc. 50:62-66.

8

Ultrasound of The Intestines

J.P. Varshney and P.S. Chaudhary

Ultrasound and survey radiography are two important diagnostic modalities regularly employed in the diagnosis of intestinal diseases. Both modalities are complementary to each other in investigating the problems related to intestines. It is always better to have plain survey radiograph of abdomen first and then ultrasound to rule out obstruction or radio-opaque foreign bodies. Wherever barium meal radiograph is indicated, it should be done after sonographic examination as barium may degrade image quality of the sonogram. Assessment of intestinal motility can be done in real time sonography.

Imaging Technique

- A fasting of 12-24 hours prior to sonography is desirable for better quality images.
- The effect of gas artefacts (present in the gastrointestinal tract) can be minimized by adopting scanning from the ventral abdomen through a cut top in the table, changing position of the patient, or putting mild pressure with probe on the abdominal wall,
- Dogs and cats are placed in dorsal or lateral recumbency.
- Site is prepared as usual by clipping/ shaving hairs and applying acoustic gel.
- Both longitudinal and transverse axis of different intestinal segments is viewed.
- Intestines (Fig.73) are viewed in sequence as duodenum, jejunum, ileum, cecum ileocolic junction (dogs)/ ileocecocolic junction (cats) and colon (ascending, transverse and descending).

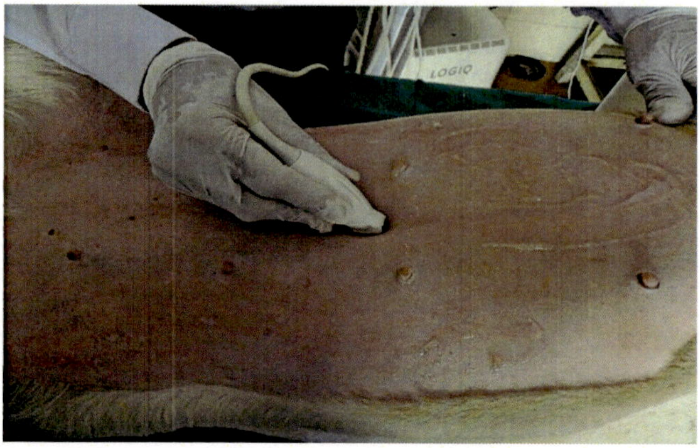

Fig. 73: Imaging of intestines

- For anal sac sonography, dogs and cats are examined either in sternal recumbency or in standing position with the tail reflected over the dorsum (Fig.74.). A linear array transducer of 5.0 to 9.0 MHz can be used. The area around anus is prepared and gel is applied. Dorsal images of anal sac are obtained by scanning the anal region.

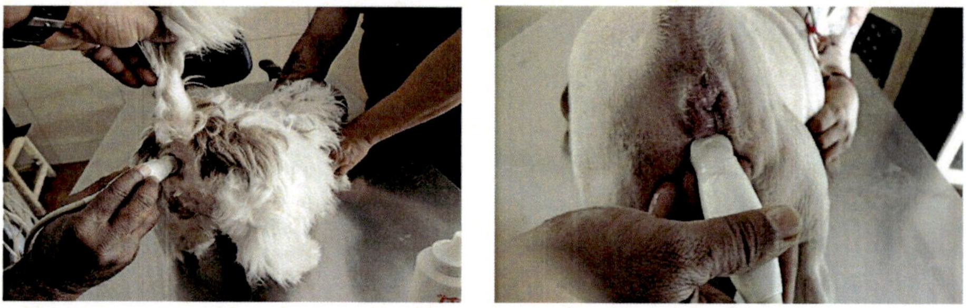

Fig. 74: Imaging of anal sac in a dog in standing position

Landmarks

- Ileum is short and is situated in the right cranial to mid quadrant of abdomen. Right kidney is lateral to ileum.
- Other landmark for ileum is transverse colon or ileo (ceco) colic junction.
- Transverse colon is immediately caudal to gastric body.
- Due to gas in cecum, identification of ileum in dogs is difficult as compared to cats.

- Ileocolic junction (dogs)/ ileocecocolic junction (cats) is medial to right kidney in the right cranial quadrant of abdomen.
- It is not always possible to identify cecum (blind sac) because of superimposition of gas filled intestinal segment. It is medial to descending colon.
- Ascending colon is short and is in right cranial abdomen.
- Transverse colon is immediately caudal to greater curvature of stomach and it lies in the right to left cranial abdomen.
- Descending colon is immediately dorsal to urinary bladder.Therefore urinary bladder serves as a land mark for identifying descending colon.

Points of Observation

- Whether the diameter is uniform or varying.
- Whether the wall is thickened or normal.
- Whether the wall layers are normal or discrete
- What is the nature of luminal contents?
- Whether peristalsis is present or not.

Ultrasonographic Features of Intestines

- Normal intestinal wall of dogs (Fig. 75A) and cats (75B) has ultrasonographically distinct five layers (from outside to inside) as follow :

Serosa	- It is thin hyperechoic layer
Muscularis	- It is thin hypoechoic layer
Sub-mucosa	- It is thin hyperechoic layer
Mucosa	- It is very prominent hypoechoic thickest layer
Mucosal surface/ Lumen interface of the bowel	- Hyperechoic layer in the centre

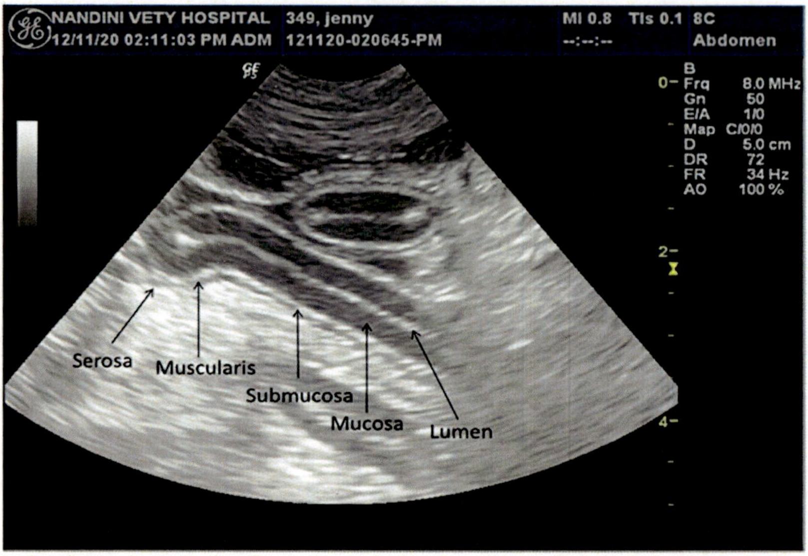

Fig. 75A: Intestinal sonogram of a dog showing different layers of intestinal wall. From outside to inside layers are thin hyperechoic serosa, thin hypoechoic muscularis, thin hyperechoic submucosa, thickest hypoechoic mucosa, and hyperechoic layer in the centre mucosal surface or lumen interface.

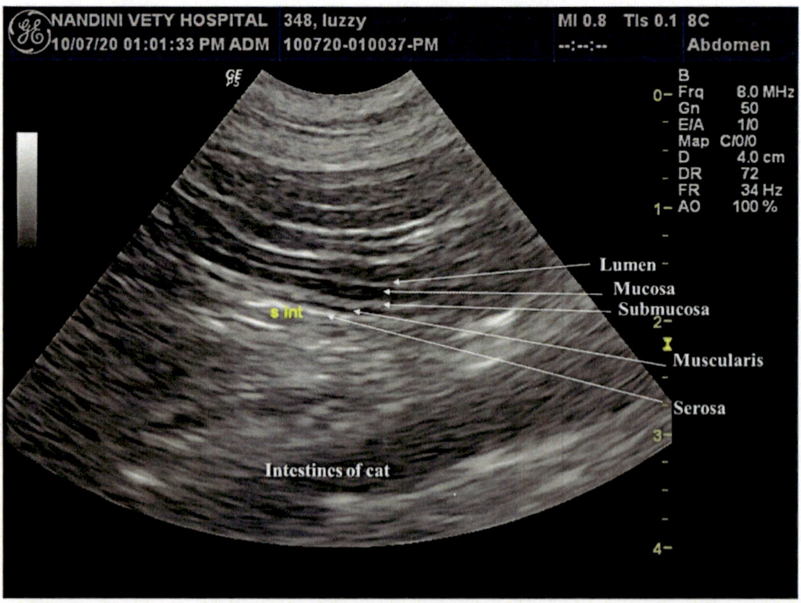

Fig. 75B. Intestinal sonogram of a cat showing different layers of intestinal wall. From outside to inside layers are thin hyperechoic serosa, thin hypoechoic muscularis, thin hyperechoic submucosa, thickiest hypoechoic mucosa, and hyperechoic layer in the centre mucosal surface or lumen interface. Intestinal layering in cats are almost similar to dogs.

- Submucosa of ileum is prominent in dogs.
- Submucosa and muscularis layer of ileum are prominent in cats. Cats have sonographically absent lumen mucosal surface.
- Mucosa, submucosa and muscularis layers of cecum of normal dogs have uniform thickness (Besso *et al.,* 2004).
- Feline cecum has a hypoechoic nodular inner layer and an adjacent hpyerechoic submucosal layer (Hehn *et al*., 2017).
- The colon has thin wall and its different layers are indistinguishable. Gas and faecal material look as hyperechoic reverberation artefact with irregularly margined, hyperechoic, partial distal acoustic shadowing material.
- Most surfaces of the anal sac tissue are surrounded by the hypoechoic external sphincter muscle. The anal sac tissue may occasionally appear as thin hyperechoic line. Anal sacs in dogs are ellipsoidal (Fig.76). In cats anal sacs are some what rounder. The normal anal sac contents of dogs appear as hypoechoic with diffuse point like hyperechoic debris. The normal anal sac contents of cats appear as more hyperechoic.

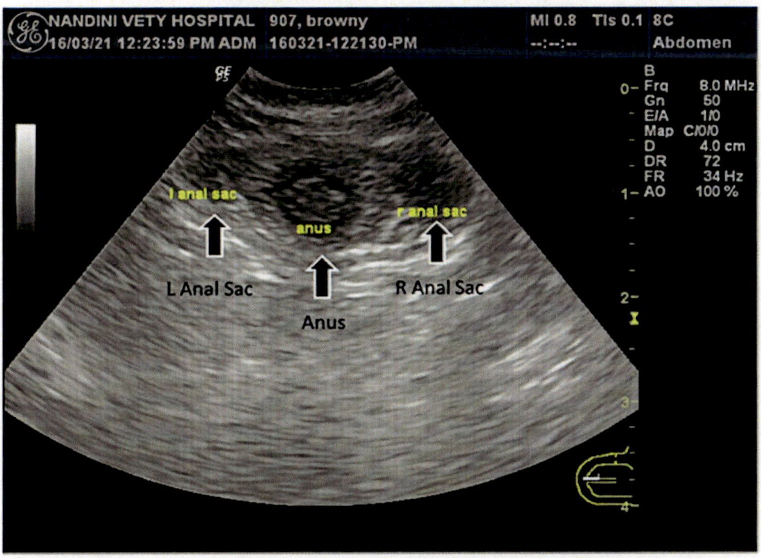

Fig.76: Anal sonogram of a crossbred male dog showing both anal sacs. Anal sacs are ellipsoidal in shape. Anal sac contents are appearing as hypoechoic with diffuse point like hyperechoic debris.

Ultrasonographic Features of Intestinal Diseases

- Lymphoma in cats appears as focal or multiple masses with thickened wall and indistinguishable intestinal layers (Grooters *et al*., 1994).

- Adenocarcinoma in cats appears as circumferential transmural thickening with a loss of normal intestinal layering.
- Intussusceptions occur in young dogs and cats. It is ultrasonographically characterized by multi-layered appearance in longitudinal axis and concentric ring appearance (Fig.77) in transverse axis (Patsikas *et al.*, 2003 a and b).

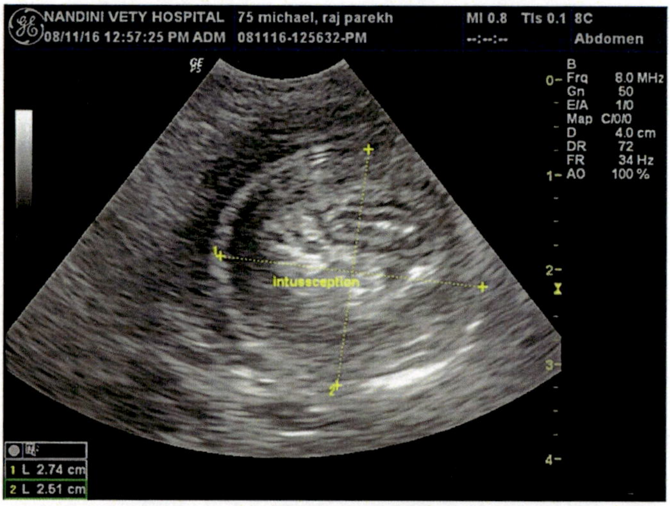

(A)

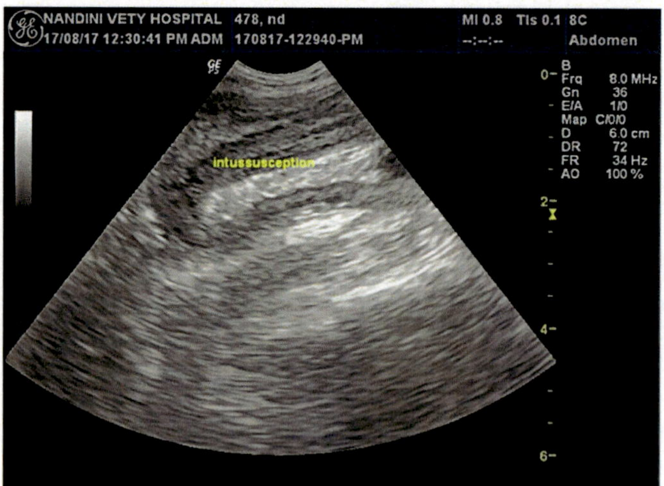

(B)

Fig. 77: Transabdominal sonograms of a dog showing concentric ring appearance of intestines in transverse axis **(A)** and multilayered appearance in longitudinal axis **(B)** suggesting intestinal intussusception.

- Large intestinal adenocarcinoma appears as nodular pedunculated mass causing annular constriction. Ultasonographically circumferential transmural thickening with loss of normal intestinal layering can be visualized.
- Mast cell tumours of colon of cats' are characterized by focal or diffuse wall thickening (Laurenson *et al.*, 2011).
- Histocytic, granulomatous and fungal colitis can cause focal wall thickening or masses.
- Eosinophilic sclerosing fibroplasia in the ileocecocolic junction and the colon of cats appear as masses or focal wall thickening with a loss of normal wall layering (Weissman *et al.*, 2013).
- Inflammatory bowel diseases (lymphocytic-plasmacytic enteritis) are usually associated with mild to moderate symmetric wall thickening (involving mucosa, submucosa and/or muscularis layer), diffuse echogenic mucosa, or presence of bright mucosal speckles (Baez *et al.*,1999; Penninck *et al.*, 2003).
- Severe colitis (inflammatory bowel disease) in dogs and cats may be associated with altered or lost wall layering; micronodular, submucosal hypoechoic and/or anechoic lesions (1 to 3 mm) representing intraparietal lymphoid follicles (Citi *et al.*, 2013).
- Ultrasonographic differentiation between colitis and large intestinal infiltrative neoplasia is very difficult and requires histopathological examination of the lesion(s).
- Anal sac tumours are generally adenocarcinoma. Anal sac tumours (Fig.78) appear as circumscribed or infiltrative masses of increased echogenicity.

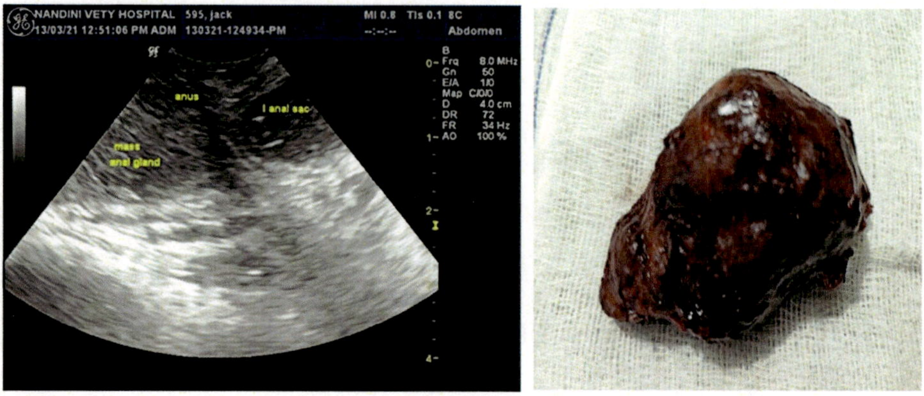

(A) **(B)**

Fig. 78: Sonogram of a dog in dorsal recumbancy showing circumscribed echogenic mass in right anal sac **(A)** suggesting a mass/tumour. The left anal sac and anus are also visible in the sonogram. Surgically removed affected gland is looking like a tumour **(B)**.

References

Baez, J.L., Hendrick, M.J., Walker, L.M. and Washabau, R.J. (1999). Radiographic, ultrasonographic, and endoscopic findings in cats with inflammatory bowel disease of the stomach and small intestine: 33 cases (1990-1997). J.Am.Vet.Med.Assoc. 215: 349-354.

Besso, J.G., Rault, D.and Begon, D. (2004). Feline cecum and ileocecocolic junction: normal ultrasonographic features and clinical applications (abstract). Vet. Radiol. Ultrasound 45:599.

Citi, S., Chimenti, T., Marchetti, V. (2013). Micronodular ultrasound lesions in the colonic submucosa of 42 dogs and 14 cats. Vet. Radiol. Ultrasound 54:646-651.

Grooters, A.M., Biller, D.S. and Ward, H.(1994). Ultrasonographic appearance of feline alimentary lymphoma. Vet. Radiol. Ultrasound 35:468-472.

Hahn, H., Pey, P. and Baril, A. (2017). Ultrasonographic, endoscopic and histological appearances of the caecum in cats presenting with chronic clinical signs of caecocolic disease. J. Feline Med. Surg.19:94-104.

Laurenson, M.P., Skorupski, K.A., Moore, P.F. and Zwingenberger, A.L. (2011). Ultrasonography of intestinal mast cell tumours in the cat. Vet. Radiol Ultrasound 52:330-334.

Patsikas, M.N. , Jakovljevic, S. and Moustardas, N. (2003 a). Ultrasonographic signs of intestinal intussusception associated with acute enteritis or gastroenteritis in 19 young dogs. J. Am. Anim. Hosp. Assoc. 39:57-66.

Patsikas, M.N., Papazoglou, L.G. and Papaioannou, N.G. (2003b). Ultrasonographic findings of intestinal intussusception in seven cats. J. FelineMed. Surg .5:335-343.

Penninck, D., Smyers, B., Webster, C.R. (2003). Diagnostic value of ultrasonography in differentiating enteritis from intestinal neoplasia in dogs. Vet Radiol Ultrasound 44:570-575.

Weissman, A., Penninck, D. and Webster,C.(2013). Ultrasonographic and clinicopathological features of feline gastrointestinal eosinophilic sclerosing fibroplasia in four cats. J. Feline Med. Surg. 15:148-154.

9

Ultrasound of The Pancreas

J.P. Varshney and P.S. Chaudhary

The pancreas is a thin and elongated 'V' shaped organ having two lobes (right and left) and body. It lies in the right cranial quadrant of the abdomen. It is difficult to visualize normal pancreas sonographically because of its echogenicity similar to that of adjacent mesentery and fat.

Ultrasonographic Technique

- Pancreas is visualized through trans-abdominal approach.
- Excessive gas in gastrointestinal tract and deep chest conformation may inhibit visualization of pancreas.
- Normal pancreas is not visible sonographically.
- Visualization of pancreas becomes difficult in obese animals.
- Dogs and cats with pancreatitis resent transducer pressure due to pain.
- It is better to fast the animal for at least 8-12 hours before ultrasonographic examination of pancreas to reduce interference of gastric contents.
- Linear or convex transducers of 7.5 to 15 MHz for small and 5 to 8 MHz for large dogs are appropriate.
- Dogs and cats can be placed in supine posture, right or left recumbent position for scanning.
- Area is prepared by shaving and application of acoustic gel as described earlier.

Landmark for Identifying Pancreas

- Pancreas lies in the right side of abdomen adjacent to stomach. Right limb of the pancreas extends caudally and parallel to the descending duodenum (Fig.79). Right limb is visualized dorsal to the duodenum when scanned from ventral abdomen with the dog in right lateral recumbency.

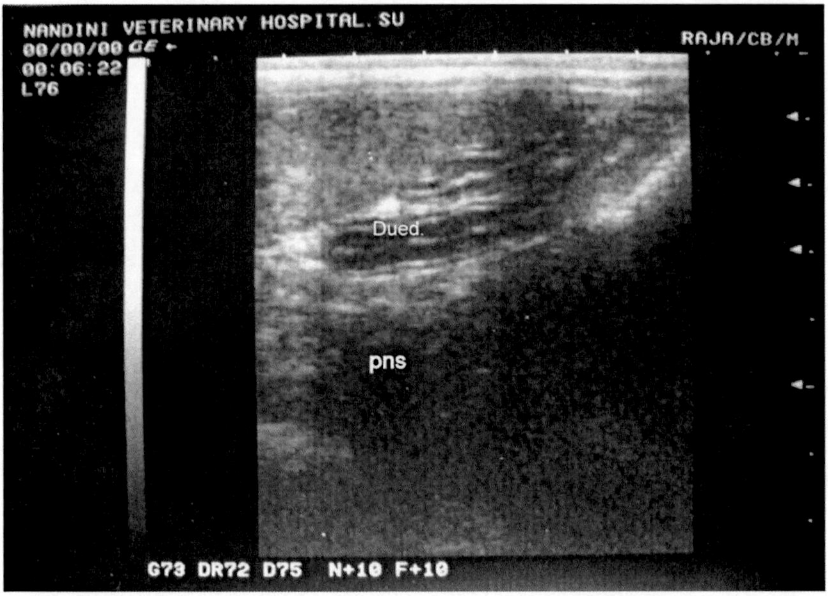

Fig. 79: Pancreatic sonogram of a dog showing right lobe of the pancreas extending caudally and parallel to the duodenum. Diseased pancreas is visualized as hypoechoic structure.

- When large amount of gas is present in gastro-intestinal tract (causing reverberation or acoustic shadowing artefacts), right kidney may be used as land mark for identifying right lobe of the pancreas.
- Left limb is associated with greater curvature of stomach and is cranial to stomach.
- Pancreas is not visible in healthy dogs and cats.
- In dogs with pancreatitis right lobe can be visualized using ventral approach placing transducer medial to the right 13th rib. Transducer is moved medial to descending duodenum to get better view of right lobe.
- The pancreatic duodenal vein in dogs can be a landmark for the right lobe.
- Right limb of pancreas in dogs is visible as triangular structure immediately adjacent to duodenum
- In cats right limb goes along the descending duodenum and then distal third curves cranially in the form of a hook. Right limb is closer to mid line position.

- Left limb of pancreas in dogs extends to the left of midline near the cranial pole of left kidney. It is difficult to visualize due to gastrointestinal contents.
- In cats left limb is larger and extends close to splenic hilum. Pancreatic duct can be visualized in cats. It can be visualized easily. The portal and splenic veins may serve as an land marks for identifying body and left limb of pancreas in cats.
- The body of the pancreas in dogs can be located at a place where left and right limbs come together. It extends caudally to the pyloric region and it is on the right and ventral to portal vein.
- The body of pancreas and pyloro duodenal junction in cats are in a mid-line position.

Ultrasonographic Features

- Generally normal canine pancreas is not identifiable sonographically as it is isoechoic or slightly hypoechoic to the surrounding mesentery.
- Normal pancreas of dogs is approximately 6.0 to 8.0 mm thick.
- Normal pancreas of cats is approximately 5.0 to 6.0 mm thick.
- Occasionally pancreas may look diffusely hyper echoic but may measure within limits.
- Feline pancreas is easily visible as discrete organ as hypoechoic (echogenicity is similar to the liver) linear structure with smooth border and a well demarcated anechoic pancreatic duct.
- The pancreatico-duodenal vein is usually not visible in cats.

Ultrasonographic Feature in Pancreatic Diseases

- Detection of pancreatitis may sometimes become difficult as pancreas looks ultrasonographically normal. So normal appearing pancreas may not rule out pancreatitis.
- The pancreas may be visualized as enlarged hypoechoic organ with round or irregular margins (Fig. 80) in cases of acute pancreatitis. Surrounding mesenteric fats is hyperechoic. Some amount of echogenic fluid in the area of inflamed pancreas may also be seen owing to peritonitis and /or fat saponification (steatitis).

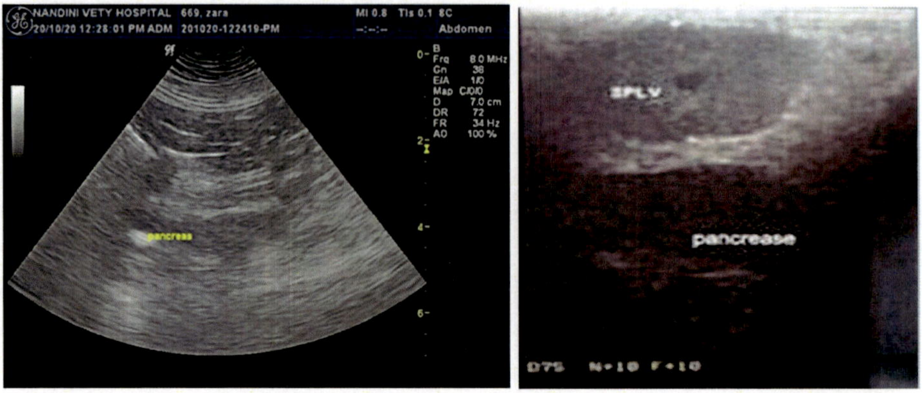

Fig. 80: Pancreatic sonogram of dogs showing enlarged hypoechoic pancreas with round or irregular margin suggesting pancreatitis

- Sensitivity of ultrasound alone in the diagnosis of pancreatic diseases in felines is comparatively low.
- In cats pancreatitis may be in association with hepatic lipidosis, inflammatory bowel disease and cholangiohepatitis.
- Necrotizing pancreatitis may be characterized by hypo to anechoic regions due to haemorrhages and necrosis. Doppler examination needs to be performed to assess blood flow in pancreas.
- Cystic lesions in pancreas are characterized by round anechoic structures associated with distal enhancement artefacts. Differentiation of cystic lesions from congenital cysts, pseudo cysts, and retention cysts is not possible sonographically.
- Pancreatic abscesses are characterized by distal acoustic shadowing, thick irregular wall and reverberation artefacts.
- Thickened hyperechoic or heterogeneous (hypo/hperechoic areas) pancreas (Fig.81) is the indicative of chronic pancreatitis.

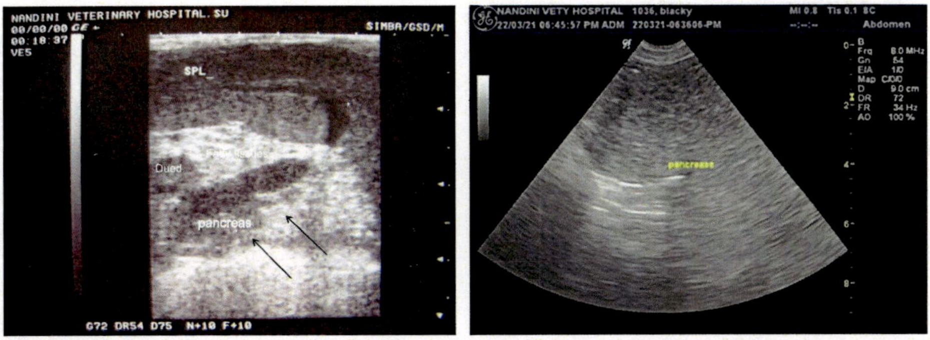

Fig. 81: Pancreatic sonogram of dogs showing hyperechoic (arrows) or heterogeneous pancreas suggesting chronic pancreatitis.

- In cats, ductal dilation may also be seen in chronic pancreatitis. Or it may be related with aging.
- Tiger stripe appearance of pancreas owing to multiple anechoic areas due to oedematous fluid in interlobular septae in dogs and cats is suggestive of pancreatic oedema due to hypoalbuminaemia or portal hypertension (Lamb, 1999).
- Sonographic differentiation of pancreatic neoplasia, abscess, necrosis, nodular hyperplasia (Fig. 82) or acute inflammatory changes is difficult. If a single lesions is large (> 2 cm diameter), there is likelihood of neoplasia.

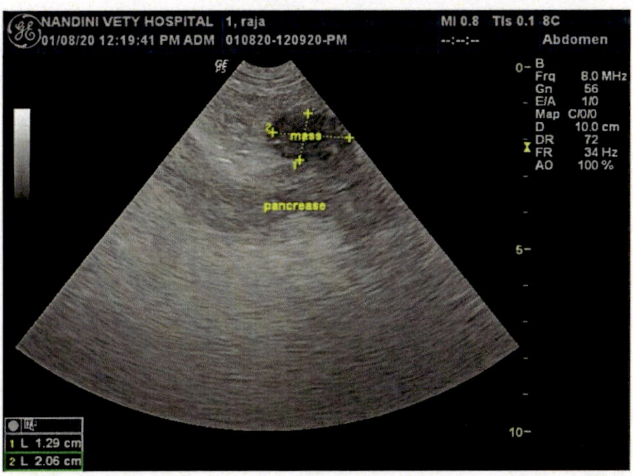

Fig. 82: Transabdominal sonogram of a dog showing hypoechoic pancreas and an anechoic 1.29 x 2.06 cm rounded single lesion in pancreas suggesting a mass. It is difficult to differentiate tumour, abscess, nodular hyperplasia and acute inflammatory changes on the basis of sonogram only. The size of the lesion is large, there may be a possibility of a neoplasm.

References

Lamb, C.R. (1999). Pancreatic oedema in dogs with hypoalbuminemia and portal hypertension. J .Vet. Intern. Med. 13:498-500.

Suggested Further Readings

Mannion, P. (2006). Diagnostic Ultrasound in Small Animal Practice. Blackwell Science Ltd. Oxford, U.K.

Nyland, T. G., Mattoon, J. S. and Herrgesell, E. J.(2002) Pancreas. In: Small Animal Diagnostic Ultrasound, 2nd edn, W. B. Saunders Co., Philadelphia, pp 144-157.

Varshney, J.P., Chaudhary, J.P., Deshmukh, V.V. and Sutaria Prajwalita (2011). Pancreatitis associated with clinical babesiosis in dog. J. Canine Dev. Res. 7: 74-76.

10

Ultrasound of The Urinary Tract

J.P. Varshney and P.S. Chaudhary

The urinary tract is the body's drainage system. It includes kidneys, ureters, urinary bladder and urethra. Ultrasound is a most preferred imaging tool for the diagnosis of diseases of urinary tract not only in humans but also in dogs and cats. Little adipose tissue in urinary system of dogs makes the contrast between different planes and anatomical structures poor.

Kidneys

Canine kidneys are bean shaped paired organ, surrounded by adipose tissues, situated in retroperitoneal space. While feline kidneys are oval in shape.

Landmarks for Identifying Kidneys

- Cranial pole of left kidney of dogs is close to greater curvature of stomach and dorsomedial to craniodorsal extremity of spleen (Fig. 83).

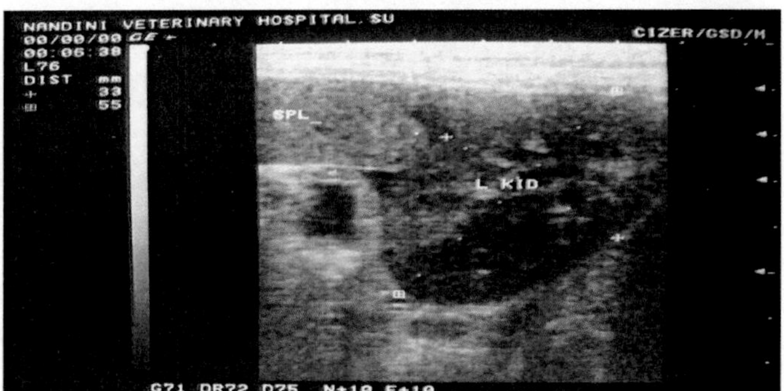

Fig. 83: Sonogram of a dog showing left kidney in the vicinity of the spleen

- Right kidney of dogs is more cranial than left one.
- Right kidney of dogs is situated within renal fossa of the caudate lobe of liver. In cats retroperitoneal fat separates right kidney from the caudate lobe.

Assessing normal Kidney size in dogs

- Ratio of left and right kidney to the length of L5 and L6 is 1.3 to 2.7 (Barell *et al.*, 2012).
- Ratio of kidney length to aortic diameter width is 5.5 to 9.1 (Mareschal *et al.*, 2008).

Scanning Technique

- Site is prepared by clipping or shaving the area and applying acoustic gel as usual.
- First left kidney is scanned. Then moving in clockwise fashion scanning of urinary bladder, proximal urethra and then right kidney is done.
- Kidneys are imaged in sagittal, dorsal and transverse planes.
- In dorsal or sagittal plane, kidneys are visualized from medial to lateral; and dorsal to ventral. In transverse plane kidneys are scanned from cranial to caudal.
- It is easy to locate left kidney.
- It may be difficult to image right kidney especially in deep chested dogs due to its more cranio-dorsal location in the abdomen.
- In such cases lateral approach through 11th or 12th intercostal space may be helpful.
- Scanning of right kidney may be affected by gas in gastrointestinal tract.

Ultrasonographic Features of the Kidney

- In sagittal plane renal sinus, cortex and medulla can be visualized.
- Ultrasonographic features of the normal kidney of the dog and cat are shown in the Fig.84 and 85 .
- Renal medulla is least echogenic (Fig. 86).
- Renal cortex is little more echogenic than medulla (Fig.86).
- Renal sinus is more echogenic with hyperechoic fat (Fig.86).
- Corticomedullary distinction is identifiable.
- Renal cortex is slightly hyperechoic to the liver.
- Renal medulla is homogeneous and has coarse echotexture.
- In renal pelvis small amount of fluid can be seen occasionally.

- Width of renal pelvis may be around 2 mm in dogs and around 1.6 mm in cats.
- Linear measurements of kidneys (length -L, width- W and depth- D) can be recorded on the largest cross sectional sagittal and transverse images with the help of built-in calipers. The volume of kidney is then calculated by the formula as :

V (volume of the kidney) = L x W x D x 0.523 (Hricak and Lieto, 1983).

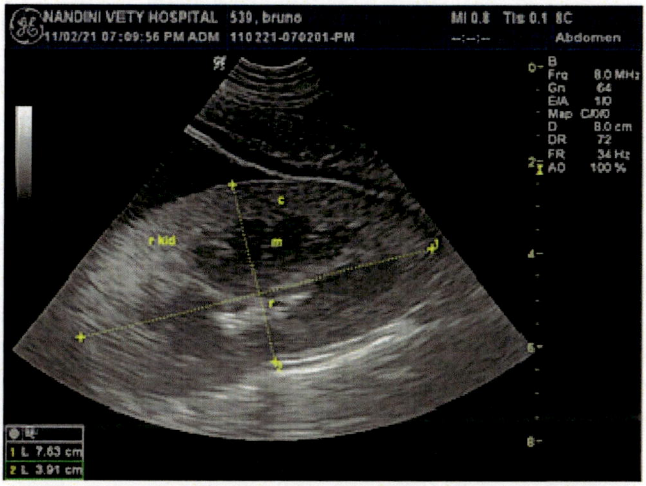

Fig. 84: Transabdominal sonogram of right kidney of an adult healthy dog in sagittal plane. Kidney is slightly bean shaped.

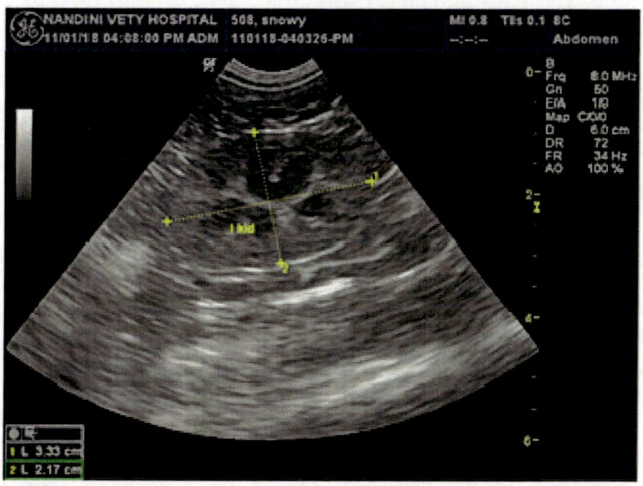

Fig. 85: Transabdominal sonogram of left kidney of an adult healthy cat in sagittal pane. Kidney is slightly oval in shape.

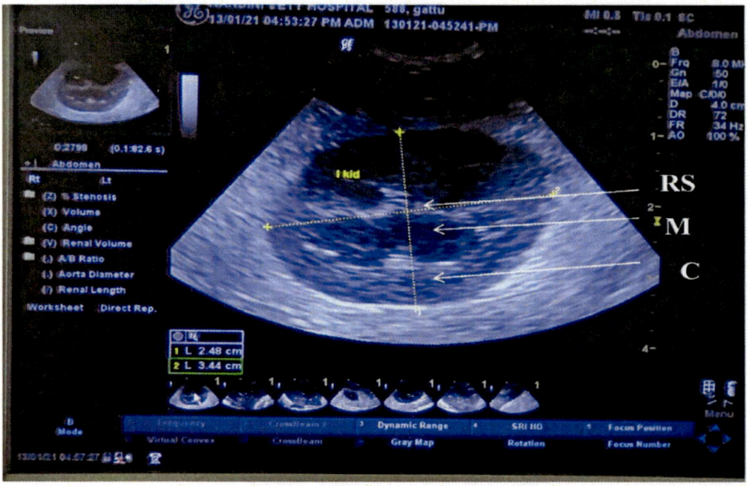

Fig. 86: Transabdominal sonogram of left kidney of an adult healthy dog in sagittal plane showing renal pelvis, cortex and medulla. Renal cortex is hyperechoic © and renal medulla is least echogenic (M) . Renal sinus is more echogenic(RS).

Sonographic Features in Kidney Diseases

- When there is only one kidney present, it may be slightly hypertrophied with normal internal architecture.
- Autosomal dominant polycystic kidney disease is inherited and more common in Persian cats (pure bred as well as Persian crosses), cairn terriers and bull terriers (McKenna and Carpenter,1980; Reichle et al., 2002). These cysts are rounded with anechoic center having smooth sharply demarcated thin wall (Fig. 87).

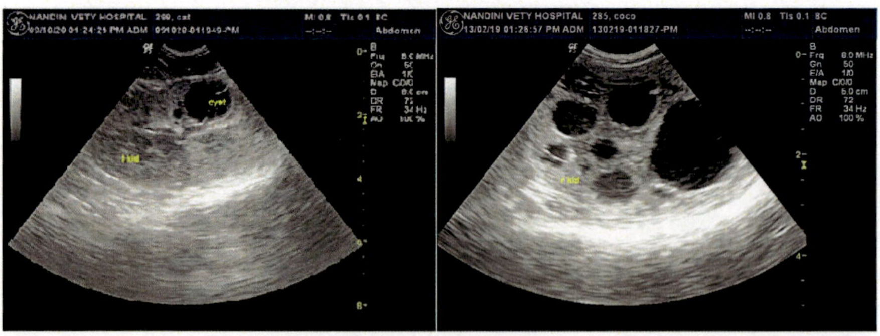

(A) **(B)**

Fig. 87: (A) Sonogram of a six year old male cat with anorexia, marked vomiting and weakness showing cyst in the left kidney suggesting Cystic kidney. The cat had category 4 renal failure (serum creatinine 16.4 mg/dl, and BUN 100 mg/dl) and marked dehydration (skin tenting test > 6 second). **(B)** Sonogram of another three year old female cat showing multiple thin walled round structures filled with anoechoic fluid in right kidney suggesting polycystic kidney

- Renal haematomas are sonographically characterized by a mixture of anechoic, hypoechoic and hyperechoic contents within renal cortex or medulla.
- Renal abscess are sonographically characterized by poorly demarcated cavity having irregular contours, sedimentation, echoes and variable degree of distal acoustic enhancement.
- Renal infarcts are sonographically characterized by well-defined wedge shaped cortical lesions. In chronic phase they are hyperechoic with focal cortical depression.
- Nephrocalcinosis (renal mineralization) is the problem of geriatric dogs and cats. It is visualized as hyper attenuating foci with distal acoustic shadowing (Fig.88 A, B and C).

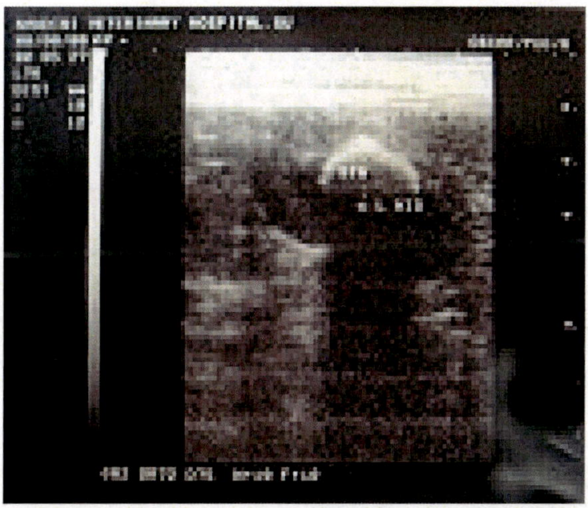

Fig. 88 A: Renal sonogram of left kidney of a male pug with urinary tract infection. The bright hyperechoic curvilinear focus with distal acoustic shadowing is a calculus.

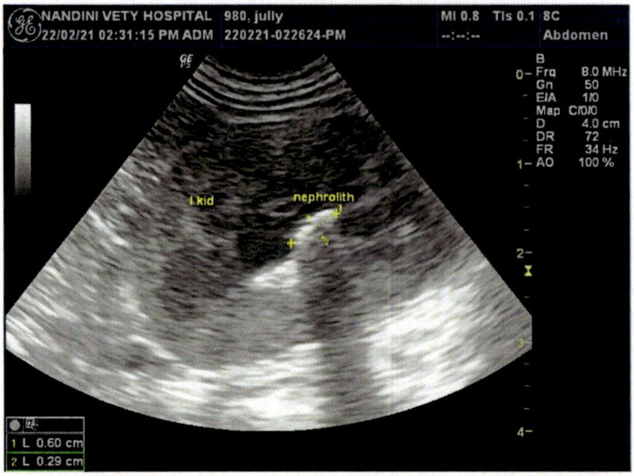

Fig. 88 B: Renal sonogram of left kidney of an another dog. The bright hyperechoic curvilinear focus with distal acoustic shadowing in left kidney is clearly visible suggesting renal lith.

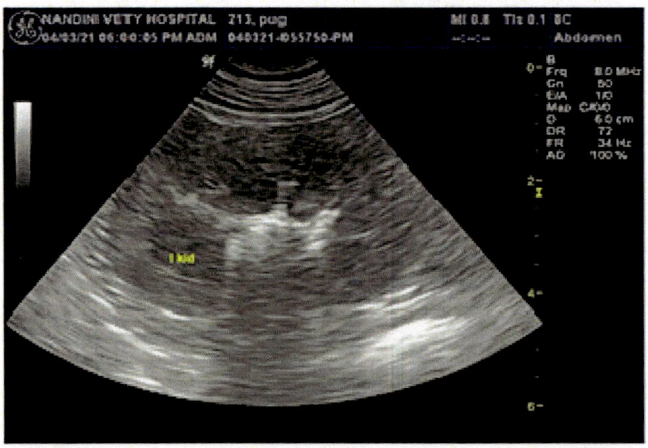

Fig. 88 C: Renal sonogram of left kidney of a nine year old male pug with mineralization of the renal pelvis. The bright hyperechoic foci of mineralization appears similar to pelvic renolith but acoustic shadowing is not as marked as in renal calculi. Appearance is also less discrete.

- Renal adenocarcinomas in German Shepherds are seen as fluid filled cavities (may be one or several) and solid tissue component infiltrating kidney protrude into cyst (Moe and Lium,1997).
- Other renal tumours (Fig. 89) may be visualized as homogeneous/ heterogeneous; hypoechoic/isoechoic /hyperechoic; regular/irregular margin; hypoechoic halo at the periphery of the cortex; hyperechoic foci or striations throughout the medulla; hypoechoic medullary or cortical nodules or masses (Konde *et al.,*1985).

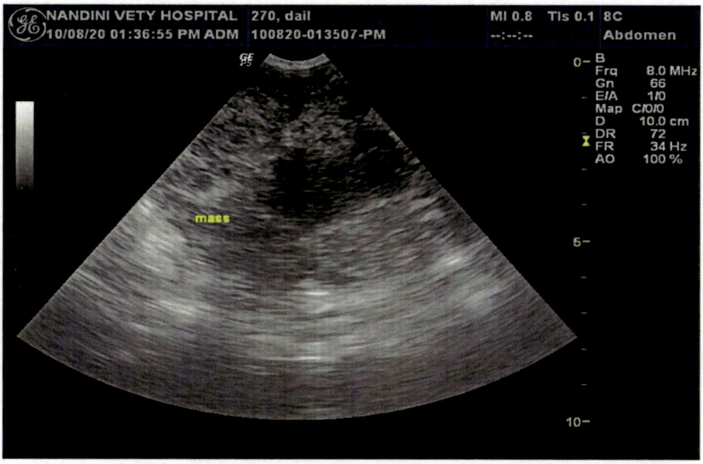

Fig. 89: Transabdominal renal sonogram of a dog showing hyperechoic irregular margined mass in the kidney suggesting tumour. For identifying the type of tumour, biopsy and histopathology is necessary.

- Renal lymphoma is a common tumour of kidney in cats and is characterized by irregularly hyperechoic enlarged kidneys with hypoechoic subcapsular thickening (Valdes-Martinez *et al.*, 2007).
- Kidneys in ethylene glycol toxicosis are ultrasonographically characterized by an increased hyperechogenicity of cortical and medullary region with circumferential hyperechoic band in medulla parallel to corticomedullary junction (medullary rim sign). This type of appearance is also seen in mineralization, necrosis, congestion, and /or haemorrhages (Konde *et al.*, 1985).
- Chronic interstitial nephritis is characterized by small, irregular and diffusely hyperechoic kidneys having no cortico-medullary demarcation.
- Detection of anechoic fluid around one or both kidneys between the renal capsule and cortex is suggestive of perirenal pseudo cysts (Ochoa *et al.*, 1999). These cysts are more common in cats.
- Pyelonephritis is sonographically characterized by mild renal enlargement with pelvic and ureteral dilation ; hyperechoic mucosal margin parallel to the wall of renal pelvis and proximal ureter (Neuwirth *et al.*,1993); hyperechoic band at corticomedullary junction; hyperechoic focal areas in medulla, patchy focal hypoechoic/hyperechoic areas in renal cortex (Neuwirth *et al.*,1993).

- In hydronephrosis renal pelvis and diverticuli are dilated and distorted (Fig. 90). Renal diverticuli appear as anechoic finger like projections extending from anechoic renal pelvis. In chronic cases of hydronephrosis renal pelvis becomes distended and parenchyma atrophied.

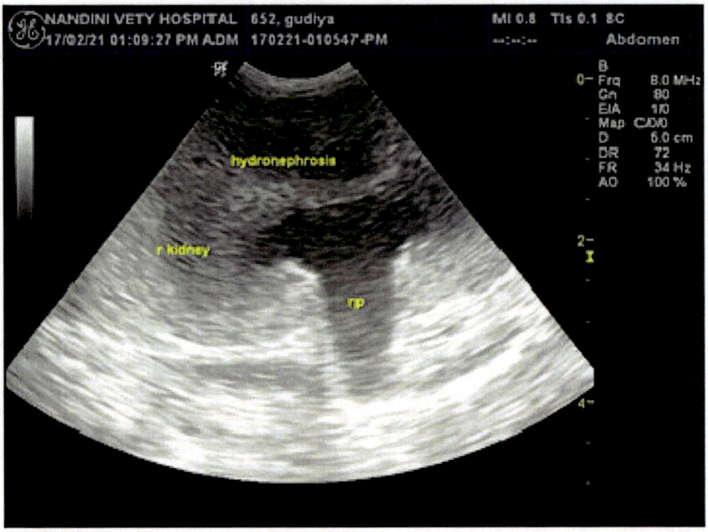

Fig. 90: Sonogram of a female 4.5 year old cat with marked dullness, vomiting and recumbency showing marked dilation of renal pelvis suggesting hydronephrosis. Biochemical investigations revealed category 4 renal failure (serum creatinine 13.8 mg/dl and BUN 78 mg/dl).

- Hydro ureters are easily visualized at renal hilus. Distended ureters can be secondary to ectopia, ureteritis, obstruction or congenital conditions (Lamb, 1998).

Urinary Bladder and Urethra

Ultrasonographic examination of urinary bladder is generally recommended in cases of haematuria, dysuria in both sexes of dogs and cats. It may reveal information about the capacity of urinary bladder, urinary wall thickness, mural or intraluminal masses, crystals/ stones.

Scanning Technique

- Site is prepared by clipping hairs and applying acoustic gel as described earlier.
- For best results bladder should be examined when it is distended as an empty or minimally distended bladder gives a false impression of bladder wall thickness.

- A convex, linear or sector transducer of 5 to 10 MHz is suitable for examining distal ureter, urinary bladder and proximal urethra.
- Intrapelvic ureter is viewed best with micro convex probe with small foot print.
- Transducer is put in long axis and then moved caudally to a level between the last 2 mammary chains to view urinary bladder in long and short axis.
- Transducer is moved further caudally to visualize trigon region.

Ultrasonographic Features of Urinary Bladder

- Urinary wall thickness is calculated on the degree of distension of urinary bladder. Urinary bladder wall in healthy dogs may vary from 1.4 to 2.3 mm depending on bladder distension (Geisse *et al.*, 1997).
- In dogs normal bladder wall is 1.0 mm thick and in cats it is 1.3 to 1.7 mm thick.
- Urine in bladder is usually anechoic (Fig.91). Nevertheless echogenic urine is not specific of urinary tract disease and may be an artifact. Side lobe (pseudo sludge) or grating lobe artifacts are the other artefacts commonly seen.
- For assessing urinary bladder volume, maximal length (from cranial pole of bladder to bladder neck), longitudinal and transverse depth are measured from maximal longitudinal (ventral to dorsal wall) and transverse images (maximum depth and maximum width) and volume is calculated as per formula described for humans (Hakenberg *et al.,* 1983) given below:

Bladder volume (ml) = L x W x (DL+DT)/2 x 0.625

L=Longitudinal diameter, W = transverse diameter, DL = depth at longitudinal diameter, DT= depth at transverse diameter.

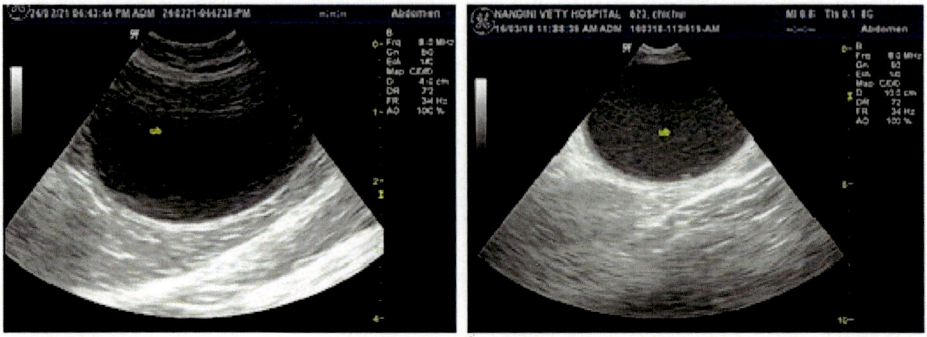

(A) Dog **(B) Cat**

Fig. 91: Trans abdominal sonograms of dog **(A)** and cat **(B)** showing urinary bladder. Urinary bladder appears as a sac containing anechoic fluid.

Diagnosis of urethral and urinary bladder abnormalities

- Ureterocele is visualized as thin walled round structure containing an anechoic fluid within the neck of urinary bladder (Stiffer *et al.*, 2002).
- Ruptured bladder is best diagnosed by positive contrast cystography. However, break in the continuity of the bladder wall and anechoic fluid in the vicinity may be visualized (Fig.92) in case of ruptured bladder.

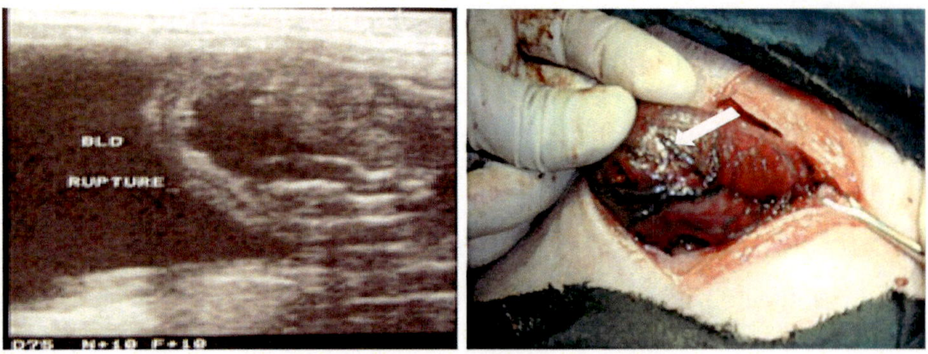

(A) **(B)**

Fig. 92: Abdominal sonogram of a dog showing break in the continuity of the bladder wall and anechoic fluid in the vicinity **(A)** suggesting urinary bladder rupture. Surgery confirmed the bladder wall rupture **(B)**

- Cystic calculi (Fig.93) are visualized as variable sized spherical and hyperechoic curvilinear interface with distal acoustic shadowing and sedimenting in the dependent portion of bladder. They can also adhere to inflamed urinary bladder wall. The calculi move within bladder lumen according to the position of the animal due to gravity.

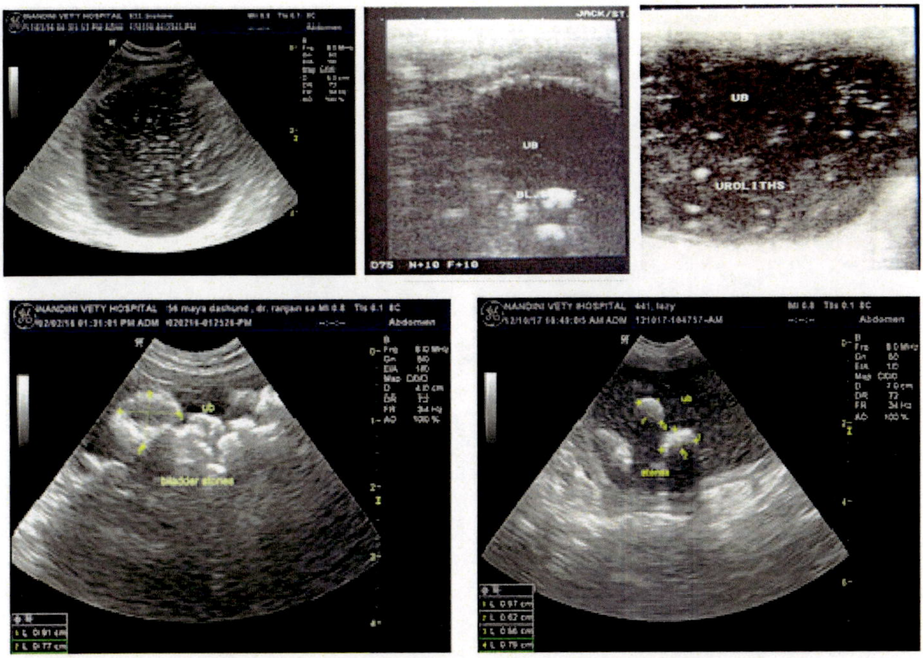

Fig. 93: Abdominal sonogram of dogs showing variable size hyperechoic material sedimenting in the dependent part of the bladder with distal acoustic shadowing suggesting crystals/calculi/cystoliths.

- Blood clots in bladder are secondary to trauma, neoplasm, infection or bleeding disorder. Sonographically (Fig.94) they are irregular in shape, hyperechoic without distal acoustic shadowing and gravity dependent (Leveille, 1998) .

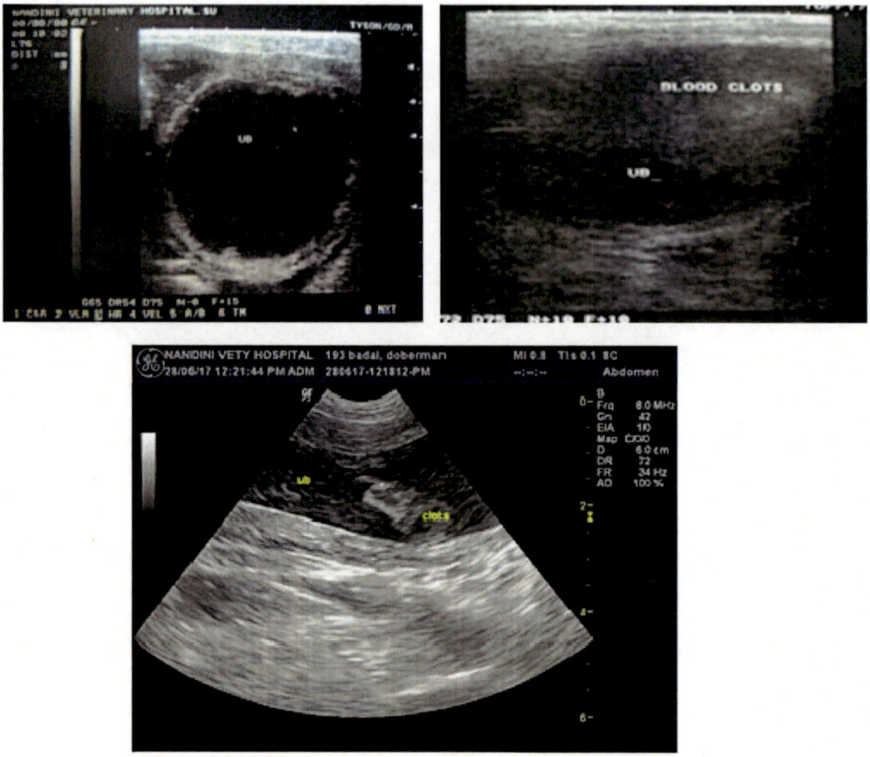

Fig. 94: Abdominal sonogram of dogs showing gravity dependent slightly hyperechoic material without distal acoustic shadowing suggestive of haemorrhage and blood clot.

- Chronic cystitis is characterized by bladder wall thickening and irregular mucosal surface (Fig.95) more pronounced cranioventrally.

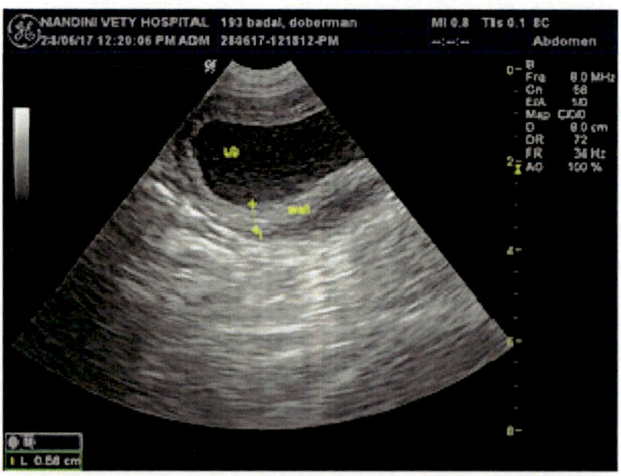

Fig. 95: Abdominal sonogram of a dog showing thickened (> 3 mm) hyperechoic urinary bladder wall suggesting cystitis.

- Polypoid cystitis is characterized by wall thickening with multiple small masses (cranio ventrally) projecting into bladder lumen. Large polyps appear pedunculated at their attachment site (Takiguchi and Inaba, 2005).
- Emphysematous cystitis is characterized by irregularly marginated hyperechoic bladder wall with acoustic shadowing and reverberation produced by the gas by gas producing organisms (E. *coli, Aerobacter, Preoteus* and *Clostridium*).
- Transitional cell carcinoma is an irregular mass with broad based attachment projecting into bladder lumen in trigone area. Sonographically it is heterogeneously hyperechoic/isoechoic/hypoechoic (Fig. 96 and 97) in relation to bladder wall (Leveille *et al*., 1992). Definite diagnosis requires ultrasound guided biopsy of the mass and its histopathology.

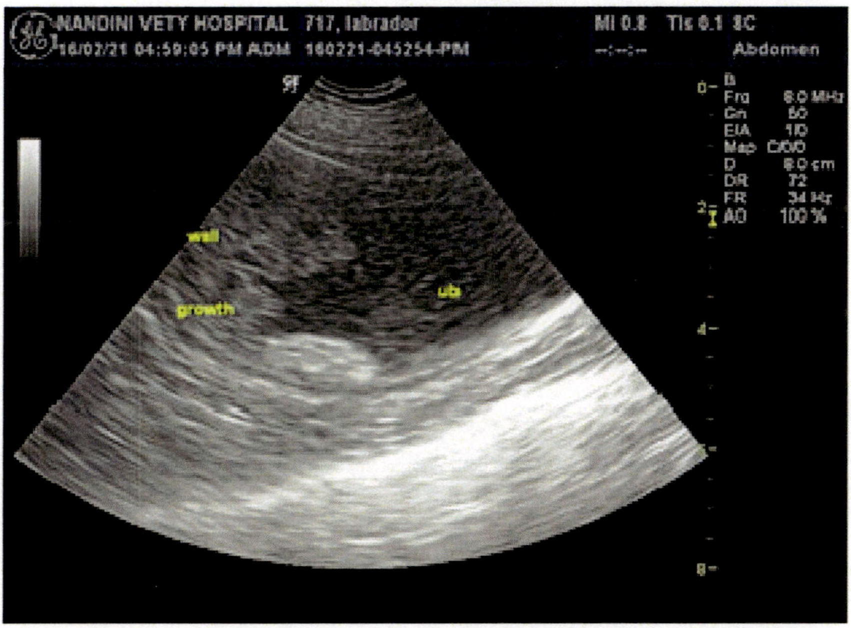

Fig. 96: Ultrasonogram of a six year old Labrador bitch with haematuria showing irregular broad based echogenic mass attached to bladder wall and projecting in to lumen of urinary bladder in trigone area suggesting the possibility of transitional cell carcinoma. Examination of urine revealed *Proteus mirabilis* >1,00,000 CFU/ml, turbidity, alkaline pH, sp. Gravity 1.015, few crystals of triple phosphate, transitional cells and protein in the urine (++++). Confirmatory diagnosis always requires histopathology of the biopsied material.

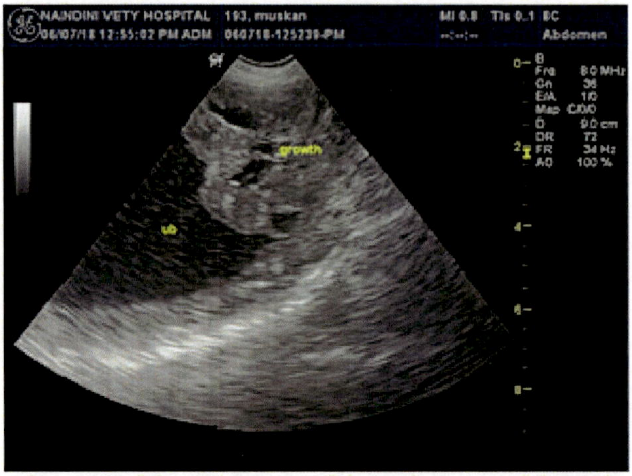

Fig. 97: Abdominal sonogram of a dog showing broad based irregular echogenic mass attached to bladder wall suggesting tumour in the urinary bladder.

- Squamous cell carcinoma is other neoplasm. Differentiation of bladder neoplasm on the basis of ultrasound is not possible. Biopsy or traumatic catheterization and histopathology is needed.
- Urethral calculi are small curvilinear hyperechoic foci with distal acoustic shadowing (Fig.98) generally seen proximal to os penis in male dogs.

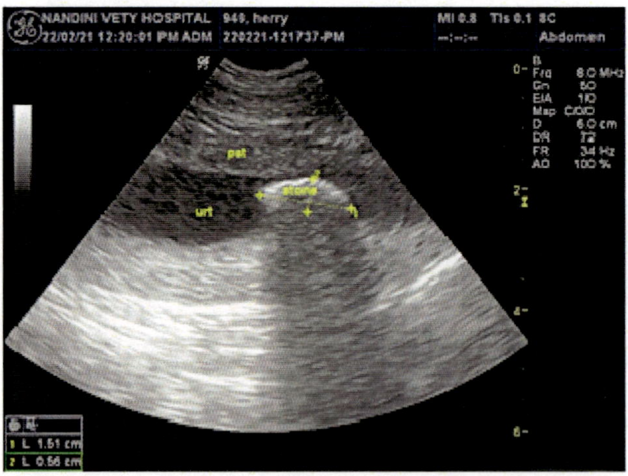

Fig. 98: Trans abdominal sonogram of a male dog showing curvilinear hyperechoic foci in the urethra with distal acoustic shadowing suggesting urethral calculi.

- Urethral transitional cell carcinoma is associated with a hypoechoic and thickened wall urethra with hyperechoic mucosal lining (Hanson and Tidwell, 1996).

Adrenals

Adrenal glands are located within retroperitoneal space near the cranial poles of the respective kidneys. Sonographic examination of adrenals is a routine procedure in human and veterinary medicine. Sagittal plane is more informative than transverse plane. A 5.0 to 7.5 MHz transducer may be used for scanning adrenals.

- Canine adrenals are long thin structures.
- The left adrenal is located craniomedial to the cranial pole of the left kidney and lateral to aorta. The phrenico abdominal artery and vein is adjacent to left adrenal.
- The right adrenal is located medial to the right kidney and caudate process of the caudate lobe of the liver.
- Adrenals of dogs (Fig.99) and cats are hypoechoic structure with hyperechoic border.
- Left adrenal is peanut shaped in small dogs and pancake or lawn chair shaped in medium or large dogs.
- Right adrenal is oval (small breed dogs) or pancake/V shaped (medium and large breed dogs).
- Width of the adrenal is an important dimension. In healthy dogs, it is generally less than 7 mm (Fig. 98 C).
- Enlarged adrenals (width > 7.0 mm) may be seen in cases of hyperadrenocorticism.
- Mineralization of adrenals is seen in adrenal neoplastic masses in dogs.
- Feline adrenals are oval or bean shaped. They are bilaterally symmetrical and hypoechoic in relation to surrounding retroperitoneal fat.
- Mineralization of feline adrenals is an incidental finding.

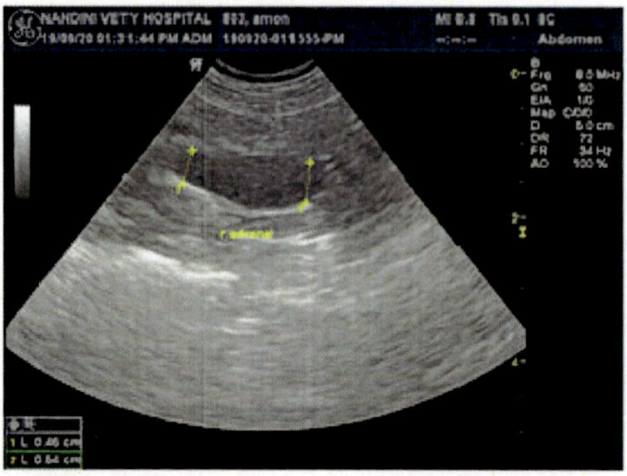

(A) Right Adrenal

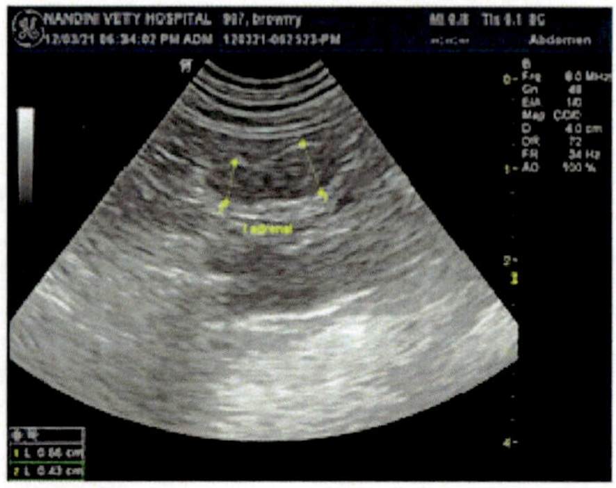

(B) Left Adrenal

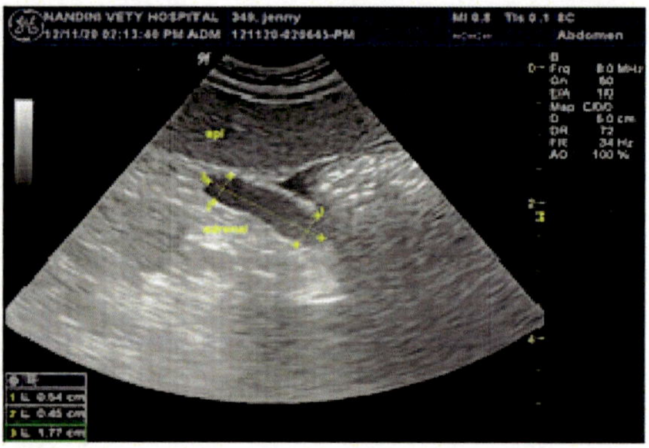

(C) Width of normal adrenal (4.2 to 6.0 mm)

Fig. 99: Sonogram of a German Shepherd dog showing adrenals as a long thin hypoechoic structure with hyperechoic border. The right adrenal **(A)** appears as pan cake shape .The left adrenal **(B)** appears as long thin structure. The width of the normal adrenal is varying from 4.2 to 6.0 mm **(C)**.

References

Barella, G., Lodi, M., Sabbadin, L.A. and Faverzani, S.A. (2012). New method for ultrasonographic measurement of kidney size in healthy dogs. J. Ultrasound 15:186-191.

Geisse, A.L., Lowry, J.E., Schaeffer, D.J. and Smith, C.W. (1997). Sonographic evaluation of urinary bladder wall thickness in normal dogs. Vet. Radiol. Ultrasound 38:132-137.

Hakenberg, O.W., Ryall, R.L., Langlois, S.L. and Marshall, V.R. (1983). The estimation of bladder volume by sonocystography. J.Urol.130: 249-251.

Hanson, J.A. and Tidwell, A.S. (1996). Ultrasonographic appearance of urethral transitional cell carcinoma in ten dogs. Vet. Radiol. Ultrasound. 37:93-299.

Hricak, H. and Lieto, R.P. (1983). Sonographic determination of renal volume. Radiol. 148:311–2. [PubMed] [Google Scholar]

Konde, L.J., Wrigley, R.H., Park, R.D. and Lebel, J.L.(1985). Sonographic appearance of renal neoplasia in the dog. Vet. Radiol. Ultrasound 26 :74-81.

Leveille, R. (1998).Ultrasonography of urinary bladder disorders. Vet. Clin. North. Am. Small Anim. Pract. 28: 799-821

Leveille, R., Biller, D.S. and Paugh, B. (1992). Sonographic investigation of transitional cell carcinoma of the urinary bladder in small animals. Vet.Radiol. Ultrasound 33:103-107.

Mareschal, A., d'Anjou, M.A. and Moreau, M. (2007). Ultrasonographic measurement of kidney-to-aorta ratio as a method of estimating renal size in dogs. Vet. Radiol. Ultrasound 48 :434-438.

McKenna, S.C. and Carpenter, J.L. (1980). Polycystic disease of the kidney and liver in the Cairn Terrier. Vet. Pathol.17:436-442.

Moe, L. and Lium, B. (1997). Hereditary multifocal renal cystadenocarcinomas and nodular dermatofibrosis in 51 German shepherd dogs. J. Small Anim. Pract.38:498-505.

Neuwirth, L., Mahaffey, M. and Crowell, W. (1993). Comparison of excretory urography and ultrasonography for detection of experimentally induced pyelonephritis in dogs. Am. J. Vet. Res.54:660-669.

Ochoa, V.B., DiBartola, S.P. and Chew, D.J. (1999). Perinephric pseudocysts In the cat: a retrospective study and review of the literature. J. Vet. Intern. Med.13:47-55.

Reichle, J.K., DiBartola, S.P. and Leveille, R. (2002). Renal ultrasonographic evaluation and computed tomographic appearance, volume, and function of cats with autosomal dominant polycystic kidney disease. Vet. Radiol. Ultrasound 43:368-373.

Stiffler, K.S., Stevenson, M.M. and Mahaffey, M.B.(2002). Intravesical ureterocele with concurrent renal dysfunction in a dog: A case report and proposed classification system. J. Am. Anim. H sp. Assoc. 38:33-39.

Takiguchi, M. and Inaba, M.(2005).Diagnostic ultrasound of polypoid cystitis in dogs. J. Vet. Intern. Med. Sci. 67:57-61.

Valdes-Martinez, A., Cianciolo, R. and Mai, W. (2007).Association between renal hypoechoic subcapsular thickening and lymphosarcoma in cats. Vet. Radiol. Ultrasound 48:357-360.

Suggested Further readings

Varshney, J.P. and Chaudhary, P.S. (2018). Polycystic kidney disease in a Persian Cat. The Blue Cross Book 38: 118-119.

Varshney, J.P. (2019). Haematuria in cats due to struvite crystalluria and its management. J Canine Dev. Resch.15: 62-65.

11

Ultrasound of The Reproductive Tract

J.P. Varshney and P.S. Chaudhary

Application of ultrasonography has become a routine practice in canine and feline medicine to detect pregnancy, to ascertain foetal wellbeing, to ascertain live/dead status of the foetus, ovarian dynamics, and to diagnose reproductive ailments (uterine, ovarian,) in females. Sonography is also being preferred in males for the diagnosis of diseases of prostate gland, cryptorchid, and testicular diseases.

Female Reproductive Tract

Landmarks

Uterus

- Uterus in bitches and queens is located between urinary bladder (Fig.100) and ventral aspect of colon. Urinary bladder and colon are used as a land mark for locating uterus. In standing position the cervix in bitches and queens is situated between bladder neck and colon (dorsal aspects of urinary bladder neck and ventral aspect of the colon) .Short uterine body is cranial to cervix. The uterine body branches in to two long uterine horns running towards the ovaries.
- It can be visualized in scanning transversely. It is difficult to visualize non-gravid or healthy uterus.

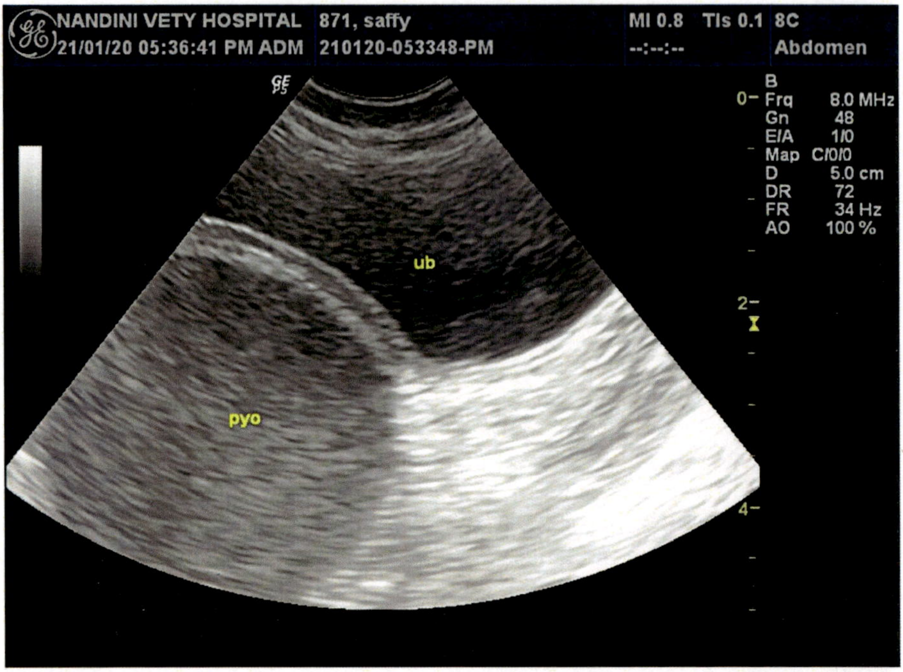

Fig. 100: Transabdominal sonogram of a bitch in dorsal recumbency showing the location of the uterus with pyometra. The uterus is anterior and ventral to the urinary bladder in this scan.

Ovaries

- The ovaries are located caudal and slightly lateral to the caudal poles of the ipsilateral kidneys

Procedure of Scanning

- An area of caudal ventral abdomen is clipped or shaved.
- A lateral approach is recommended in fatty bitches or bitches with excessive mammary development.
- Acoustic gel is applied as described elsewhere.
- No sedation is generally required.
- Linear, microconvex, curvilinear or sector transducers of 5.0 to 7.5 MHz may be used but 7.5 MHz transducer is the most appropriate as it produces high resolution images. For visualization of ovaries high frequency transducer (7.5 MHz for bitches and 10 to 15 MHz for queens).
- Normal, non-gravid uterus is often difficult to visualize.

Ultrasonographic Features

Uterus

- Usually visualizing normal or non-gravid uterus is difficult. Further it is hard to distinguish it from the intestines. A sonographic view of non-gravid and non –diseased uterus of a bitch and a queen is illustrated in the Fig.101 and Fig.102.

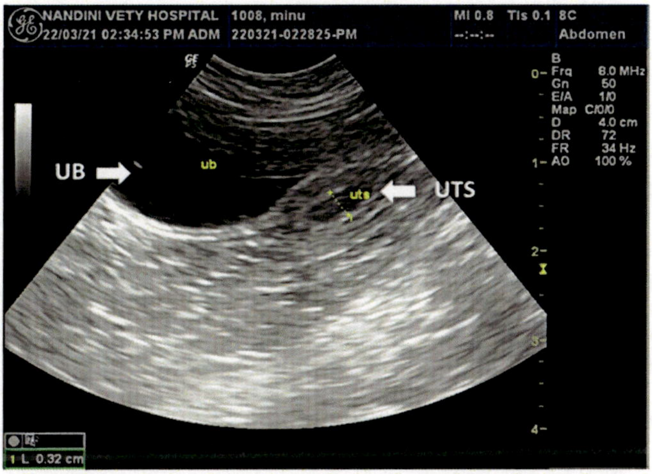

Fig. 101: Trans abdominal sonogram of a healthy eight month old non- descript bitch showing a small uterus (UT) between urinary bladder and intestine (colon).

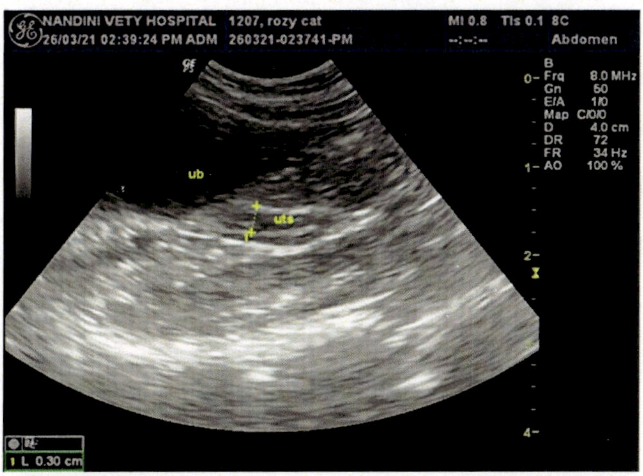

Fig. 102: Trans abdominal sonogram of a healthy eight month old Persian queen showing a small uterus between urinary bladder and intestine (colon).

- Uterine body and cervix can be visualized as continuous hypoechoic round structure.
- Anechoic urinary bladder is ventral to uterus.
- Hyperechoic crescent shaped colon is dorsal to uterus.
- Full urinary bladder serves as an acoustic window and facilitates scanning of uterus.
- Uterine cervix is slightly cranial to trigon area of bladder.
- Cervix is visualized better in sagittal view and appears as an oblique hyperechoic linear structure.
- Diameter of uterine body is smaller than the cervix. Uterine body extends up to cranial one third of bladder.
- Uterine horns are difficult to image unless enlarged during oestrus, pregnancy or due to any pathological condition.
- Uterus is composed of the mucosal, the muscular and the serosal layers. In health differentiation of endometrium and myometrium is difficult.
- Generally uterine lumen is not visible sonographically. If some fluid is present, lumen may be visible as hypoechoic to anechoic region or as a bright echogenic central area owing to the presence of intraluminal mucus.

Ovaries

- The ovaries are small structures and visualization of inactive ovaries is difficult. Appearance of the ovaries varies with the oestrus stage.
- The ovaries (Fig.103) during anoestrus look as small oval to bean shaped of homogenous echogenicity (similar to renal cortex). The ovaries are hypoechoic relative to adjacent surrounding tissues.

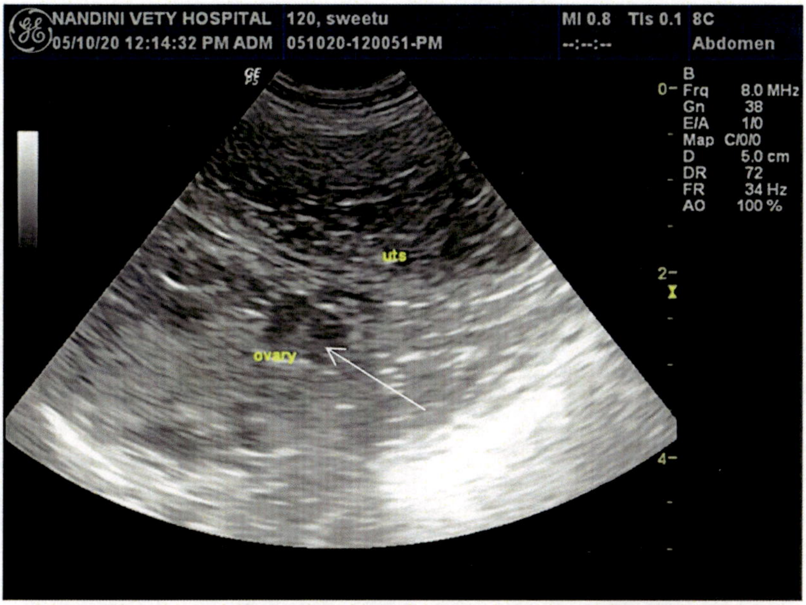

Fig. 103: Transabdominal sonogram of a bitch showing small oval shaped ovary.

- During folliculogenesis, multiple anechoic/hypoechoic cyst like structures are seen in the ovarian parenchyma.
- During luteal phase, large cystic structures are visualized.
- For ascertain ovulation serial scanning is recommended.
- Proestrus is sonographically characterized by multiple anechoic follicular cystic structures. They enlarge with the time. These structures have distinct wall and anechoic fluid with distal enhancement. The surface of the ovaries may appear irregular or lumpy.
- At the time of ovulation, anechoic fluid filled follicles become hypoechoic to hyperechoic corpora haemorrhagica. They progress over several days to hypoechoic corpora lutea.
- During diestrus, the ovaries are lobular with hypoechoic corpora lutea of variable size.
- A combination of vaginal cytology, serum progesterone estimation, LH assays, vaginoscopy, along with ultrasound is desirable for determining precise timing of ovulation.

Mammary Glands

- Healthy mammary glands of bitch have three different layers (Fig.104). The upper one is skin that is mildly echogenic and finely grained area. The middle layer is the mammary tissue (mammary parenchyma), showing a heterogenic coarse-grained structure with small areas of hyper and hypoechogenity. The third layer is of muscular tissues having medium echogenicity but slightly hyperechogenic than the parenchyma (Balaci *et al.*, 2015).

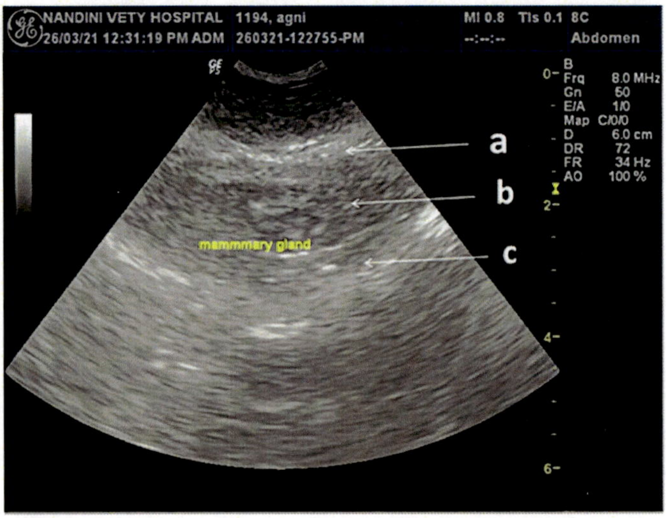

Fig. 104: Sonogram of a healthy abdominal mammary gland of an adult Labrador bitch with a micro-convex transducer of 8 MHz. White arrows indicate layers of healthy mammary gland as skin **(a)**, mammary tissue **(b)** and muscle **(c)**. The skin looks as mildly echogenic and finely grained. The mammary tissue looks as heterogeneously coarse grained structure with small areas of hyper and hypoechogenicity. The muscle layer is slightly hyperechoic than the mammary parenchyma.

Pregnancy Diagnosis

Ultrasonography has become an important tool in the diagnosis of pregnancy not only in humans but also in animals. The presence of anechoic vesicular conceptus ascertains pregnancy. Ultrasonography plays an important role in providing a definite evidence of viability of foetus as foetal heart beat can be visualized sonographically. Ascertaining the viability of foetus is otherwise very difficult. Other important uses of ultrasonography in veterinary medicine are studying foetal development, determining the sex, detecting the presence of more than one foetus and predicting the expected date of delivery.

Bitches

- Gestation period in canine is approximately 63 days (range 57 to 72 days).
- Pregnancy in bitches can be diagnosed by abdominal palpation, relaxin testing, radiography and ultrasonography. Each method has different time frame.
- Pregnancy diagnosis by abdominal palpation is possible in cooperative bitches at 28 to 30 days after ovulation. It is sometimes difficult to palpate and confirm pregnancy in large bitches and bitches with few pups in cranial abdomen.
- Radiographic diagnosis is possible at 42 to 50 days after first mating. Accurate counting of puppies is feasible at about day 55 after first breeding.
- Relaxin is a hormone produced by canine placenta. Relaxin pregnancy test can diagnose pregnancy in bitches as early as 21 to 28th day post breeding. False negative results are seen. Repeat testing is required after 7 to 10 days in such cases or other tests may also be performed.
- Nowadays ultrasound examination is being increasingly conducted to diagnose pregnancy, foetal liveability, gestation age, foetal sex, variables of foetal development, and prediction of date of whelping.
- Confirmation of pregnancy is possible as early as 17 days after LH surge in bitches and 11-14 days after mating in queens. The gestational sac (entirely yolk sac) appears as discrete, anechoic sphere within uterine lumen.
- At 30days post breeding, pregnancy can be confirmed in routine practice.
- It is not accurate in counting the number of puppies.
- Live and dead status of puppies can be ascertained by determining heart beat.

Ultrasonographic Feature of Pregnancy

- Gestational development of foetal structures is diagrammatically represented in the Fig.105 A and sonograms of different stages of pregnancy are shown in Fig.105 B.

Gestational Development of Foetal Structures

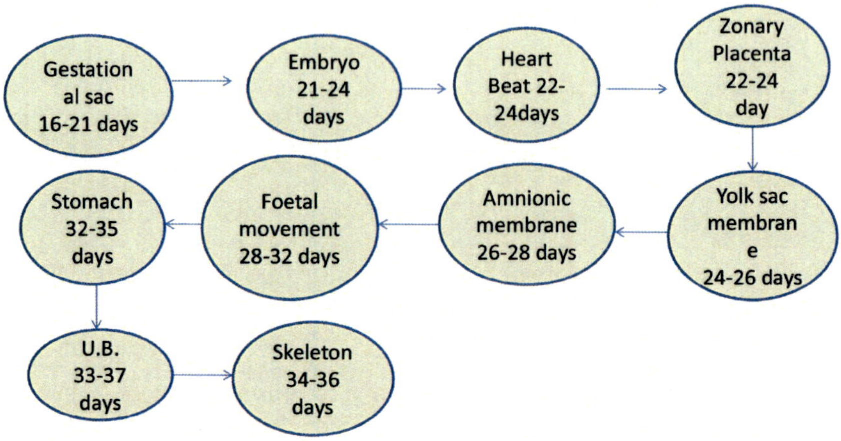

Fig. 105 A: Diagrammatic representation of gestational development of foetal structures in dogs as detectable by ultrasonography.

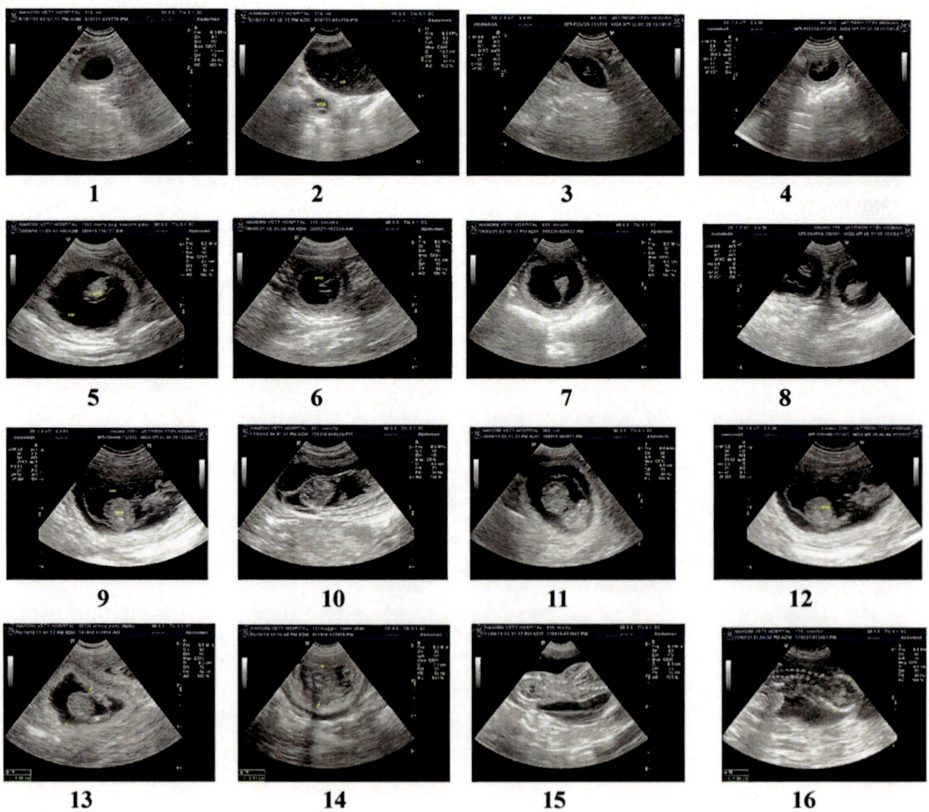

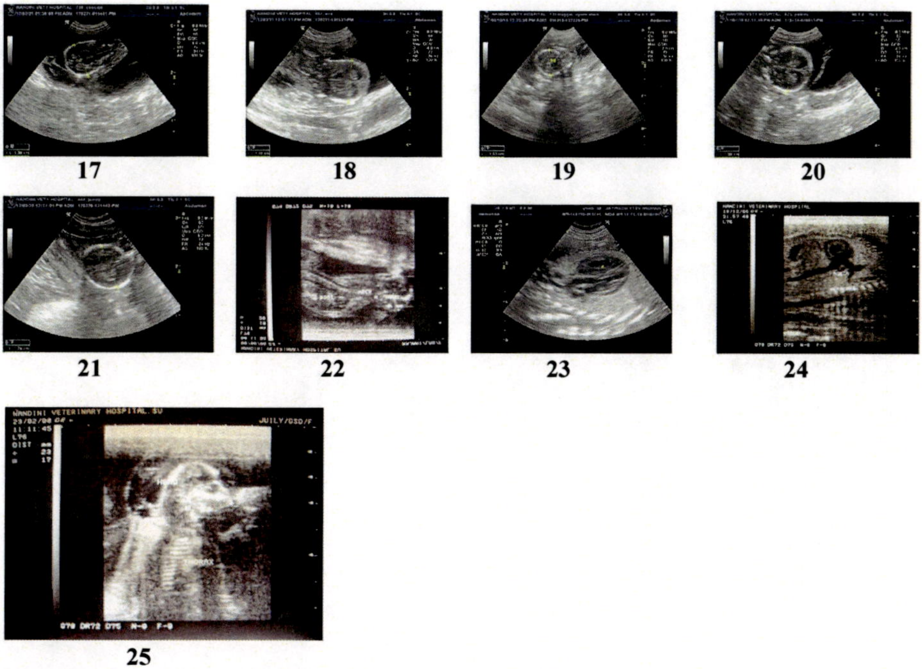

Fig. 105 B: Sonograms of different stages of pregnancy in bitch. The sonograms were taken at different days post mating.

1. (17th day) **2.** (18th day) **3.** (19th day) **4.** (20th day) **5.** (21st day) **6.** (22nd day) **7.** (23rd day) **8.** (26th day) **9.** (27th day) **10.** (28th day) **11.** (29th day) **12.** (30th day)**13.** (32nd day)**14.** (33rd day) **15.** (38th day) **16.** (39th day)**17.** (40th day)**18.** (41st day) **19.** (42nd day) **20.** (43rd day) **21.**(47th day) **22.** (55th day) **23.** (60th day) **24.** (61st day) and **25.** (62nd day).

- The gestational sac (entirely yolk sac) may be visualized as discrete, anechoic sphere within uterine lumen by 17 days after LH surge in bitches and by 11-14 days after mating in queen.
- Embryo is visible around day 21 of gestation as small echogenic structure close to endometrium in bitches (Fig.106).

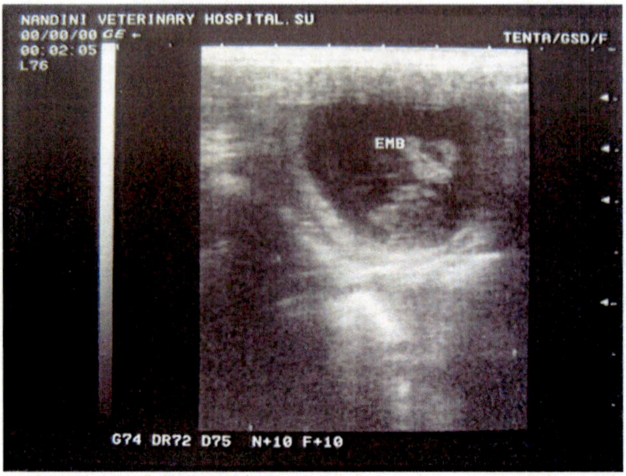

Fig. 106: Trans abdominal sonogram of a bitch showing small echogenic structure close to endometrium suggestive of an embryo

- Around 25-26 days gestational sac becomes more oval (Fig.107) and the embryo is distinctly bipolar and larger and begins to move away from endometrium.

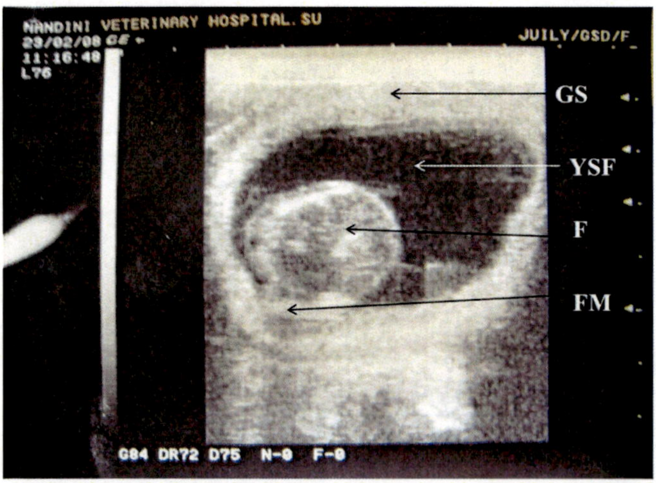

Fig. 107: Transabdominal sonogram of a bitch around 25-26 day pregnancy showing oval shaped hyperechoic gestational sac **(GS)**, containing echogenic foetus **(F)** separated from uterine wall by anechoic yolk sac fluid **(YSF)**.

- Embryo has bipolar shape by day 28th and head region can be identified as having anechoic area by day 30.
- Foetal heart (Fig.108) can be detected as early as 29th day of gestation (Helper, 1970).

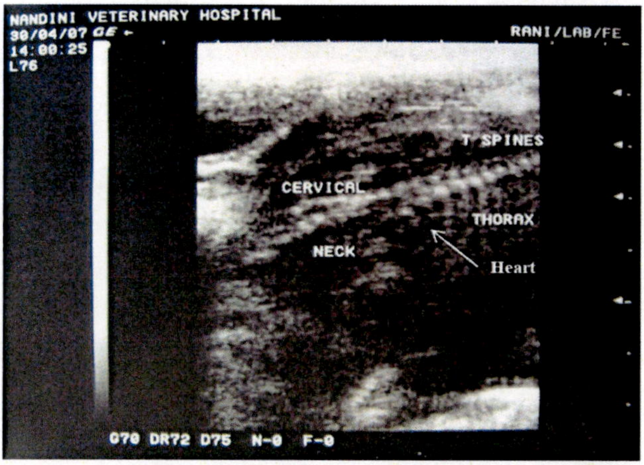

Fig. 108: Trans abdominal sonogram of a pregnant bitch showing heart of the foetus. Foetal ribs are appearing as hyperechoic with distal acoustic shadowing. The heart is visualized as anechoic structure surrounded by echogenic lung tissue.

- Limb buds are identifiable at 32 to 34 day of gestation.
- Stomach is the first abdominal organ develops around 33 days and then bladder around 34 days (Aissi, 2008).
- The crown-rump length remains less than length of placental girdle until day 36.
- Foetal skeleton (Fig.109) is seen by day 34 of gestation.

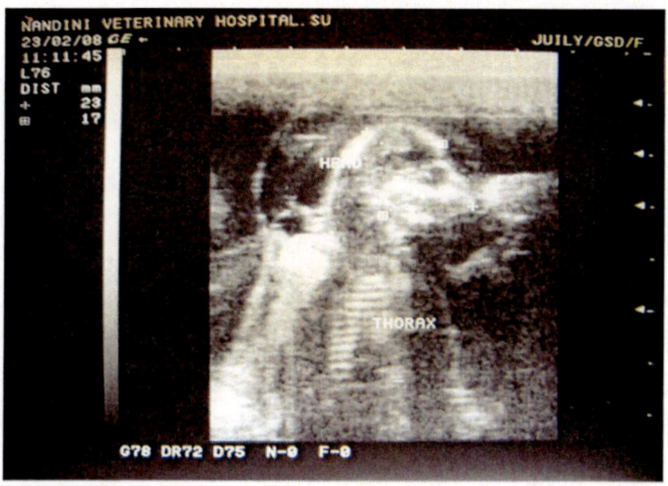

Fig. 109: Trans abdominal sonogram of a pregnant bitch showing skeleton of the foetus.

- Foetal bones look hyperechoic. Bones of head appear first.
- Generally by day 38 to 40 trunk diameter exceeds to that of head.
- Kidneys are only visible within last 20 days of gestation when imaged with 5.0 MHz transducer (Yeager *et al.,* 1992).
- Intestines are detectable between 57 to 63 days of pregnancy.

Determining Gestation age

- Gestation age can be determined by appearances of certain organs (stomach around day 33, bladder around day34 and kidneys within last 20 days).
- It can also be calculated as follows with the accuracy of ± 2 days (Son *et al.,* 2001; Kutzler *et al*., 2003; Luvoni and Beccaglia, 2006)

(a) For pregnancy <40 days

Gestation Age (GA) = (6 x GSD or ICC) + 20

Where GSD= Gestational sac diameter

ICC= Inner chorionic cavity diameter

(b) For pregnancy >40 days

Gestation Age = (15 x BPD or HD) +20

Where BPD = Biparietal diameter

HD = Head diameter

Predicting Whelping

- Whelping can be predicted by measuring at least three parameters (diameter of gestational sac or chorionic cavity, crown-rump length, abdominal diameter at the level of stomach and liver, biparietal diameter after mid gestation) for two or more foetuses.

Determining Foetal Sex

- It is based on appearance of external genitalia in foetus in uterus in a specific position.
- Foetal sex identification is possible between 55 to 58 days of gestation (Gil *et al*., 2015)

Sonographic Features of Pregnancy Ailments

(a) Foetal Abortion

- Echogenicity of amniotic and allantoic fluid is increased with an increase in echogenic particle.
- Absence of heart beat and thickening of uterine wall are other features of foetal abortion (Concannon *et al.*, 2003).

(b) Resorption of Embryo- If foetus dies before 35 days of pregnancy, complete resorption of foetus takes place. The following changes have been reported in cases of resorption of embryo (Concannon *et al.*, 2003).

- Reduced volume of conceptus
- Increased echogenicity of embryonic fluid (free floating particles are also seen in allantoic fluid).
- No embryonic heart beat.
- Disintegration of embryonic mass.
- Inward bulging of uterine wall due to collapse of conceptus.

(c) Foetal Abnormalities

- Foetal abnormalities viz. hydrocephalus, foetal anasarca, herniation of the ventral abdominal wall and foetal monsters can be diagnosed by identifying changes in the anatomical appearance of the foetus (Poffenbarger and Feeney, 1986).

(d) Foetal Distress

- Foetal distress or hypoxia is suggested by foetal heart rate less than twice the maternal heart rate (Zone and Wanke, 2001).
- Absence of heart beat, absence of foetal movement, reduced volume with increased echogenicity of foetal fluid, and accumulation of gas within foetal stomach/other cavities, or in the uterus are suggestive of foetal death (Matton and Nyland, 1995).

Queens

- Gestational period in cats varies from 58 to 67 days.
- Ultrasonography is commonly used in queens for the diagnosis of pregnancy, its monitoring, and evaluation of foetal viability and to estimate the date of parturition.

- Trans abdominal ultrasonography is the preferred approach for pregnancy diagnosis in felines.
- Transducers of 7.5, 10, or 12.5 MHz. may be used for pregnancy diagnosis in queens.
- Early features of feline pregnancy are an enlarged uterus, gestational sacs and foetal poles recognizable at 4th, 11th and 15th day respectively.
- Pregnancy of 3 weeks or more can be reliably diagnosed using ultrasonography. By this time foetal vesicles are easily detected.
- Foetal heart beat can be detected at day 23 to 25th of gestation.
- Foetal morphology is recognizable at day 26.
- Foetal membranes are seen at as early as 21 days of gestation.
- Generalized foetal movements are seen as early as day 28.
- Foetal movements are detected at 34 to 36 days of gestation.
- Gender of foetus can be determined between 38 to 43 days of gestation.
- Stage of pregnancy can be evaluated by measuring the length of embryonic vesicle, or crown-rump length of the embryo from day 11 to 17 respectively.
- Limbs, neural tube and stomach are visible from day 19, 20 and 26 respectively. These parameters can be used to date gestation.

Ultrasonographic Features of Foetal Development in Queens

- Sonograms of different stages of pregnancy in queens are shown in Fig.110.

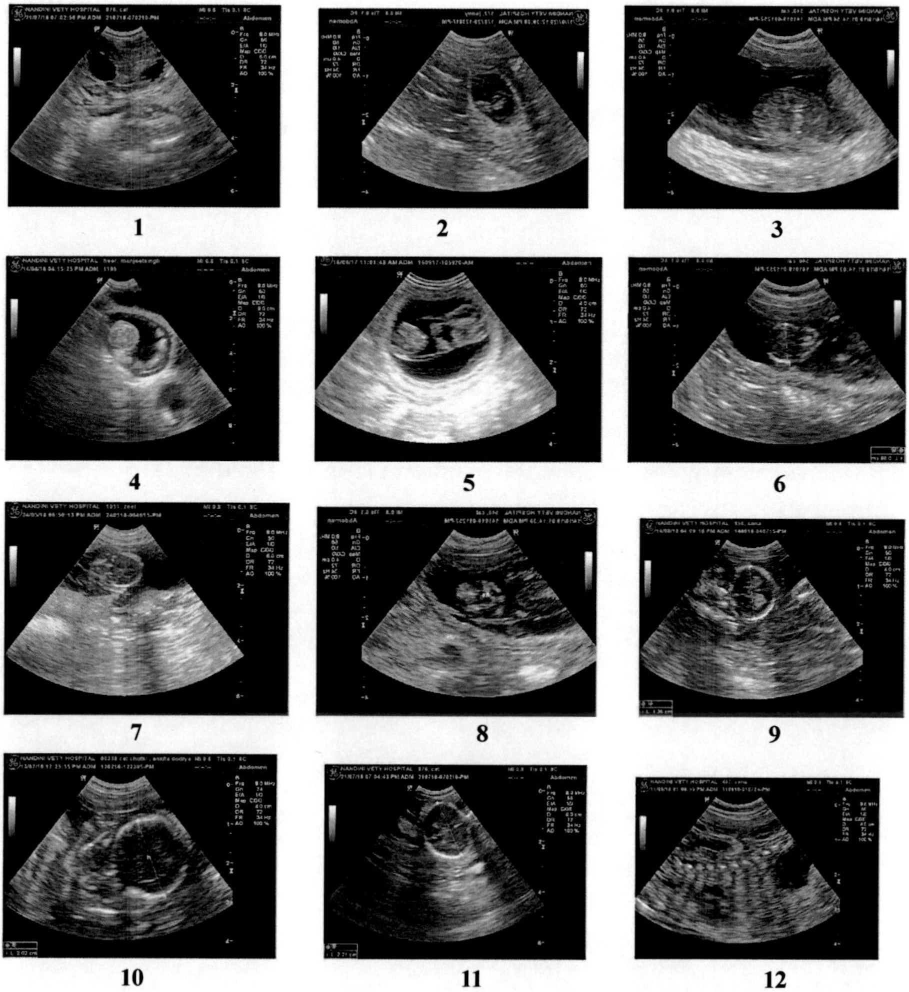

Fig. 110: Sonogram of different stages of pregnancy in queens. The sonograms were taken at different days post mating. **1.**(18th day) **2.** (22nd day) **3.** (25th day) **4.** (27th day) 5. (30th day) **6.** (34th day) **7.** (37th day) **8.** (39th day) **9.** (40th day) **10.** (50th day) **11.** (53rd day) and **12.**(58th day)

Ultrasonographic Features in Diseases

(A) **Uterus**

- Ultrasonographic evaluation of the uterus can provide information regarding thickness of uterine wall, presence/absence of cystic structures, luminal size and its contents, and position of uterus and its symmetry.
- Emphysematous pyometra is sonographically characterized by homogenously hypoechoic wall and echogenic fluid with gas in the

lumen. Intraluminal gas changes its position with several positional changes of the bitch (Mattei et al., 2018).

- Uterus masculinus (persistent Mullerian duct) is a vestigial embryological remnant of the paramesonephric duct system in male dogs. Sonographically, it may appear as single or two horn-like, tubular or cylindrical structures, originating from the craniodorsal aspect of the prostate gland extending cranially. Concomitant prostatomegaly and urinary infection may also be seen (Lim *et al.*, 2015).
- Cystic endometrial hyperplasia/pyometra are characterized by endometrial thickening and focal anechoic structures in uterine wall (dilated cystic glands and tortuous glandular ducts).
- Anechoic fluid accumulation in uterine lumen is suggestive of hydrometra, mucometra, or pyometra (Fig. 111 and 112).

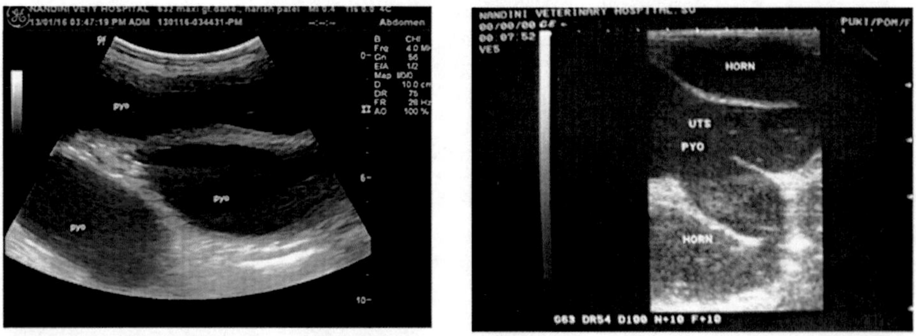

Fig. 111: Trans abdominal sonogram of bitches showing anechoic fluid accumulation in uterine horns suggesting hydro/muco/pyometra.

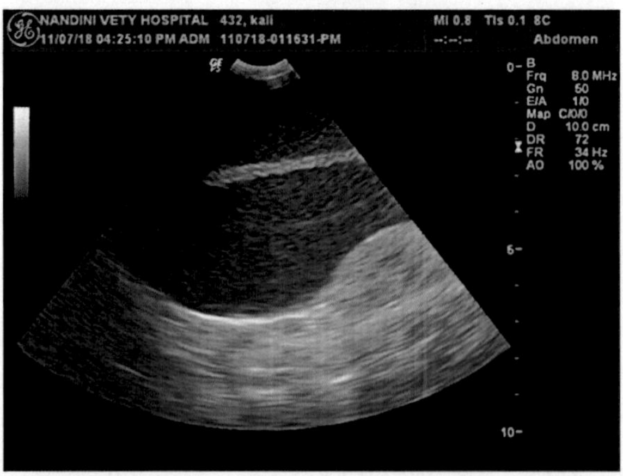

Fig. 112: Trans abdominal sonogram of a queen cat showing anechoic fluid accumulation in uterine horns suggesting hydro/muco/pyometra.

- Resorption of foetus (Fig.113 A) and retention of placental tissue (Fig. 113 B) can be visualized as intraluminal focal hyperechoic image (s).

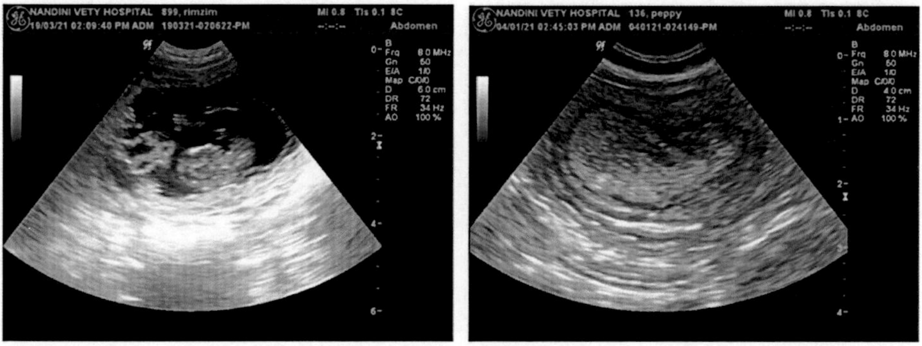

(A) (B)

Fig. 113: Abdominal sonogram of bitches showing foetal resorption **(A)** and retained sac **(B)**. Foetal resorption and retained sac appears as intraluminal focal hyperechoic images.

- Thin uterine wall and anechoic luminal contents are indicative of hydrometra or mucometra. While pyometra has wall thickening (Fig.114 and 115).

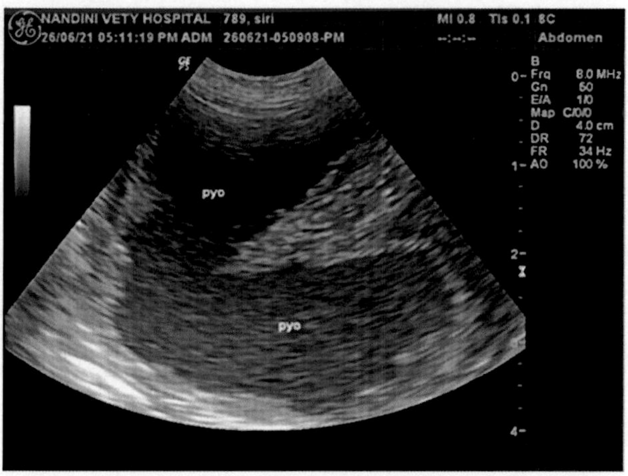

Fig. 114: Abdominal sonogram of a bitch showing anechoic luminal contents with thickened uterine wall suggesting pyometra.

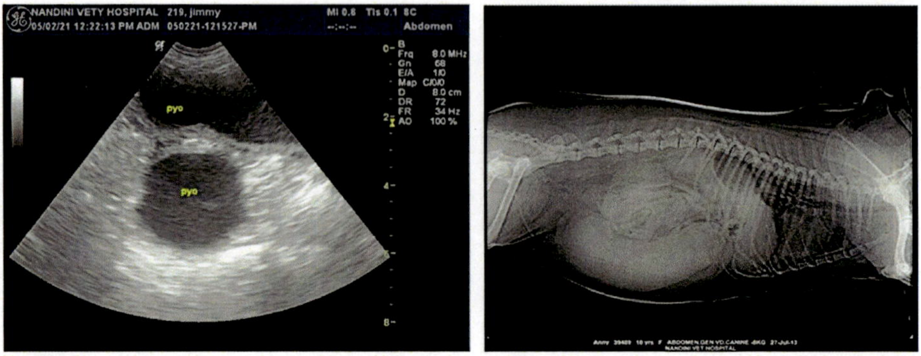

(A) (B)

Fig. 115: Abdominal sonogram of a bitch showing thickened uterine wall with anechoic fluid in the lumen **(A)** suggesting pyometra. Abdominal x-ray of the bitch also confirmed uterine distension with fluid **(B)**.

- In cases of stump pyometra the uterine remnants can be visualized just cranial to pubis between urinary bladder and colon.
- Uterine tumours have different echogenicity from that of surrounding tissues and may project in the lumen (Fig.116).

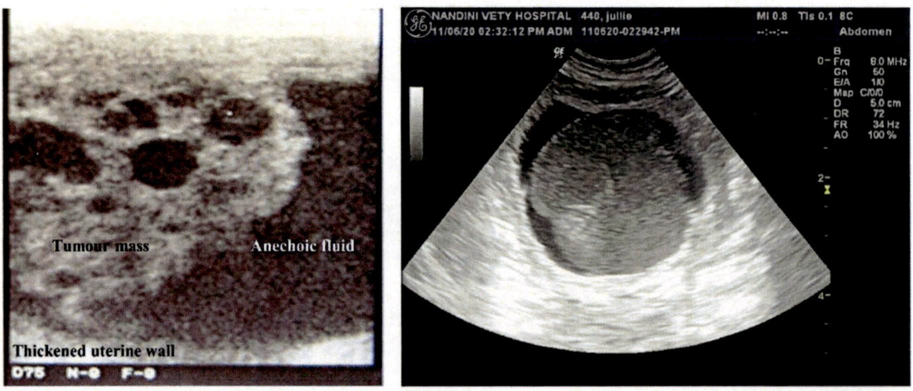

(A) (B)

Fig. 116: (A) abdominal sonogram of a bitch showing hyperechoic mass projecting into uterine lumen, thickened hyperechoic uterine wall and anechoic fluid in the uterine lumen suggesting tumour with pyometra. Sonogram **(B)** of another bitch is also showing hyperechoic large mass with peripheral anechoic fluid in the uterus and thickened uterine wall suggesting a tumour in the uterus

- Though ultrasound may be used to diagnose retained placenta (Fig.117), it is very much subjective whether placenta is retained and therefore not very reliable.

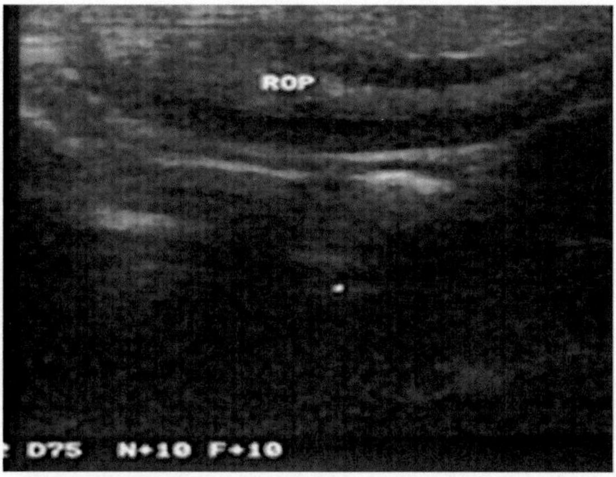

Fig. 117: Sonogram of a recently whelped bitch showing uterine lumen with hyperechoic contents suggesting retained placenta.

(B). Ovaries

- Cystic ovaries are cystic lesions within ovaries having anechoic fluid surrounded by thin wall and distal acoustic enhancement (Fig.118). They may be single, unilateral, bilateral or multiple in numbers and of varying size (very small to quite large).

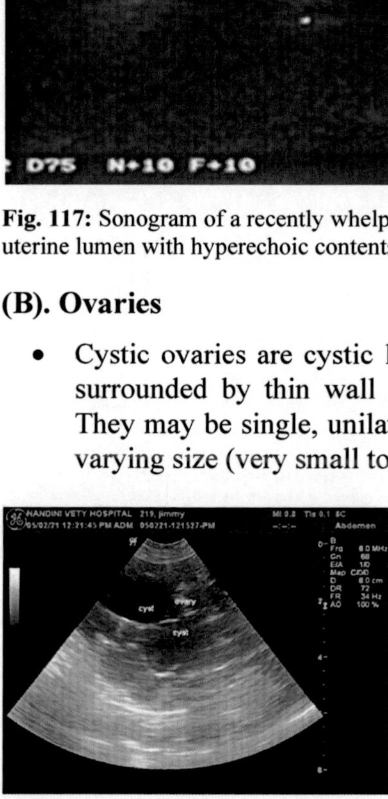

(A)

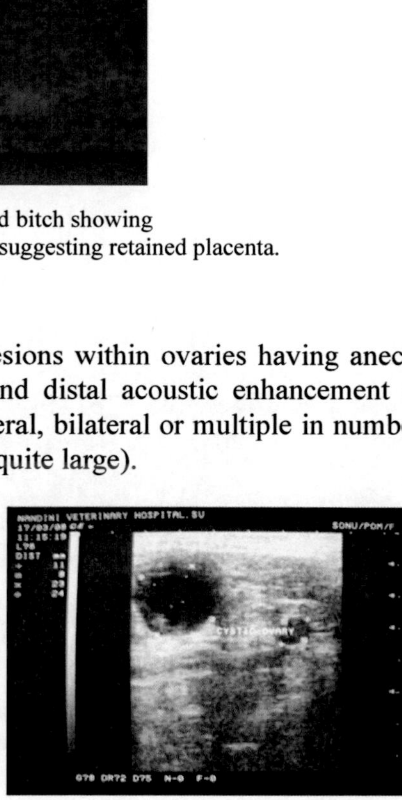

(B)

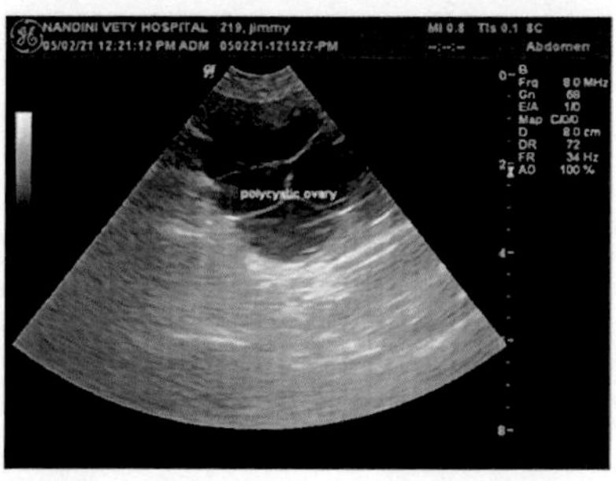

(C)

Fig. 118: Abdominl sonogram **(A, B, C)** of bitches showing cystic ovaries. Cystic lesions within ovaries are sonographically characterized as anechoic fluid surrounded by thin wall and distal acoustic enhancement

- Thick wall of solitary luteinizing cysts may differentiate them from follicular cysts.
- Ovarian tumours are the mass of variable size with complex internal architecture in one or both ovaries. Malignant tumours may have multicystic structure with irregular margins and ascites.

Vaginal Passage

- Growth in the vaginal passage appears as hyperechoic mass (Fig.119).

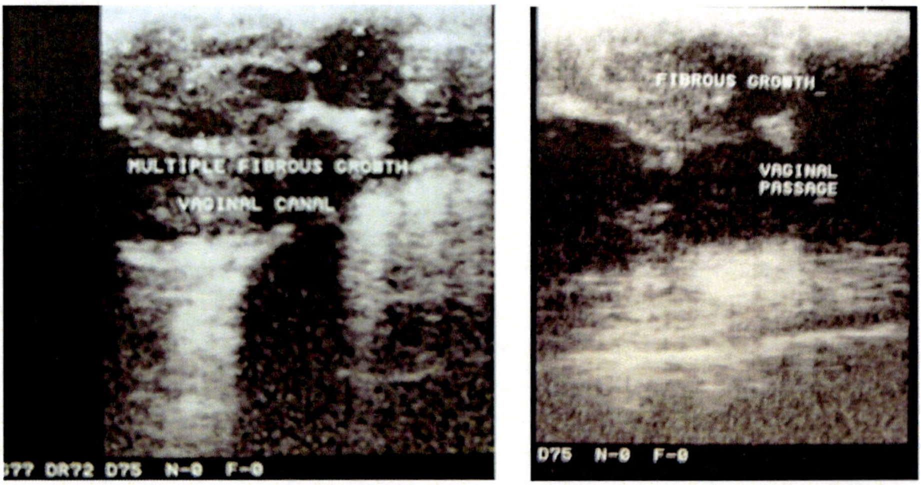

Fig. 119: Sonograms of a bitch showing hyperechoic mass in the vaginal passage

Mammary Glands

- Inflamed mammary parenchyma may appears either as hypoechogenic or hyperechogenic as compared to that of healthy tissues. Layering architecture may be lost. In some cases multiple hyperechogenic septa, alternating with hypo-echogenic areas and acoustic artefacts may be seen. (Balaci *et al.*, 2015).

Male Dogs and Cats

Prostate Gland

The prostate is a bilobed glandular structure located caudal to the neck of urinary bladder in male dogs. Diseases of the prostate are common in intact male dogs. Prostatic hyperplasia and cysts are most common while prostatic neoplasia and abscess are rare. Prostatic carcinoma is rare in tom cats.

Imaging Techniques

- The dog is placed in lateral or dorsal recumbency.
- Canine prostate is visualized caudal to trigon area and are located surrounding the proximal urethra.
- Feline prostate is not a discrete macroscopic structure. Hence not visualized sonographically.
- Canine prostates are visualized by placing sector transducer cranial to pubis and directing the beam caudally. Urinary bladder is a land mark for identifying prostate glands.
- After having basic dimension, the prostatic size is calculated as follows (Kamolpatana et al.,1999) :

  Prostatic volume (cm^3) = {(L+W+D)/2.6}+1.8

  L= Length (cranio-caudal diameter)\

  W=Width (transversal latero-lateral diameter)

  D= Depth (dorso-ventral diameter)

Ultrasonographic Features of the Prostate in Health and Diseases

- The prostate has homogeneous echo dense pattern.
- The normal prostate is a symmetrical structure of uniform echotexture (Fig.120). It is relatively echogenic structure and is hyperechoic to the spleen, liver and kidneys. In castrated males, it is small and hypoechoic.

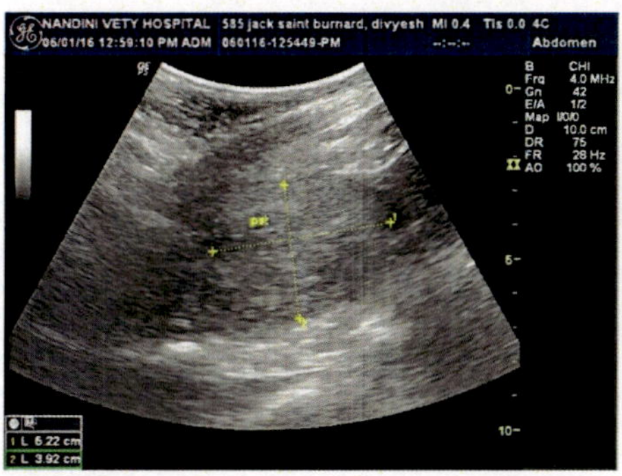

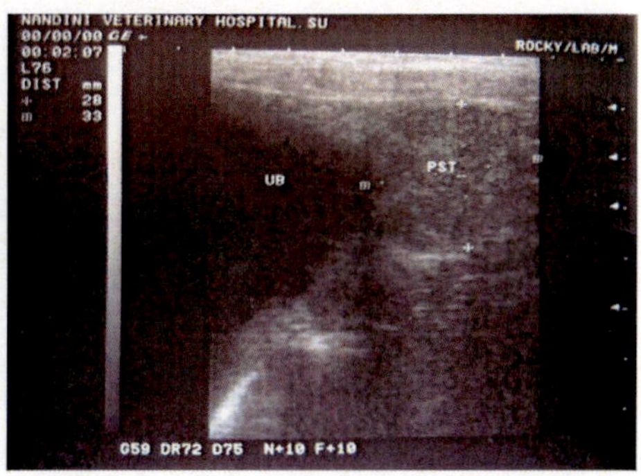

(A) **(B)**

Fig. 120: Abdominal sonogram of adult male healthy Saint Bernard **(A)** and Labrador **(B)** showing echotexture of normal prostate. The normal prostate is a symmetrical structure of uniform echotexture (slightly hypoechoic).

- Its homogenous echo pattern is lost (Fig.121) when there is inflammation, hyperplasia or neoplasia of prostate. Focal to multifocal areas of hyperechoic and /or hypoechoic tissue become apparent.

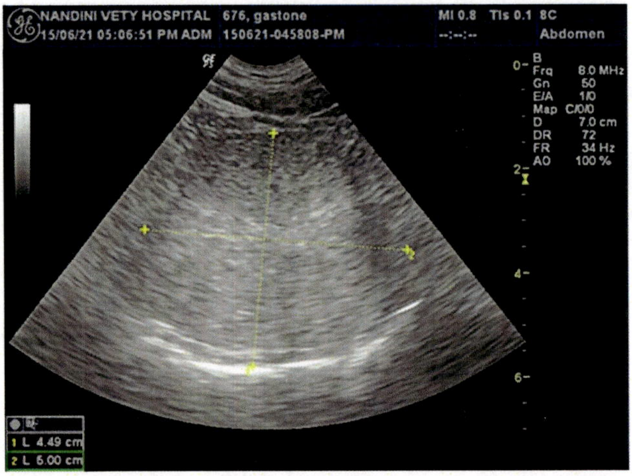

Fig. 121: Sonogram of prostate gland of a 12 year old male Labrador with haematuria and constipated bowel showing prostatomegaly (30 x 30.6 mm) with smooth contours and multiple hyperechoic areas suggesting prostatic hyperplasia. Prostate specific antigen level was very low (0.01 ng/ml).

- Unlike the human prostate, the canine prostate affected by BPH is furthermore characterized by cystic degeneration.
- These prostatic cysts are classified as retention cysts (intra parenchymal and typically linked to BPH) or paraprostatic cysts (outside the gland and unrelated to BPH).
- Prostatic cysts (Fig.122) or prostatic abscessization (Fig.123) is sonographically characterized by anechoic or hypoechoic areas (Levy and Mimouni, 2013).

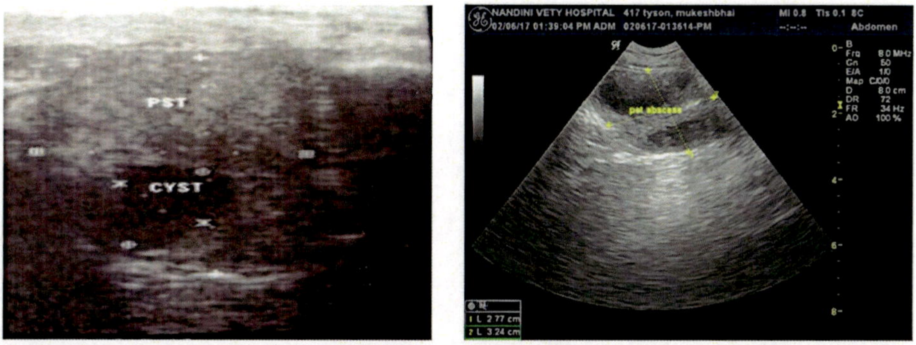

Fig.122: Abdominal sonograms of dogs showing a hypoechoic area in prostate gland suggesting prostatic cyst or abscess

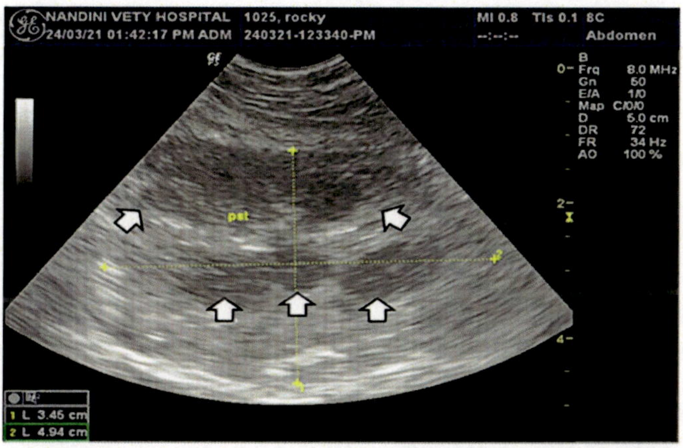

Fig. 123: Abdominal sonogram (sagittal) of a male dog showing multiple large thick-walled anechoic structures (arrow) with moderate posterior acoustic enhancement deep to cavitation lesion suggesting prostatic abscesses.

- In chronic prostatitis or prostatic tumours, hyperechoic area (Fig.124) underlined by shadow cone (calcification) may be visualized.

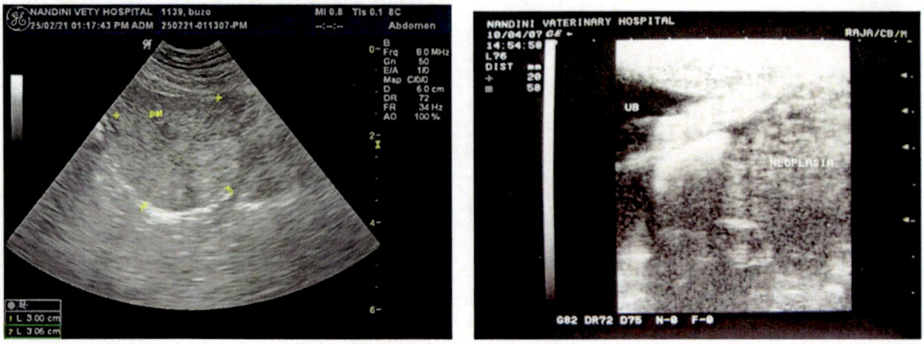

Fig. 124: Abdominal sonogram of dogs showing a hyperechoic area underlined by shadow cone in prostate gland suggesting either chronic prostatitis or prostatic tumour.

- Prostatic biopsy/aspiration is needed for definite diagnosis of prostatic diseases. Ultrasound guided aspiration (Fig.125) is done for cytological/ cultural examination of the prostatic aspirate.

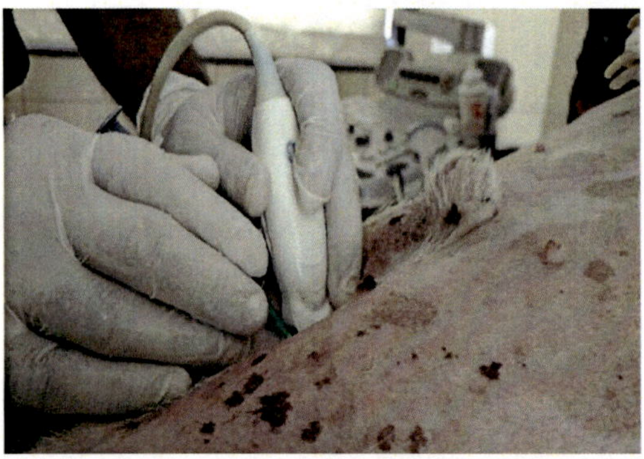

Fig. 125: Ultrasound guided aspiration of the prostate gland

Scrotum and Testis

- Scrotum and testis are also imaged sonographically (Fig.126).
- Animals are restrained in standing position or dorsal recumbency.

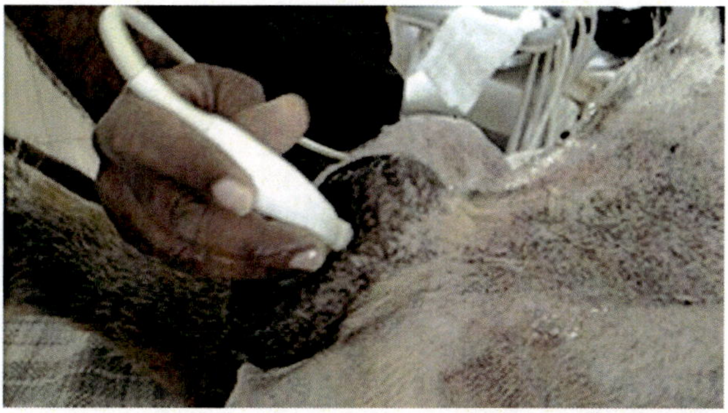

Fig. 126: Showing sonography of testicles using a transducer of 6 MHz

- Normal testicular parenchyma is homogenous with coarse medium echo pattern (Fig.127). Mediastinum testis appears as a bright echogenic line in the centre.

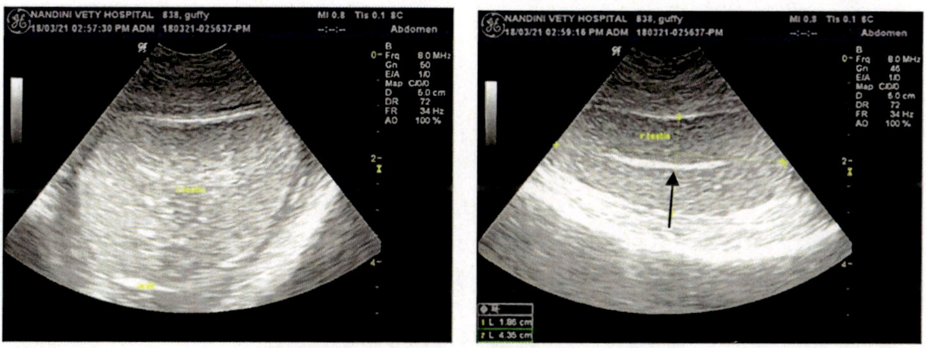

(A) **(B)**

Fig. 127: Scrotal sonograms (Longitudinal axis) of an adult healthy dog **(A)** left testicle, **B-** right testicle) showing homogenous compact hyperechoic echotexture of the testis. The bright echogenic line in the centre of the sonogram of right testis **(B)** represents mediastinum testis.

- The epididymis are less echogenic (Fig.128) than testicular parenchyma.

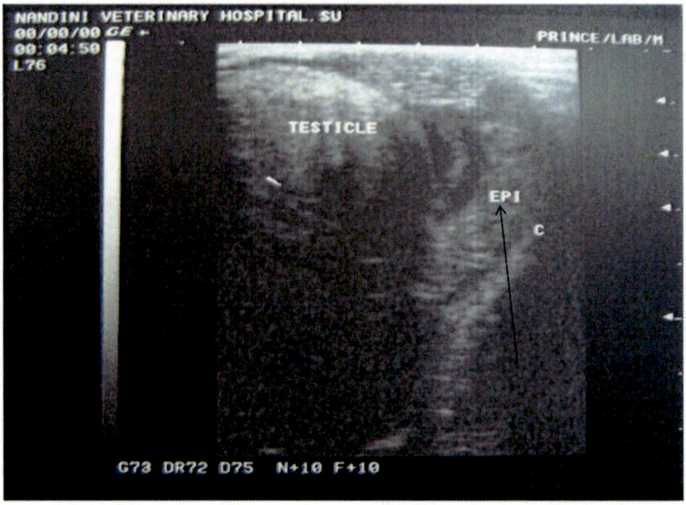

Fig. 128. Scrotal sonogram of an adult male dog showing testicle, epididymis and cord. The epididymis (black arrow) is less echogenic than the testicular parenchyma.

- The scrotal septum appears as highly echogenic line between two testicles.
- The scrotal skin appears as a thick hyperechoic image encircling testicles.
- The inflamed testicles lose their coarse medium echo pattern and appear as mildly hypoechoic (Fig.129).

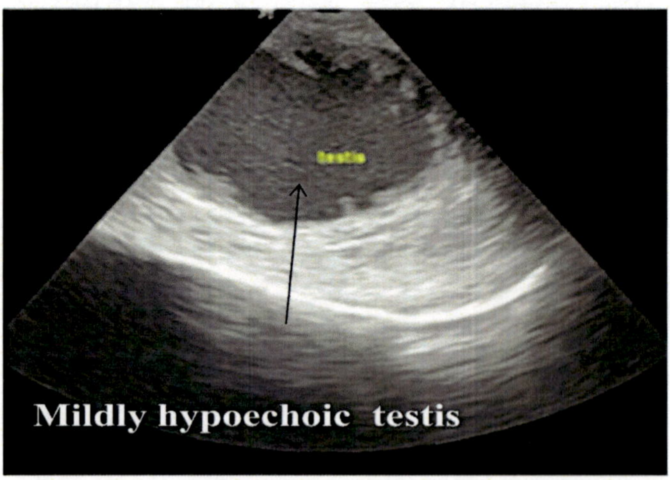

Fig. 129: Testicular sonogram of a male German Shepherd with testicular trauma showing hypoechoic testicle suggesting inflammation of the testicle.

- Ultrasonography of the abdomen, inguinal region and pre scrotal area is helpful in identifying scrotal tissue in cases of retained testis (Fig.130). The sensitivity of sonography in localizing undescended testes has been reported to be up to 97% (Dogra *et el.* 2003)

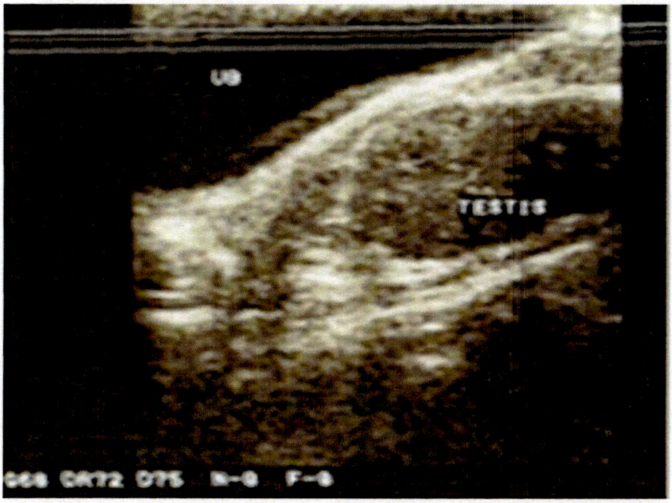

Fig. 130: Sonography of the inguinal region of a male dog showing the presence of a structure having homogenously coarse echo texture similar to the testis in the inguinal area suggesting retained testicle.

- Seminomas, interstitial cell tumour and sertoli cell tumours are the most common testicular tumours. Exact diagnosis of testicular tumours is based on histopathological examination of the fine needle aspirate or post-surgical tissue. Nevertheless scrotal ultrasound plays a significant role in differentiation of normal or abnormal testis and getting ultrasound guided fine needle aspirate for histopathology.
- Testicular cysts appear as anechoic with no internal vascularity but with posterior acoustic enhancement.
- Seminomas and interstitial cell tumours show mixed echogenic pattern, whereas sertoli cell tumour may show hypoechoic pattern (Fig.131).

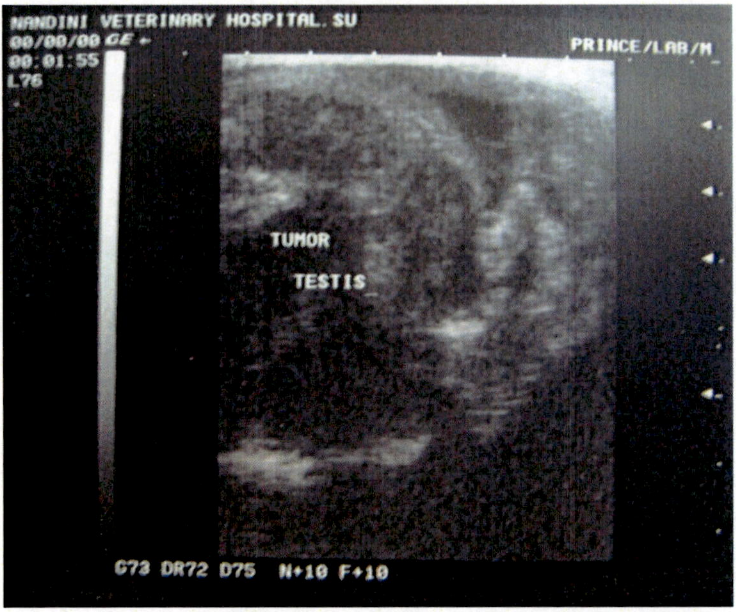

Fig.131: Testicular sonogram of a dog showing hypoechoic pattern suggestive of tumour.

- Hydroceles have typical anechoic areas (Fig.132).

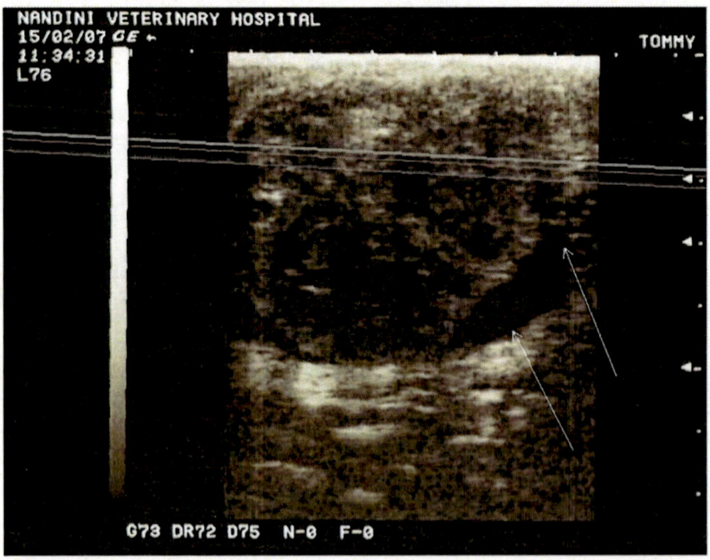

Fig. 132. Scrotal sonogram of a dog showing an anechoic fluid accumulation (arrows) suggestive of hydrocele.

- Infectious testicular lesions may have both hypoechoic and hyperechoic patterns. Diagnosis of testicular torsion can be facilitated with colour Doppler. Ultrasonography is also being used to measure testicular size.

Penis

- Veneral granulomas are common in both male and female dogs. They appear as mixed echogenic irregular masses on the penis (Fig.133) and female genitalia.

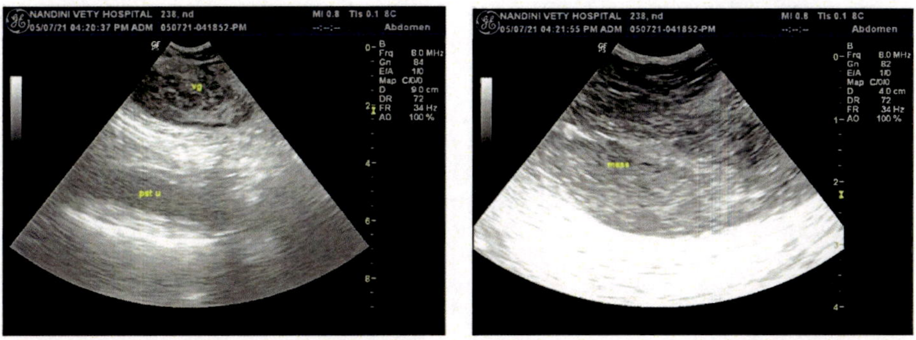

Fig. 133: Transabdominal sonogram of a male non-descript dog with swelling on penis showing mixed echogenic irregular mass on glans penis suggesting veneral granuloma.

References

Aissi, A. (2008). Aspects of ultrasonographic diagnostics of pregnancy in bitches depending on the first mating. Vet. World 1: 293-295.

Balaci, I.M., Ciupe, S., Pop, A.R., Parlapani, L., Arion, A., Vasiu, I., Purdoiu, R., Papuc, I. and Groza, I. S. (2015). Ultrasonographic findings of mastitic and normal mammary gland in bitches. Bull. UASVM Vet. Med. 72: 110-116.

Concannon, P.W., England, G., Verstegen, J. and Linde-Forsberg, C. (2003). Ultrasonographic imaging of reproductive tract of the bitch. Int.Vet.Inform.Service (www.ivis.org). Ithaca, NewYork, USA.

Dogra, V.S., Gottlieb, R.H., Oka, M. and Rubens, D.J. (2003). Sonography of the scrotum. Radiol. 227:18–36. 29.

Gil, E.M.U., Garcia, D.A, A., Giannico, A.T. and Drsci, T.R.F. (2015). Use of B- mode ultrasonography for sex determination in dogs. Theriogenology 84: 875-879.

Helper, L.C. 1970. Diagnosis of pregnancy in the bitch with an ultrasonic Doppler instrument. J.Am.Vet. Med. Assoc.156:60-62.

Kamoplatana, K., Johnston, G.R. and Johnston, S.D. (1999). Determination of canine prostatic volume using trans abdominal ultrasonography. Vet. Radiol. Ultrasound 36: 226–230.

Kutzler, M.A., Yeager, A.E., Mohammed, H.O. and Meyers, W.V.N. (2003). Accuracy of canine parturition date prediction using foetal measurements obtained by ultrasonography. Theriogenol 60: 1309-1317.

Levy, X. and Mimouni, P. (2013). Echographie de la prostate. Pratique. Vet. Comp. Anim. 109: 42–45.

Lim, C.K., Heng, H.G., Hui, T.M., Thompson, C.A. and Childress, M.O. (2015). Ultrasonographic features of uterus musculinus in six dogs. Vet. Radiol. Ultrasound. 56:77-83.

Luvoni, G.C. and Beccaglia, M. (2006). The prediction of parturition date in canine pregnancy. Reprod. Domest. Anim. 41, 27-32.

Mattei, C., Febbi, M. and Hansson, K. (2018). Radiographic and ultrasonographic findings in a dog with emphysematous pyometra. Acta.Vet.Scand. 60:67. https://doi.org/10.1186/s13028-018- 0419-z

Mattoon, J.S. and Nyland, T.G. (1995). Ultrasonography of the genital system: In: Veterinary Diagnostic Ultrasound. Nyland, T.G. and Mattoon, J.S.(Eds), W.B. Saunders, USA.pp146-148.

Poffenbarger, E. and Feeney, D. (1986). Use of gray-scale ultrasonography in the diagnosis of reproductive disease in the bitch: 18 cases (1981-1984). J. Am.Vet. Med. Assoc. 189: 90-95.

Son,C.H., Jeong,K.A., Kim.J.H., Park, I.C., Kim, S.H. and Lee, C.S. (2001). Establishment of the prediction table of parturition day with ultrasonography in small pet dogs. J. Vet. Med. Sci. 63 : 715-21

Yeager, A.E., Mohammed, H.O., Meyers-Wallen, V.,Vannerson, L. and Concannon, P.W. (1992). Ultrasonographic appearance of the uterus, placenta, foetus, and foetal membranes throughout accurately timed pregnancy. In: Gil, E.M.U., Garcia, D.A.A., Giannico, A.T. and Froes,T.R.(2015).Use of B-mode ultrasonography for foetal sex determination in dogs. Theriogenol, 84: 875–879.

Zone, M.A. and Wanke, M.M. (2001). Diagnosis of canine foetal health by ultrasonography. J. Reprod. Fertility 57: 215-219.

Further Reading

Mannion, P. (2006). Diagnostic Ultrasound in Small Animal Practice. Blackwell Science Ltd a Blackwell Publishing company, Oxford OX4 2DQ, UK

Varshney, J.P., Deshmukh, V.V. and Chaudhary, P.S. (2010). Acute prostatitis in German shepherds-A report of two cases. Intas Polivet 11:90-93.

12

Ultrasound of The Thyroid and Parathyroid

J.P. Varshney and P.S. Chaudhary

Ultrasound has been used to image thyroid and parathyroid glands. It can assist in the diagnosis of hyperthyroidism and hyperparathyroidism in dogs and cats. Recently it has also been used to differentiate cases of primary hypothyroidism or euthyroid syndrome.

Landmarks for Identifying Thyroid and Parathyroid Glands

- Thyroid gland in dogs and cats has two lobes located on either side of the trachea on the ventral side of the neck.
- Landmarks for the identification of both thyroid lobes are the medially located trachea and laterally located common carotid arteries, ventrally located sternothyroid muscles and dorsally located esophagus for the left lobe (Wisner *et al.*, 1991, Wisner and Nyland, 1998).
- There are four parathyroid gland in each thyroid.
- Parathyroids are very small and may be around 2-3 mm in diameter.
- Parathyroids can be located on the cranio-dorsal edge or caudal aspects of thyroid.

Imaging Techniques

- Dogs and cats are placed in dorsal recumbency with straight neck and the nose extended parallel to the table.
- Because of superficial location (1.5-2.0 cm below the surface of the skin) of thyroids, a 10 MHz transducer can serve the purpose.
- High frequency transducer is placed in transverse plane on larynx to visualize right thyroid gland (Fig.134).

- Transducer is taken caudally keeping trachea in the centre.
- Jugular vein, carotid artery are visible lateral to trachea.
- Thyroid glands are visualized in cross section in-between trachea and carotid artery.
- By rotating the transducer slowly 90 degrees thyroid gland can be visualized in sagittal plane.
- Left thyroid has similar land marks. It is slightly more caudal and oesophagus is lateral or dorsal to left thyroid.

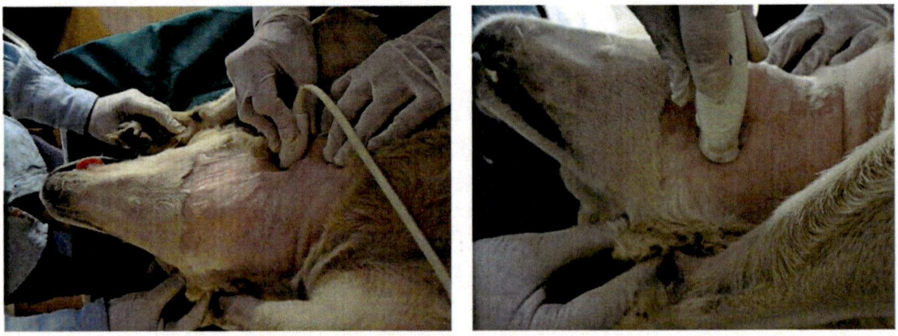

Fig. 134: Imaging of thyroid glands in dogs

Ultrasonographic features of Thyroid and Parathyroid Glands

- Ultrasonographically thyroids (Fig.135) have finely granular echotexture isoechoic to muscle. The lobes are hypoechoic relative to the surroundings. They appear as homogeneous, well delineated structure with hyperechoic capsule (Wisner et al.1991, Wisner and Nyland ,1998).

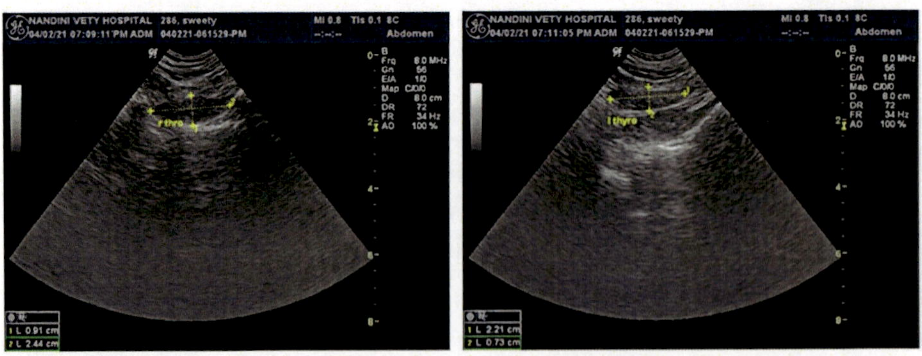

(A) Right Thyroid **(B) Left Thyroid**

Fig. 135: Sonogram of thyroid glands (long axis) of an adult dog. Thyroid have finely granular echotexture isoechoic to muscle and appear as homogeneous, well delineated structure with hyperechoic capsule. The measurement of right and left thyroid gland revealed their size as 2.44 x 0.91 cm and 2.21 x 0.73 cm respectively.

- The shape, echogenicity and size of thyroid lobes are variable.
- In sagittal plane thyroid appears as fusiform in shape.
- In transverse plane thyroid looks oval or triangular.
- The long axis of thyroid is parallel to the long axis of the neck.
- Parathyroids are hypoechoic round structure appear as embedded within thyroid tissue (Fig.136). Usually there are four parathyroid glands. Two of these are associated with each thyroid lobe. Caudal one is embedded within thyroid tissue and cranial one is outside capsule but embedded within fascia. Parathyroids are less echogenic than thyroids.

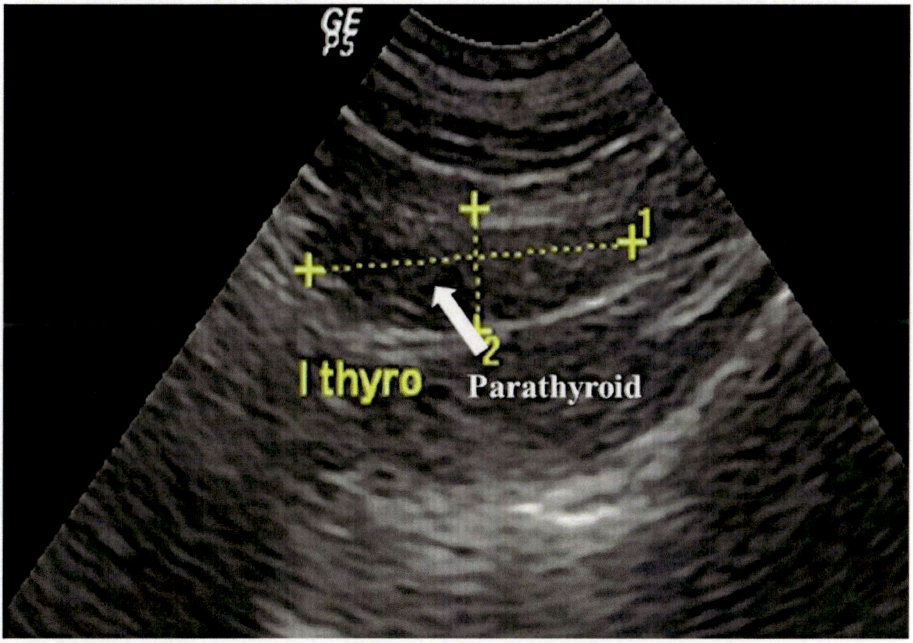

Fig. 136: Sonogram showing normal canine thyroid and parathyroid glands. Long axis view of the gland showing fusiform thyroid gland surrounded by well-defined hyperechoic capsule. The cranial parathyroid gland appears to be embedded within thyroid tissues as relatively more hypoechoic structure (white arrow).

Ultrasonographic Features of Thyroid and Parathyroid Glands in Diseases

- Thyroid hyperplasia and neoplasia are common endocrine abnormality.
- Thyroid carcinoma presents as highly vascular large mass located more caudally.

- Colour Doppler examination is more valuable in scanning thyroid with carcinoma.
- Hyperplastic thyroid lobes in cats are marginated and slightly hypoechoic to normal thyroid.
- Thyroid adenomas in cats have uniform or mottled echotexture. They may be focal or involve entire lobe.
- Thyroid glands in cases of primary hypothyroidism may have hypoechoic parenchyma compared to the overlying sternothyroid muscle, non-homogeneous parenchyma, an irregular outline of the lobe, decreased size of the lobe or a more rounded shape of the lobe on transverse images (Bromel *et al.*, 2005).
- In euthyroid dogs, thyroid glands appear sonographically normal.
- Hyperparathyroidism may be due to hyperplasia, adenoma or adenocarcinoma.
- Adenoma or adenocarcinoma are single large (>3 mm) nodule hypoechoic to thyroid.

References

Bromel, C., Pollard, R.E. and Kass, P.H. (2005). Ultrasonographic evaluation of thyroid gland in healthy, hypothyroid and euthyroid golden retrievers with non-thyroidal illness. J.Vet. Intern. Med. 19:499-506.

Wisner, E.R., Mattoon, J.S., Nyland, T.G. and Baker, T.W. (1991). Normal Ultrasonographic anatomy of the canine neck. Vet.Radiol.Ultrasound 32:185-190.

Wisner, E.R. and Nyland, T.G. (1998).Ultrasonography of the thyroid and parathyroid glands. Vet.Clin.North Am.Small Anim. Pract. 28:973-91.

13

Ophthalmic Ultrasound

J.P. Varshney

Ophthalmic or ocular ultrasound can provide important diagnostic information that is readily not available with other diagnostic techniques. Ocular ultrasound is emerging as an important diagnostic modality in veterinary ophthalmology.

Ocular Sonographic Anatomy

- Sonographic anatomy of eye consists of cornea, anterior chamber, lens, iris, cilliary body, posterior chamber (vitreous), posterior wall of the globe, retrobulbar tissues and optic nerve. The choroid, retina and posterior sclera are seen as single structure.
- Visualization of posterior chamber is difficult.
- The optic, iris, and cilliary body are not always visualized.

Indications for Ophthalmic Ultrasound

- Ophthalmic ultrasound is an important tool for diagnosing eye conditions those escape identification during routine ophthalmic examination specially when there is opacity of the eye (cornea, aqueous humour, lens, or vitreous humour).
- It is useful in the diagnosis of cataract and evaluation of post cataract surgery.
- Ophthalmic ultrasound is being used to measure anterior chamber depth (including axial distance from cornea to the anterior capsule of the lens), thickness of the lens (from anterior capsule to posterior capsule of the lens), depth of vitreous chamber (from posterior capsule of the lens to the posterior pole of the eye), and axial length of the eye (from cornea to posterior pole of the eye) (Gonzalez *et al.*, 2001).
- Ophthalmic ultrasound is commonly indicated for the diagnosis of retinal detachment, ocular tumour, ocular haemorrhages, foreign body, or lens dislocation.

Ophthalmic Ultrasound Techniques

- Dogs and cats are placed in sternal recumbency. They are restrained manually and eye lids are held open.
- Generally no sedation or anaesthesia is required. Anaesthesia or sedation should be avoided to decrease the likelihood of prolapse of nictitans.
- Anaesthetic eye drops (proxymetacaine hydrochloride or 0.5% proparacaine hydrochloride or 2% lidocaine) are instilled in the eyes.
- Sonographic examination is conducted after 5 minutes with the help of an ophthalmic ultrasound unit equipped with a high frequency transducer.
- Direct contact with cornea or an immersion technique (ultrasound gel is applied in more quantity. It acts as a standoff pad between eye and transducer) may be used to examine the eyes. After the sonographic examination, eyes should be flushed with water to decrease the potential irritation from the gel.
- A high frequency transducer (8 to 20 MHz) is ideal for ophthalmic examination (Martin *et al.*, 2010).
- Sector probes with small head surface (foot print) are preferable to large linear array probes.
- Transducer is positioned in longitudinal position.
- Scanning is done in horizontal (coronal), sagittal (vertical) or oblique sagittal planes.

Ultrasonographic Features of Normal Eye Components

- Sonogram of normal eye is shown in Fig.137.
- The cornea is sonographically visualized as hyperechoic lines in B mode sonography.
- The anterior chamber is visualized as a space between the cornea and anterior lens face, filled with anechoic fluid (aqueous humour).
- Anterior and posterior capsules of the lens are visualized as two parallel hyperechoic lines in B mode. This facilitates identification of the lens.
- The nucleus of the lens is an anechoic area.
- The vitreous chamber is deep to the lens and is filled with vitreous fluid. That is anechoic.

- The posterior pole of the eye or posterior wall of the globe (the retina, the choroid, and the sclera) is visualized as hyperechogenic convex structure in B mode.
- The retrobulbar tissues are echogenic.
- The optic disc can be visualized as slightly thickened echogenic area in posterior globe. It is slightly more echogenic than the wall.
- The optic nerve may be visualized caudal to optic disc as funnel shape structure relatively hypoechoic linear band, in relation to the adjacent retro bulbar tissue, surrounded by echogenic fat.

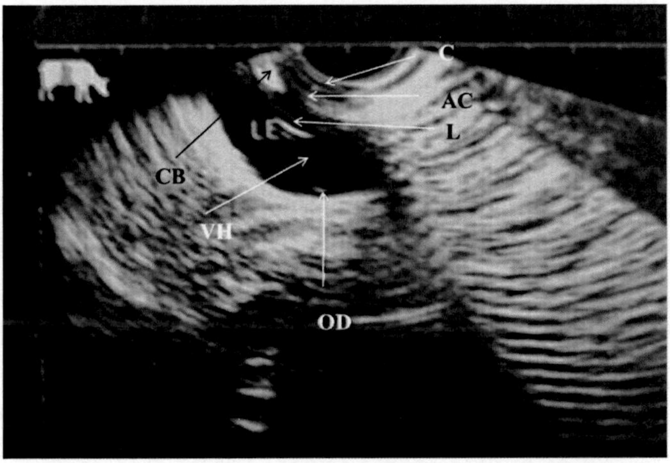

Fig. 137: Sonogram of the normal canine eye. **C**= cornea (hyperechoic line), **AC** = anterior chamber (space between cornea and lens filled with anechoic fluid), **L**== lens (two parallel hyperechoic lines), **CB**= cilliary body (hyperechoic echotexture)), **VH**= vitreous chamber (deep to the lens filled with anechoic fluid), **OD**= optic disc (echogenic area in posterior globe).

Ultrasonographic Features of Ocular Diseases

- Hyphema in anterior chamber is visualized as echogenic change in the normal anechoic anterior chamber.
- Hypopyon is also characterized by echogenic change in the normal anechoic anterior chamber.
- Cataract is usually identified on clinical examination. Sonographically it is associated with thickening of anterior and posterior surface of the lens. An Early stage of cataract (cortical) is sonographically characterized by hyperechoic lines within the lens and echogenic anterior and posterior cortices. Asymmetric nucleus with increased echogenicity is seen in

nuclear cataract. In morgagnian cataract, anterio-posterior thickness of the lens is reduced and the capsule becomes wrinkled.

- Haemorrhagic clot in vitreous chamber is visualized as amorphous echogenic heterogeneous mass. It is difficult to distinguish clot sonographically from other echogenic irregular lesions.
- Retinal detachment can be focal or along entire surface. Sonographically it is visualized as thin echogenic lines (either freely movable or attached at optic disc/or at serrate) within vitreous humour. Complete retinal detachment may show typical morning glory sign in a longitudinal plane attached to optic disc with thicker and more echogenic retinal membrane (Dar et al., 2013).
- Choroidal melanomas vary in size and shape. Small choroiodal melanoma may appear as uniform moderately echogenic. Large choroidal melanomas may appear as heterogeneously echogenic.
- Metallic foreign bodies appear as highly echogenic with reverberation artefact or posterior acoustic shadowing (Dziezyc *et al.*, 1987).

Sheep and Goat

- Hypopyon appears sonographically as a hyperechoic mass in the anterior chamber (Tookhy and Tharwat, 2013).
- Severe iridocyclitis (in acute cases of infectious keratoconjunctivitis) shows increased hyperechoic thickening of the cilliary body (Tookhy and Tharwat, 2013).

References

Dar, M., Tiwari, D.K., Patil, D.B. and Parikh, P.V. (2014). B- scan ultrasonography of ocular abnormalities: a review of 182 dogs. Iranian J.Vet.Resch.15:122-126.

Dziezyc, J., Hager, D.A. and Millichamp, N.J.(1987). Two dimensional real time ocular sonography in the diagnosis of ocular lesions in dog. J. Am .Anim. Hosp. Asso. 23: 501.

Gonzalez, E.M., Rodríguez, A. and Garcia, I. (2011). Review of ocular ultrasonography. Vet. Radiol. Ultrasound, 42:485-495.

Martins, B. C., Rodrigues Jr, E. F., Souza, A. L. G., Almeida, D. E., Brito, F. L., Canola, J.C., Brooks, D.E. and Laus, J.L. (2010). A and B mode ultrasonography in preoperative evaluation of lens and posterior segment of dogs eyes with cataract. Pesquisa Veterinária Brasileira 30:121-126.

Tookhy, O.E. and Tharwat, M. (2013). Clinical and ultraonographic findings of some ocular conditions in sheep and goats. Open Vet. J. 3:11-16.

14

Ultrasound of The Brain and Nervous System

J.P. Varshney

Sonography of the nervous system in dogs dates back to 1972 when it was employed in experimental studies. Thick bony cage of the brain limits the sonographic evaluation of the brain. It has an important place in human paediatric medicine. Sonography of the brain and the nervous system is not very common in veterinary medicine.

Indications for Sonography of Brain and Nervous System

- Paediatric sonography of the brain in premature children is an important speciality in human medicine to ascertain intraventricular or intraparenchymal haemorrhages and periventricular leucomalacia.
- Peri-intraventricular haemorrhage has been reported to occur naturally in puppies also.
- It can be used to measure the size of the lateral ventricles in cases of hydrocephalus.
- It can play an important role in evaluating the extent of tumour in the brain.
- Another important indication of sonography is to take ultrasound guided biopsy of brain lesions.
- Vascularity of the brain lesions can be determined with Doppler ultrasound.
- Transcranial ultrasonography is indicated in the diagnosis of hydrocephaly, lissencephaly, cysts, Chiari-like lesions, Dandy Walker syndrome, encephalitis, trauma and tumours.
- Ultrasonography can also be used in cases of stroke.

- Peripheral nerves can also be scanned for determining the extent of nerve injury in trauma cases, and their healing process. Neurological sonography is also used to examine neuroma formation, and detecting the involvement of nerves in tumour, granuloma or other lesions.
- Ultrasonography is being used to evaluate spinal cord in cases of trauma and diagnosing intramedullary and extra medullary lesions.

Techniques

- Convex transducer of 3.0 to 6.0 MHz and linear transducer of 7.0 to 10.0 MHz have been used for scanning the brain.
- Linear transducers of 5-10 MHz are suitable for neonates and /or opened rostral fontanelle.
- High resolution micro-convex transducer of 2 to 6 MHz is suitable for adults of small breeds with closed fontanelle.
- Open fontanelle, closed rostral fontanelle, temporal (above zygomatic arch) and sub occipital arch are the windows for scanning the brain.
- Bregmatic fontanelle can serve as sonographic window in pups of 3-4 week age
- Head area is clipped; shaved and acoustic gel is applied.
- Sedation is not always necessary.
- Dogs are positioned in sternal decubit or sitting position on the table.
- Low frequency probe has shown success in evaluating dilated lateral ventricles
- High frequency probes are preferred for most application.
- Vertebrobasilar system is imaged from the foramen magnum.
- Brain scanning is done using B- mode, colour Doppler and Pulse Doppler.
- Brain is examined in sagittal, transverse and dorsal planes.
- A high frequency probe (7.5 to 10 MHz) is suitable for scanning peripheral nerves. Compression should be avoided during scanning of nerve.
- Ultrasonographic examination of the spinal cord requires a dorsal or dorsolateral laminectomy. A ventral slot technique or dorsal or

hemilamenectomy are performed for the spinal cord sonography. A 7.5 to 10 MHz transducer is suitable for spinal sonography.

Ultrasonographic Features

- Variable cerebral echogenicity is considered normal when it is iso-echogenic or hyper-echogenic to thalamus (Fukushima *et al.*, 2000).
- Cerebrospinal fluid in ventricular system is anechoic.
- The choroid plexus is hypoechoic.
- The lateral ventricles in day old puppies look like slit.
- Peripheral nerve is usually identified by its hyperechoic surface and its location. In sagittal plane sciatic, tibial and peroneal nerves have hyperechoic near and deep surfaces. Internal area has multiple linear echo densities. The nerve fascicles of peripheral nerves on sonography in short axis appear as hypoechoic surrounded by hyperechoic connective tissues resembling to a honeycomb appearance.
- Spinal cord dura mater is hyperechoic while parenchyma is hypoechoic or may have variable echogenicity. Subarachnoid space appears as anechoic. In the centre of spinal cord an echogenic line is seen as in humans. Fat and connective tissues in ventral epidural space look as lobular echoes. Surrounding bone has a bright hyperechoic surface with distal acoustic shadowing.

Ultrasonographic Features in Diseases

- Hydrocephalus is characterized by enlargement of ventricular system and atrophy or hypoplasia of surrounding nervous tissues.
- Brain tumours in man are hyperechoic.
- The oedema surrounding tumour is also hyperechoic.
- Traumatic spinal cord appears as hyperechoic.
- The hall mark of peripheral nerve entrapment is hypoechoic enlargement at and proximal to the level of entrapment.
- Nerve trauma may occur due to compression, traction, laceration, or surgical transection.
- Nerve compression and traction injuries to nerve appear as abnormally hypoechoic and enlarged on sonography.

- After laceration or transection, a traumatic neuroma appears as hypoechoic enlargement of variable size.
- Haematoma causing secondary compression of the nerve appear as hypoechoic and heterogeneous.
- With complete nerve transection, retraction occurs between two severed nerve endings.
- Peripheral nerve tumours may have variable appearance. Large tumours have cystic regions.

Reference

Fukushima, U., Miyashita, K. and Okano, S. (2000). Evaluation of intracranial pressure by transcranial Doppler ultrasonography in dogs with intracranial hypertension. J. Vet. Med. Sci.62:353-355.

15

Ultrasound of Muscles, Tendons Joints and Bones

J.P. Varshney and P.S. Chaudhary

Imaging of muscles, tendons, joints and bones is not common practice in canine and feline medicine. However, scanning of tendons and ligaments is extensively done in race horses to see their fitness. Adhesions, ruptures/ tears and inflammation of tendons and ligaments can be detected by sonographic imaging of these structures. These structures are relatively superficial so a high frequency linear or curvilinear transducer (7.5 to 13.0 MHz) is used to scan these structures. For scanning of joints acoustic window is relatively small so micro convex or sector probes are more appropriate.

Muscles

Imaging Techniques

- Animal is kept in standing position and restrained.
- Area of the muscle (to be scanned) is cleaned and shaved.
- Acoustic gel is applied.
- Transverse and longitudinal scanning is done.

Ultrasonographic Features

- Sonographic examination of muscles is not common in veterinary practice .However; it is being practiced in human medicine.
- Normal muscle is very vascular so it is sonographically visualized as hypoechoic with hyperechoic lines due to fascia and fibrous tissues throughout the muscle belly.
- Irregular linear pattern is suggestive of muscle rupture.
- Early haemorrhages in the muscle appear anechoic. When thrombus is formed the lesion becomes hyperechoic.

- Lipomas are characterized by increased echogenicity.
- Sarcomas nay be hypoechoic.
- Sonography has been used to measure subcutaneous fat and muscle thickness in beef animals.
- Sonography has also been employed in studying muscle atrophy and hypertrophy.
- Subcutaneous oedema appears as cobble stone layer with anechoic fluid (Fig.138)

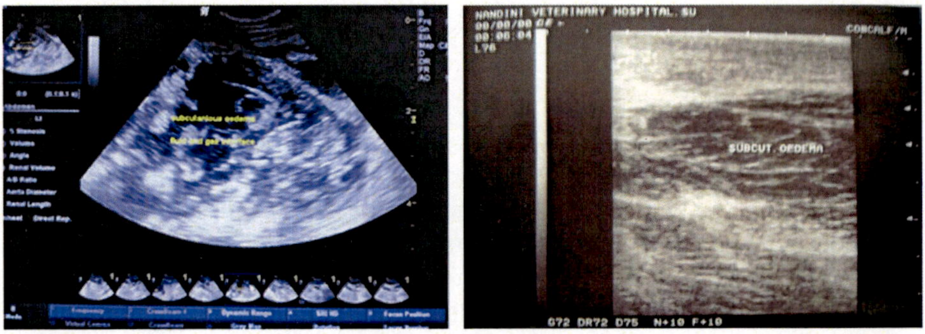

Fig. 138: Sonogram of the dogs with soft swellings showing cobble stone appearance layering with anechoic fluid collection suggesting subcutaneous oedema.

Tendons/Ligaments

- Because of large fibrous tissues, tendons are visualized as relatively hyperechoic structure with distal acoustic shadowing. When transducer is placed parallel to the long axis of the tendon, it is visualized as a rectangular structure having linear arrangement of fibres surrounded by hyperechoic peritendon. Normal tendon has a lenticular, fibrillar pattern with distinct margins.
- Ligaments are also having large amount of fibrous tissues so they also appear hyperechoic with linear pattern of fibres. Because ligaments are small structure in small animals and have close association with adjacent soft tissues, their differentiation becomes difficult except patellar ligament. It is visualized as linear hyperechoic structure with well-defined hyperechoic margins and central parallel linear echoes. Use of ultrasonography in the diagnosis of cruciate ligament rupture has been attempted in few cases. But it is not an accurate technique.

Imaging Techniques

- Animal is kept in standing position and restrained.
- A 2-3 cm strip on palmer aspect of the limb (metacarpus /metatarsus area) from accessory carpal or tarsal bone to below the fetlock is cleaned and shaved.
- On lateral side of the limb a measuring tape is fixed with 0 mark at distal aspect of accessory carpal/tarsal bone to locate the position of the lesion.
- Superficial digital flexor tendon (SDFT), deep digital flexor tendon (DDFT), inferior check ligament (ICL) and suspensory ligament can be examined.
- Transverse and longitudinal scanning is done (Fig.139).

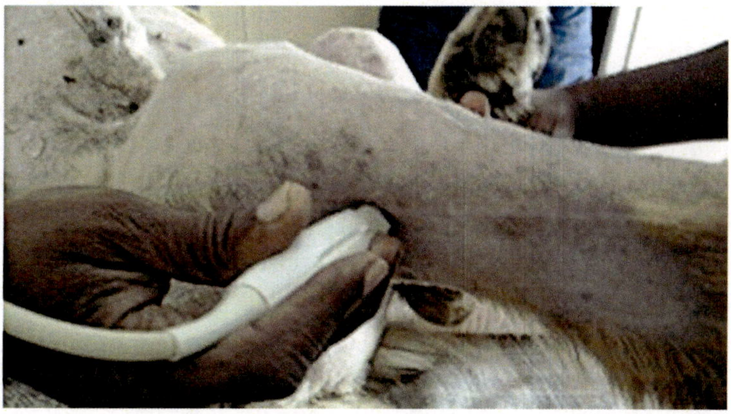

Fig. 139: Sonography of the tendon

Ultrasonographic Features

- Sonography is commonly used in equines to detect and evaluate tear in tendons and ligaments of the legs.
- Normal tendon shows lenticular, fibrillar pattern with distinct margins.
- Sagittal plane sonograms are characterized by small intense internal linear echoes. The acoustic impedance interface between two tendons is reflected by intermittent line.
- Normal linear echo pattern is lost when a tendon or ligament is diseased.
- Hypoechoic changes within the tendon indicate acute injury.
- Hyperechoic changes within the tendon indicate chronic injury.

- Superficial digital flexor tendinitis is characterized by a central hypoechoic region, known as a core lesion (normal echogenicity – grade 0, mild hypoechoic- grade 1, moderate hypoechoic-grade2, and severe hypoechoic- grade 3).
- The striated (or 'fibrillar') pattern of tendons in the longitudinal image are a good indicator of the quality of the tendon repair.
- Palmar or planter flexor tendon ligament complex consists of a hypoechoic superficial digital flexor and more echogenic deep digital flexor.
- Ultrasonographic mean grey scale (MGS) measurements have been introduced to quantify the damage and healing.

Joints and Bones

Bones are highly reflective to ultrasound beams (about 50% returns back to transducer and 50% is absorbed in bone dense material). It leads to formation of a hyperechoic line with a strong distal acoustic shadow.

- In humans, sonography has been used to examine the hip, the knee, and shoulders and to assess abnormal fluid accumulation adjacent to bones in osteomyelitis.
- Ultrasonography can provide early and additional information about bone healing. A delayed and non-union of the fractured end can be diagnosed earlier by sonography.
- Sonography is also used to examine joints and margin of the bones around the joints both in small and large animals.
- In horses, it is being used to evaluate navicular bursa, interphalangeal joints, joint spaces and navicular bones. Bursa and joint spaces are sonolucent.

Pitfalls in Musculoskeletal Ultrasonography

- Improper contralateral comparison.
- Inadequate angle of the transducer.
- Inadequate colour Doppler interrogation.
- Misinterpreting normal vessels as manifestation of the disease.
- Misinterpreting normal musculoskeletal anatomy as manifestation of the disease.

- Anisotropy- Echogenecity of muscles, tendons, ligaments and nerves is variable and also depend on the angle of insonation.
- Under use of real time dynamic imaging capabilities.
- No proper training of the operator.

Suggested Further Reading

Dickie, A. (2006). Imaging of the musculoskeletal system. In: Diagnostic Ultrasound in Small Animal Practice. Mannion, P, (ed.). Blackwell Science Limited, Oxford, U.K.

16

Cardiac Ultrasound

Neetu Saini and J.P. Varshney

Cardiac ultrasound is also known as echocardiography and it has a very important place in the diagnosis of cardiac diseases of the humans as well as animals. Echocardiography is an imaging of the heart using ultrasound. The diagnosis of congenital heart diseases, shunts, complex malformations, valvular heart diseases, different cardiomyopathies, endocarditis, pericardial effusion, cor pulmonale and cardiac tumours has been possible by cardiac ultra ultrasound that was otherwise difficult. Cardiac ultrasound is playing a very significant role in the diagnosis of occult heart diseases that otherwise remains undiagnosed by routine thorough clinical examination, electrocardiography and even laboratory tests. M-mode imaging and colour Doppler imaging have further improved our diagnostic skill in an early diagnosis of cardiac diseases. A thorough cardiac examination cannot depend solely on any single diagnostic modality but requires detailed clinical examination, survey radiography, electrocardiography, echocardiography as well as evaluation of cardiac biomarkers.

Basically three modes (real time B-mode, M-mode and Doppler) of echocardiography are used to evaluate heart in routine practice. M-mode measurements and all standard real time B-mode imaging planes from right and left side of thorax are obtained.

Real-time B- mode Cardiac Ultrasound

- It is used to examine heart, blood vessels, soft tissues and thoracic organs.
- It can provide some anatomical information.
- Real time B –mode cardiac ultrasound can detect chamber enlargement, hypertrophy, abnormal valve, dilation of great vessels.
- Diagnosis of blood flow abnormality and functional cardiac disorders is not possible by real time B mode cardiac ultrasound.

M-mode Cardiac Ultrasound

- It is oldest form of cardiac ultrasound and was introduced into veterinary medicine around late 1970s.
- M-mode imaging facilitates dimensional analysis of heart chambers, thickness of the ventricular wall, motion of the heart and valves.
- Assessment of ventricular function is made easy on the basis of left ventricular fractional shortening (FS %), velocity of circumferential fibre shortening (Vcf), systolic time interval and mitral valve E-point to septal separation (EPSS).
- It provides clean images of cardiac borders than that of 2-D mode.
- M-mode views are obtained from right parasternal acoustic window.
- When measuring free wall thickness of left ventricle, papillary muscle within left ventricle is avoided.
- From the measurements of wall thickness and dimensional analysis of chambers, indices of contractility of ventricle are determined. Fractional shortening (FS) is an important index of ventricular contractility. Other indices are the mitral valve "E" point to septal separation (EPSS), ratio of the left ventricular internal dimension in diastole (LVIDd) to the left ventricle free wall dimension in diastole (LVFWd) and ratio of the left ventricular internal dimension in systole (LVIDs) to the left ventricular free wall dimension in systole (LVFWs).

Doppler Ultrasound

- It is comparatively new form of echocardiography.
- It has revolutionized cardiac imaging. The information available through Doppler imaging is complementary to real time B- mode and M-mode imaging.
- Doppler ultrasound provides information about blood flow through heart chambers, along vessels, across valves and its disturbances as well as velocity of blood flow.
- Doppler echocardiography has ability to assess the severity of the valvular dysfunction.
- In literature normal peak velocity of blood flow across the tricuspid, mitral, pulmonic and aortic valves in dogs has been mentioned as 90 cm/sec, 110 cm/sec., 120 cm/sec and 150 cm/sec respectively.

- Atrio-ventricular valvular insufficiency can be detected by Doppler ultrasound performed from the left parasternal position.
- The pulmonic valve insufficiency can be detected by Doppler ultrasound performed from the right parasternal position. While aortic valve insufficiency can be detected from left parasternal position.

Stress Cardiac Ultrasound

- Stress cardiac ultrasound or stress echocardiography is becoming important in the diagnosis of occult cardiovascular abnormalities.
- Detection of occult cardio-vascular abnormalities associated with poor performance particularly in racing horses assumes great significance. Hence application of stress cardiac ultrasound is very valuable in equine medicine.

Contrast Cardiac Ultrasound

- Not used commonly.
- Occasionally used to detect cardiac malformations.
- It is most sensitive to detect even small right to left shunts.
- Common echo contrast agents are based on fluid filled micro-bubbles
- Saline or dextrose mixed with few drops of patient's blood, agitated just before intravenous injection, is used for studying right heart and pulmonary arteries.
- For studying left heart more advanced contrasts are required (liquids/ suspensions containing micro bubbles based on albumin micro-encapsulated particles or galactose micro-particles).

Indications for Cardiac Ultrasound

- Evaluation of cardiac chamber (atrium, ventricles) size.
- Evaluation of ventricular wall thickness.
- Evaluation of ventricular wall movement (hypo or hyperkinetic)
- Evaluation of configuration of valve and their motion
- Evaluation of the proximal great vessels.
- Detection of pericardial effusion.
- Detection of pleural effusion.

- Evaluation of pulmonary artery hypertension.
- Evaluation of blood flow velocities through mitral, tricuspid, aortic and pulmonic valves.
- Identification of mass lesions within heart and its surroundings.

Limitations of Cardiac Ultrasound

- Technical expertise is very much essential.
- Casual interpretations may be catastrophic.
- Results of echocardiography are dependent on the skill and understanding of the echo cardiographer.
- Images are highly dependent on the quality of ultrasound equipment and patient characteristics.
- Air free contact between probe and chest wall is essential for good quality images.
- Image artefacts are very common.

Imaging Procedure

- Modern ultrasound machines have the facility of real time B-mode, M-mode and Doppler examination (Fig.140).

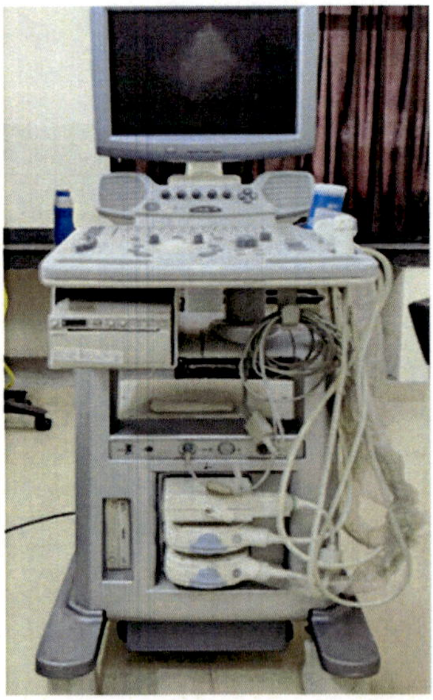

Fig. 140: GE Logic P5 Echocardiographic machine with B-mode, M-mode and Doppler facility.

- Advances in ultrasound machines have made it possible to display 2-D, M-mode or Doppler images simultaneously.
- Acoustic window for examination of heart is small because of narrow rib spaces and the surrounding lungs.
- Sector or phased array transducers with small foot print are ideal for cardiac ultrasound.
- For large dogs transducers of 3 to 3.5 MHz are recommended.
- For small dogs transducers of 5.0 to 7.5 MHz are suitable.
- For Doppler examination lower frequency transducers are appropriate.
- No sedation is generally required except for uncooperative dogs. Sedatives may have effect on cardiac rate, contractility and size. Therefore effects of sedative should be kept in mind while analysing the results of cardiac ultrasound examination if sedative has been given. Light tranquilization with buprenorphine (0.0075 -0.01 mg/kg IV) and acepromazine (0.03 mg/kg IV) may be considered for uncomfortable dogs. Uncooperative cats can be tranquilized with butorphanol (0.2 mg/kg IM) and acepromazine (0.1 mg/kg IM); or with acepromazine (0.1 mg/kg IM) followed in 15 minutes by ketamine (2.0 mg/kg IV).
- Area between costochondral junction and the sternum on both left and right thorax is clipped or shaved to provide parasternal windows (Fig.141). Acoustic gel is liberally applied to facilitate the contact of transducer.

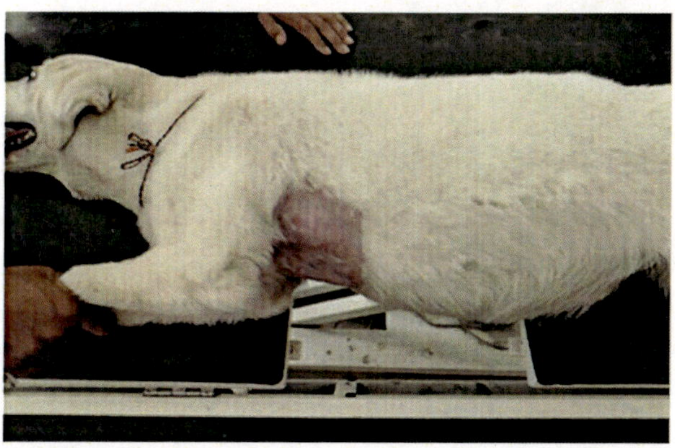

Fig. 141: Showing an area to be shaved and prepared for echocardiography

- Scanning can be done in lateral recumbency, sternal recumbency, standing or sitting positions as per condition of the patient.

- Dogs/cats are placed in right and left lateral recumbent positions. Dogs / cats with heart failure and severe respiratory distress are uncomfortable in lateral recumbency. Hence such patients should be examined in other positions.
- For better contact of transducer with acoustic windows, special table with cut out top (Fig.142) is recommended.

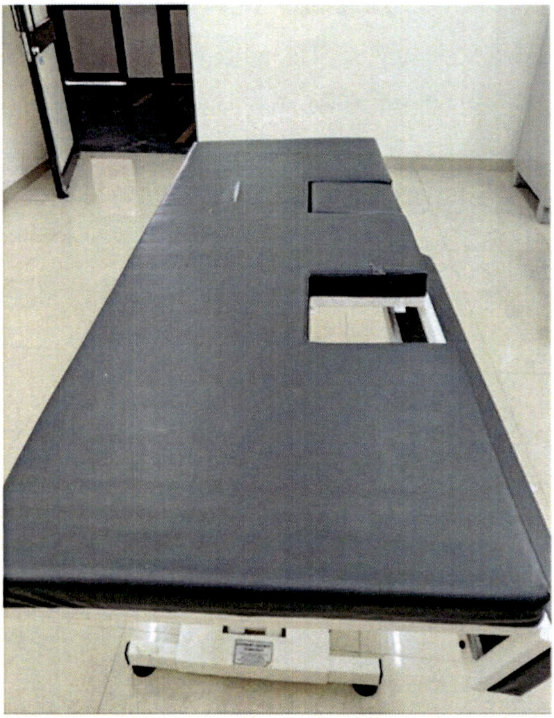

Fig. 142: Echocardiography table with cut out top to facilitate better contact of transducer with the scanning site.

- Standing, sitting or sternal positions are the other positions for the ultrasound examination of the heart.
- There are four important acoustic windows for examination of the heart viz. i. right parasternal acoustic window between 3rd and 6th intercostal spaces on the right side (Fig.143), ii. ventral window (between sternum and costochondral junction), iii . left caudal or apical parasternal window (Fig.144) at 5th to 7th intercostal space close to sternum over cardiac apex and iv. left cranial parasternal window (3rd /4th intercostal space between sternum and costochondral junction or apex beat).

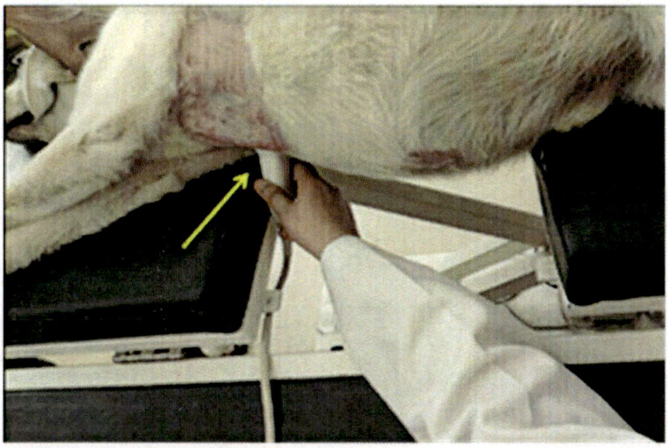

Fig. 143: Showing right parasternal acoustic window for long axis view (arrow indicates the positioning of the transducer).

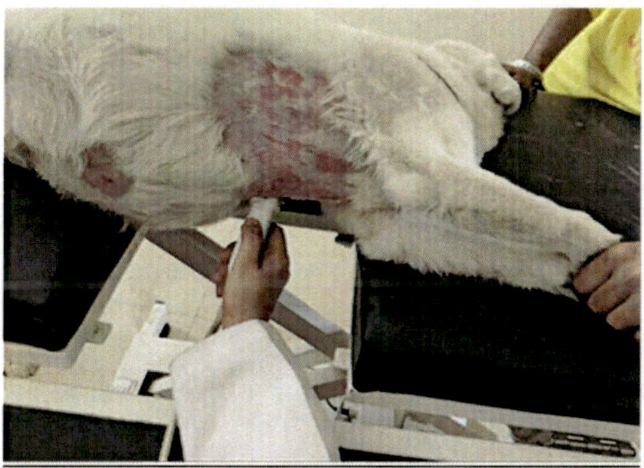

Fig. 144: Showing left apical parasternal window (transducer is placed at the apex of the heart).

- The standard protocol for echocardiographic examination is to examine the heart first from right parasternal location (patient in right lateral recumbency), then proceed to left caudal, and left cranial parasternal locations (left lateral recumbency or left side dependent).
- Examination is done in long axis (index marker of the probe is directed towards the base of the heart) and in short axis (index marker of the probe is directed towards the head of the patient) views. For long axis view, imaging is done in the long axis of the heart (from base to apex). For short axis view, imaging is done following the width of the heart.
- From each location several different views need to be taken.
- M-mode examinations are generally carried out from right parasternal approaches.

- Echocardiographic examination should be conducted in combination with electrocardiography.

Normal Visualization

Right Parasternal Window

- Long- axis views (Fig.145) - Beam is directed parallel to long axis of the heart. Views of both atria and ventricles; and atrioventricular valves are obtained. By angling ultrasound beam in cranial direction (slight clockwise rotation), left ventricle outflow tract (left ventricle, aortic valve and aortic root) and left ventricular inflow and outflow tracts are visualized. In nut shell the following can be visualized from right parasternal long axis view.
  - Four chamber view
  - Left ventricular outflow tract
  - Left ventricular inflow and outflow tracts.

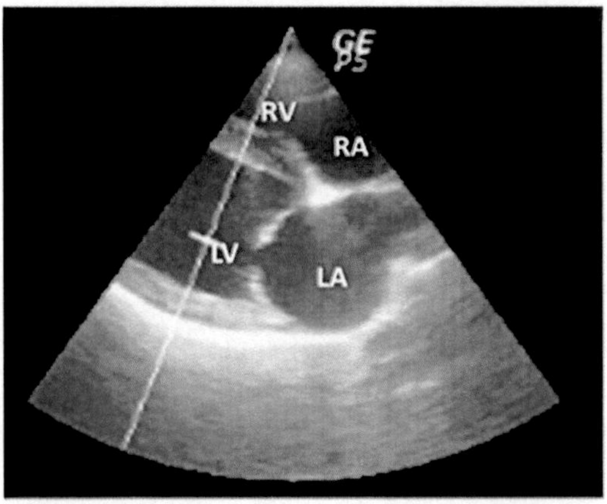

Fig. 145: Right parasternal long axis view showing both atria and ventricles

- Short –axis views (Fig.146, 147,148 and 149) -From long axis position transducer is rotated 90 ° in anticlockwise direction (orientation of the ultrasound beam is perpendicular to the long axis of the ventricles). Cardiac apex, the papillary muscles, chordae tendineae, mitral valve, aortic root, left atrium (M-mode) and main pulmonary artery are visualized. In nut shell the following cardiac parts can be visualized from right parasternal short axis view.

- Papillary muscle
- Chordae tendineae
- Mitral valve
- Aortic valve
- Pulmonary arteries

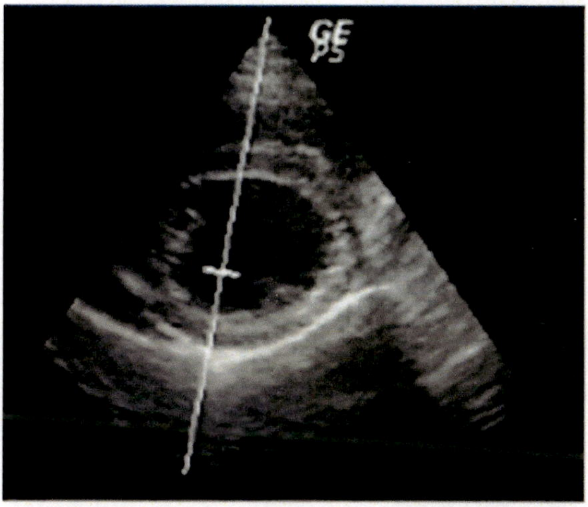

Fig. 146: Right parasternal short axis view at the level of chordae tendineae

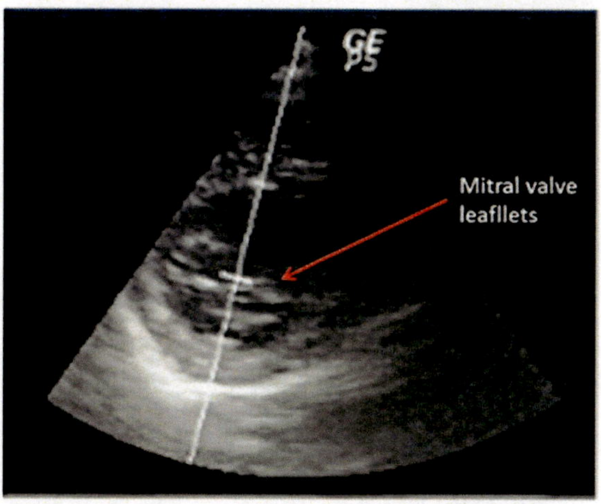

Fig. 147: Right parasternal short axis view at the level of mitral valve

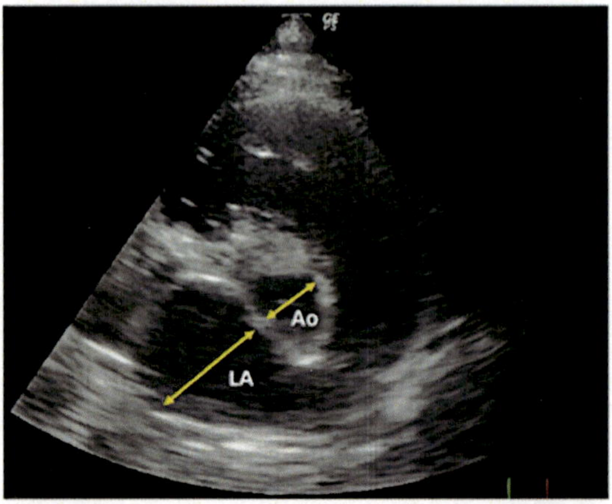

Fig. 148: Right parasternal short axis view at the level of aorta to measure left atrium and aorta.

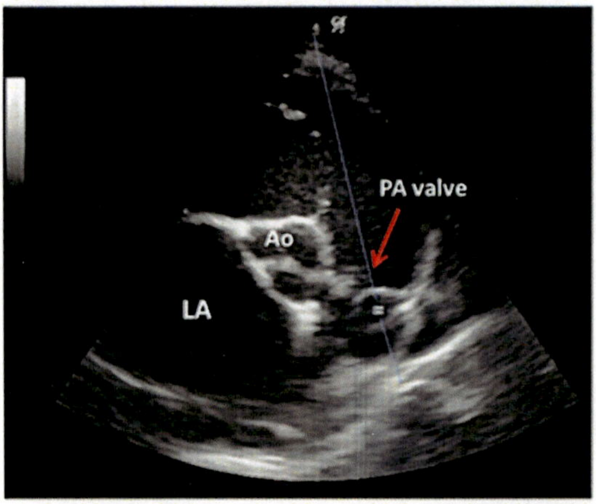

Fig. 149: Right parasternal short axis view at the level of pulmonic artery (PA) valve (arrow).

Left Caudal Parasternal Window

- Transducer is placed over the cardiac apex. Ultrasound beam is directed parallel to the long axis of the heart almost perpendicular to sternum. Beam is rotated in left caudal to right cranial direction towards base of the heart. Images of left ventricle and atrium are visualized on the right side and of right ventricle and atrium on the left side. By tilting the beam slightly cranially, left ventricle out flow tract is visualized. In nut shell the following can be visualized from left caudal parasternal view.

- Four chamber view
- Five chamber view (both atria, both ventricles and aorta)

Left Cranial Parasternal Window

- For the left cranial parasternal window, the transducer is placed in the third or fourth intercostal space between the sternum and the costochondral junction. Both long and short axis views should be taken. In nut shell the following can be visualized from the left cranial parasternal window.

Long Axis View

- Aorta
- Left ventricle

Short Axis View

- The aorta showing left ventricular inflow and out flow tracts.

M-mode Echocardiography

- Measurements of left atrium/aorta ratio; thickness of the left ventricle free wall and interventricular septum; the internal dimensions of the right and left ventricle in diastole and systole; and comparison of the aorta and main pulmonary artery are made using M- mode.
- Image of cardiac structures is in one dimensional plane.
- M mode image is produced from right parasternal long axis view (Fig. 150 A) or right parasternal short axis view (150B) by putting the cursor over the structures to be viewed.

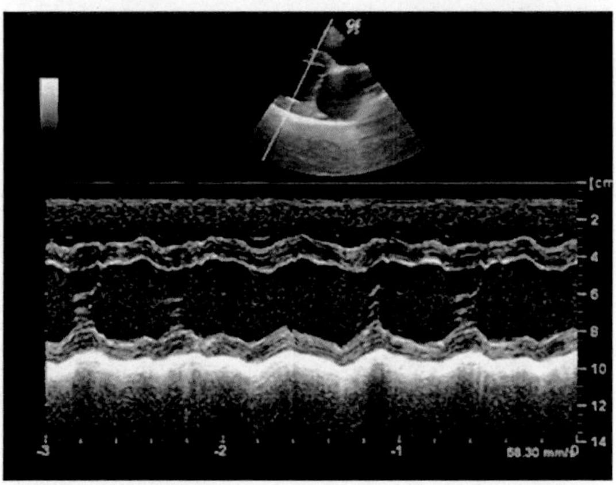

Fig. 150A: M-mode echocardiographic image (long axis view) in a healthy dog.

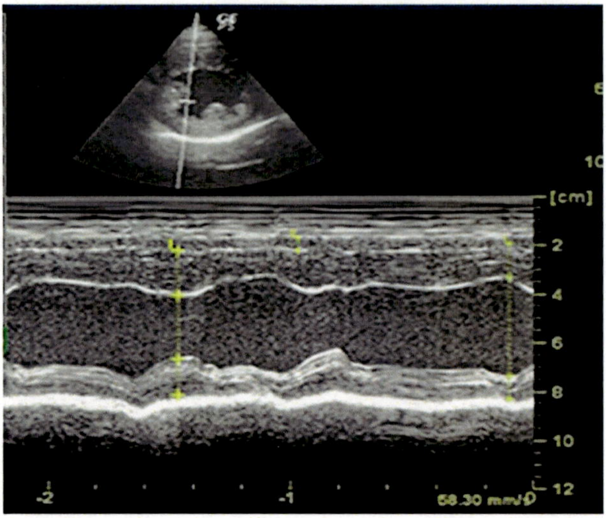

Fig. 150 B: M-mode echocardiographic image (short axis view) in a healthy dog

- Dimensions of LVIDs, LVIDd, IVSs, IVSd, LVPWs and LVPWd are taken as shown in the Fig 151.

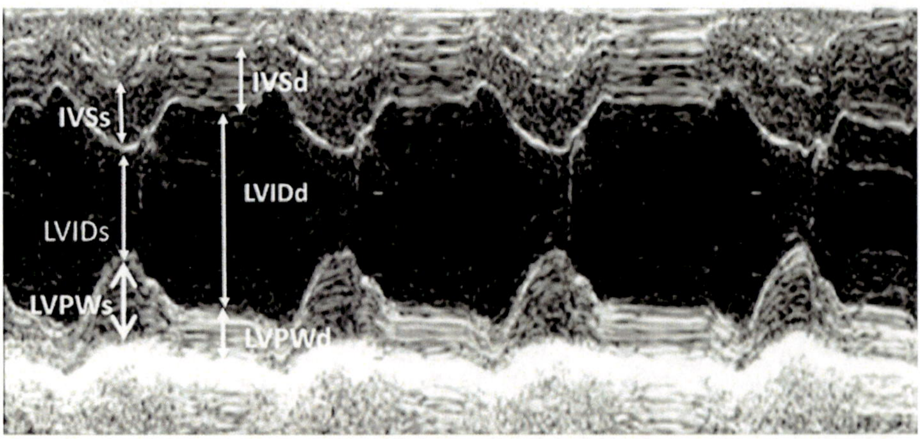

Fig. 151: Dimensions of the left ventricle in M-mode view

- By placing cursor perpendicular to the left ventricle in right parasternal long axis view at the level of chordae tendineae, right ventricle is visualized at the top, followed by interventricular septum, the left ventricle and left ventricle posterior wall at the bottom of the image.

- Similarly, left ventricle image can be taken by putting the cursor in the middle of left ventricle (in between chordae tendineae) in right parasternal short axis view (Fig. 150B).
- By placing cursor over tips of mitral valve, M shape image of the left ventricle is produced in M mode.
- The M shape has 2 peaks (Fig.152). 1st peak of M is called "E" point indicating early diastolic filling and 2nd peak of M is called as "A" point indicating atrial contraction.

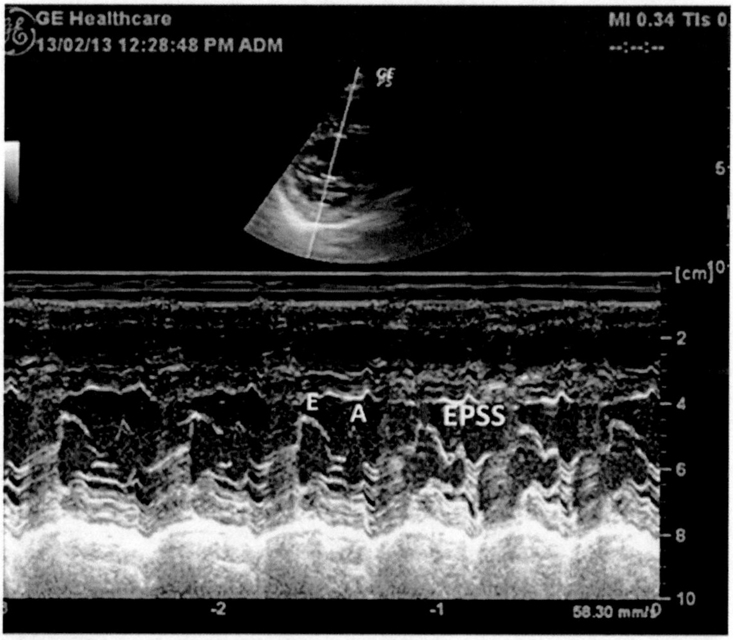

Fig. 152: Right parasternal short axis view at the level of mitral valve to measure "E" point to septal separation (EPSS)

- In normal heart "E" is bigger than "A"

Doppler Echocardiography

- It is used to determine blood flow at different valves.
- Left apical five chamber view is used to determine aortic blood flow. The pulse Doppler gate is placed inside the aortic valve as shown in figure (Fig.153). Measurements are taken at peak aortic valve velocity (Ao in m/sec) and aortic valve pressure gradient is measured from Bernoulli's equation i.e. 4x (v^2).

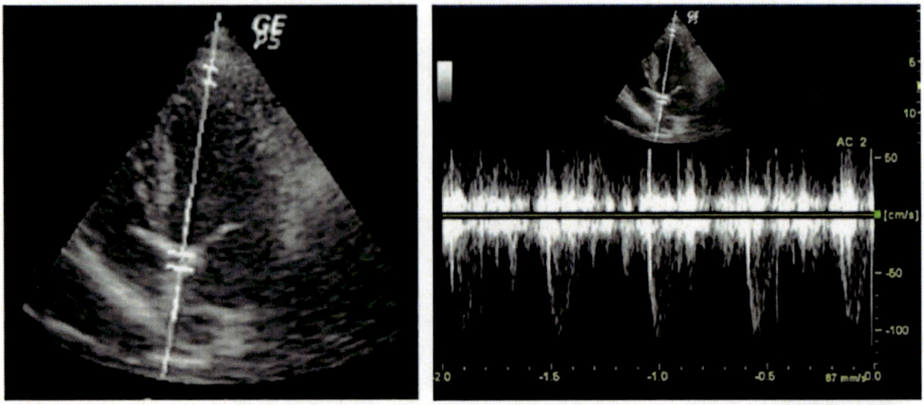

(A) **(B)**

Fig. 153: Showing position of transducer for Aortic blood flow **(A)**, Pulse wave Doppler at aortic valve **(B)**

- Left ventricular outflow tract is recorded from apical five chamber view. The PW gate is positioned in between aortic valve opening and anterior mitral valve leaflet as shown in Fig.154A.

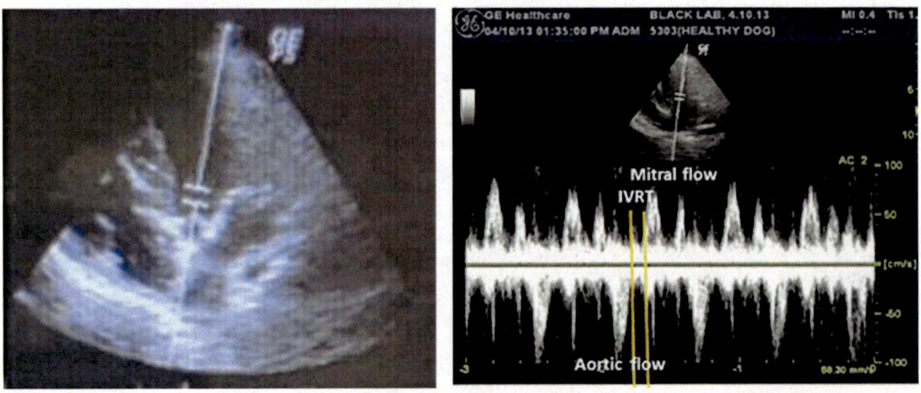

(A) **(B)**

Fig.154 (A,B): Showing Left ventricular out flow tract **(A)**. Pulse wave Doppler at left ventricular out flow tract (LVOT). The time interval from end of aortic flow to the beginning of mitral valve inflow indicated by vertical lines **(B)** shows isovolumetric relaxation time (IVRT).

- Myocardial performance index (MPI) or Tei index is calculated as follows:

MPI = IVRT+ IVCT÷ LVET

Where MPI = Myocardial performance index

IVRT = Isovolumetric relaxation time

IVCT = Isovolumetric contraction time

LVET = Left ventricular ejection time

- Mitral valve flow is recorded from left apical four chamber view. The sample volume is taken by placing the gate at tips of mitral valve leaflets when they are wide open i.e. during diastole (Fig. 154 C and D).

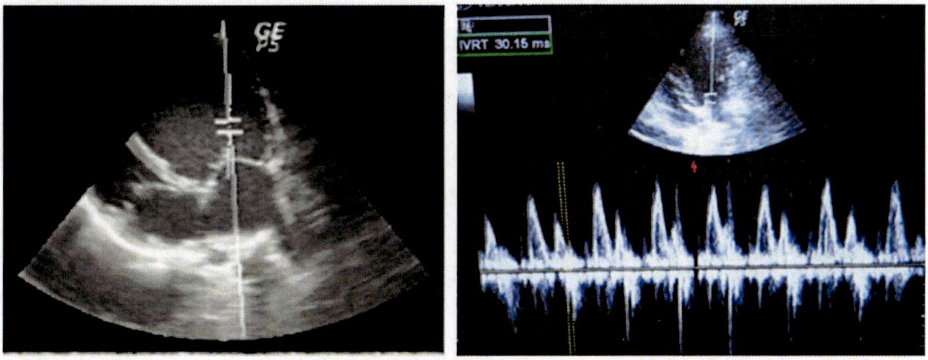

(C) **(D)**

Fig. 154 (C,D): Showing left apical four chamber view for mitral valve flow **(C)**. Pulsed wave Doppler image at mitral valve **(D)**

Two peaks are recorded above the baseline in form of M during diastole. First peak corresponds to early diastolic filling (E wave). Second arm of M corresponds to filling due to atrial contraction (A wave).

Mitral valve Deceleration time (M DecT) is the time from the point of maximal E velocity along its deceleration slope to the baseline. It is one of the important parameter for echocardiographic assessment of the diastolic functions.

MV E Vel (mitral valve peak E velocity), MV A Vel (mitral valve peak A velocity, and MV Dec T (mitral valve deceleration time) are recorded.

Mitral valve E: A ratio is greater than 1 in healthy dogs.

- Tricuspid valve flow (Fig.155) is recorded from left apical four chamber view. The sample volume is taken by placing the gate at tips of tricuspid valve leaflets when they are wide open i.e. during diastole.

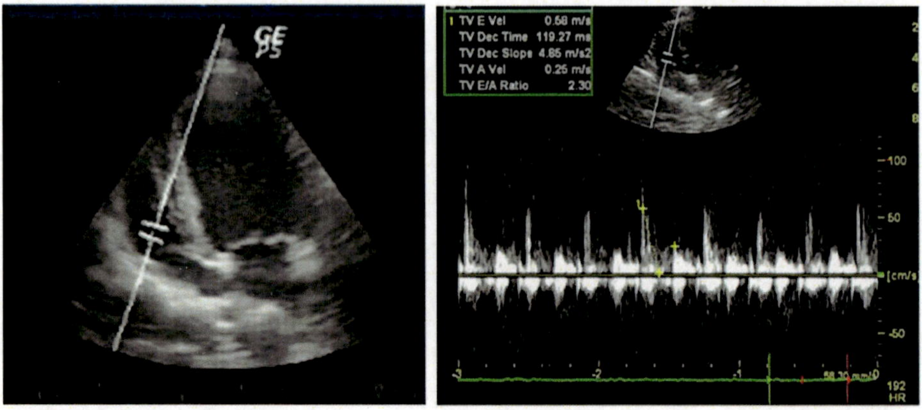

(A) (B)

Fig. 155: Showing left apical four chamber view for tricuspid valve flow **(A)**. Pulsed wave Doppler image at tricuspid valve **(B)**.

Two peaks are recorded above the baseline in form of M during diastole. 1st peak corresponds to start of diastole (E wave) and 2nd peak corresponds to filling due to atrial contraction (A wave).

TV E Vel (tricuspid valve peak E velocity), TV A Vel (tricuspid valve peak A velocity), TV Dec T (tricuspid valve deceleration time) and E:A ratio are measured.

- Pulmonary artery flow is recorded from the right parasternal short-axis plane at level of aorta and pulmonary artery. The sample volume is taken distal to the valve within the pulmonary artery (Fig.156).

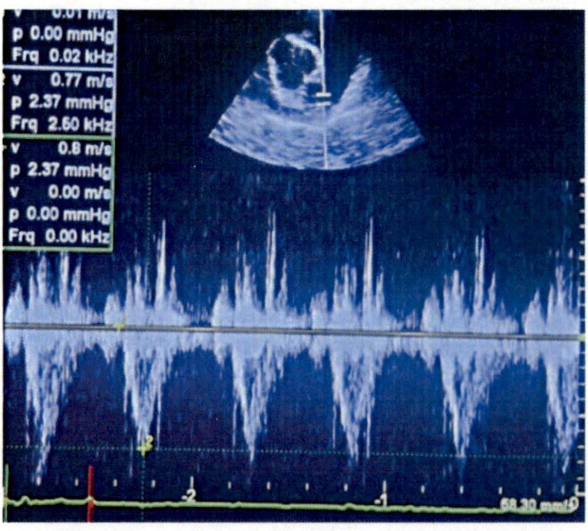

Fig. 156: Pulse Doppler at the level of pulmonic valve

PV Vel (Peak Pulmonary valve velocity, m/sec) is measured. PV Pressure gradient is determined using Bernoulli"s equation i.e. 4x (v^2) and expressed as mm Hg.

Where v^2 = Velocity of flow of blood at pulmonic valve.

- In Doppler images velocity and time are displayed on the y-axis and on the x-axis respectively.
- Blood flow towards and away from the transducer is displayed above and below the base line respectively.
- Localisation of abnormal blood flow and discriminate laminar and turbulent blood flow can be made with Pulse wave Doppler.
- Very high velocities at depth (stenosis of aortic or pulmonic valves) can be measured with continuous wave Doppler.
- Pulsed-wave Doppler measures at a specific location using a gate while continuous-wave Doppler measures indiscriminately along its path.
- Colour-flow Doppler is based on the pulsed-wave Doppler signal and produces a colour-coded image of the mean blood flow velocities.

Echocardiographic Measurements

The measurement values of LVIDd, LVIDs, LVWd, LVWs,

IVSd, IVSs, LA and Ao are expressed in mm or cm.

Left atrium: Aortic root ratio (LA:Ao)

- Measurements of diameter of left atrium and aorta (a line is drawn through middle of aortic valve leaflet and continued through left atrium in straight line) are taken during diastole in right parasternal short axis at the level of left atrium and aorta on frozen B- mode image.
- Ratio is automatically calculated by the machine.
- LA: Ao ratio in normal dogs is less than 1.5.
- It increases in left atrial enlargement and mitral regurgitation.

Fractional shortening (FS %)

- Following measurements (3 in diastole and 3 in systole) are taken in right parasternal short axis at the level of chordae tendineae on frozen M-mode image from leading edge to leading edge. The following six measurements of the left ventricle are taken.

- Left ventricular internal diameter at end diastole (LVIDd)
- Left ventricular internal diameter at end systole (LVIDs)
- Interventricular septum at end diastole (IVSd)
- Interventricular septum at end systole (IVSs)
- Left ventricular posterior wall thickness at end diastole

  (LVPWd) or left ventricular free wall thickness at end diastole (LVFWd)
- Left ventricular posterior wall thickness at end systole (LVPWs) or left ventricular free wall thickness at end systole (LVFWs)

- On the basis of the LVIDd and LVIDs measurements in M-mode, the End diastolic volume (EDV), End Systolic volume (ESV) are calculated according to the Teichholz formula by the ultrasound machine's computer software. The end diastolic volume index (EDVI, ml/m^2) and end systolic volume index (ESVI, ml/m^2) are normalised to body surface area (BSA). Fractional shortening (FS %) is calculated using the formula reported by Bonagura (1983).

Fractional shortening (FS %) = LVIDd-LVIDs ÷ LVIDd x 100

- It is automatically calculated by the machine.
- FS% is an estimate of myocardial functioning. Its value in normal healthy dogs is more than 25 %. Breed variations are there.
- The value of FS % is decreased in dilated cardiomyopathy.
- All parameters are automatically calculated by the machine.

Ejection Fraction (EF %)

- Following measurements (2 in diastole and 2in systole) are taken in right parasternal long axis view (4 chamber view) on frozen B-mode image.
  - Left ventricular internal dimension at end diastole (LVIDd)
  - Left ventricular internal dimension at end systole (LVIDs)
- Ejection fraction is automatically calculated by the machine.

  LV End Diastolic Volume (EDV) = $7x(LVIDd)^3 \div (2.4+LVIDd)$

  LV End systolic Volume (ESV) = $7x(LVIDs)^3 \div (2.4+LVIDs)$

  Ejection Fraction (EF %) = EDV – ESV ÷ EDV x100

EDVI (ml/m^2) = EDV÷ BSA (m^2)

ESVI (ml/m^2) = ESV ÷ BSA (m^2)

- Its value in normal healthy dogs is more than 50 %.
- The value of EF is decreased in dilated cardiomyopathy.

Echocardiographic Values in Healthy Labrador Retriever Dogs

M-mode echocardiographic values of different indices of healthy Labradors are given in the Table no.1 (Saini *et al.*, 2017).

Table 1: Echocardiographic values of Healthy Labrador retriever dogs

M Mode Echocardiographic parameters	values
LVIDd (cm)	3.56±0.07
LVIDs (cm)	2.41±0.05
IVSd (cm)	1.12±0.03
IVSs (cm)	1.36±0.04
LVPWd (cm)	0.85±0.02
LVPWs (cm)	1.17±0.02
FS%	31.81±0.57
EF%	60.53±0.84
LA (cm)	2.55±0.05
Ao (cm)	2.15±0.04
LA/Ao	1.20±0.02
EPSS (cm)	0.47±0.02

The values of different Doppler parameters of healthy Labradors are given in the Table no.2 (Saini *et al.,* 2020)

Table 2: Values of Doppler parameters of Healthy Labrador dogs

	Doppler Parameters	Values
Mitral valve	M E (m/s)	0.87±0.02
	MA(m/s)	0.64±0.02
	M E/M A	1.41±0.03
	M V DecT (ms)	145.08±5.29
Tricuspid valve	T E m/sec	0.62±0.02
	T A (m/sec)	0.46±0.01
	T E/T A	1.38±0.03
	T V Dec T (ms)	199.80±8.37
Aortic valve	AoV max(m/s)	1.08±0.02
	Ao Pressure (mmHg)	4.75±0.16
Pulmonic valve	PA V max (m/s)	1.00±0.02
	PA pressure (mmHg)	4.13±0.15

Echocardiographic Findings in Heart Diseases

• Patent Ductus Arteriosus (PDA)

Small shunts

- Associated with mild dilatation of pulmonary artery and mild increase in left ventricular end-diastolic dimension

Large shunts

- Associated with volume overload in lung
- Dilation of main pulmonary artery and left atrium;
- Dilation of left ventricle.
- Eccentric hypertrophy may be visualized in left ventricle.
- Right ventricular hypertrophy is seen in some cases with pulmonary hypertension.
- M-mode examination may reveal eccentric hypertrophy of left ventricle (as indicated by an increased end-diastolic dimension of left ventricular with normal septa and an increased thickness of left ventricle), left ventricular overload and variable fractional shortening (it may remain normal or increased). In case of myocardial failure fractional shortening is decreased), and enlargement of the left atrium and aortic root. Detection of abnormal blood flow (turbulent flow) within main pulmonary artery by Doppler sonography is of diagnostic value.

• Pulmonic Stenosis

- Pulmonic stenosis causes right ventricle pressure over load leading to concentric hypertrophy. Changes are proportional to the degree of obstruction.
- Severe cases may show increased thickness of the interventricular septum, right ventricular free wall. Size of moderator band of the right ventricle may be increased.
- Detection of turbulent flow distal to obstruction in Doppler examination.
- Post stenotic dilatation in pulmonary artery.
- Changes in peak flow velocity and pressure gradient across pulmonic valve in Doppler examination.
- Velocity of blood flow across the pulmonic valve may be accelerated in systole.

- **Pulmonic Insufficiency (Fig.157)**
    - Dilation of right ventricle
    - Dilation of pulmonary outflow tract
    - Dilation of main pulmonary artery
    - Absurd septal motion
    - Detection of partial opening of pulmonary valve during diastole on M-mode echocardiography
    - Detection of incomplete coaptation of pulmonary semilunar valve during ventricular diastole on 2-D echocardiography
    - Detection of turbulence proximal to pulmonic valve during ventricular diastole on Doppler echocardiography

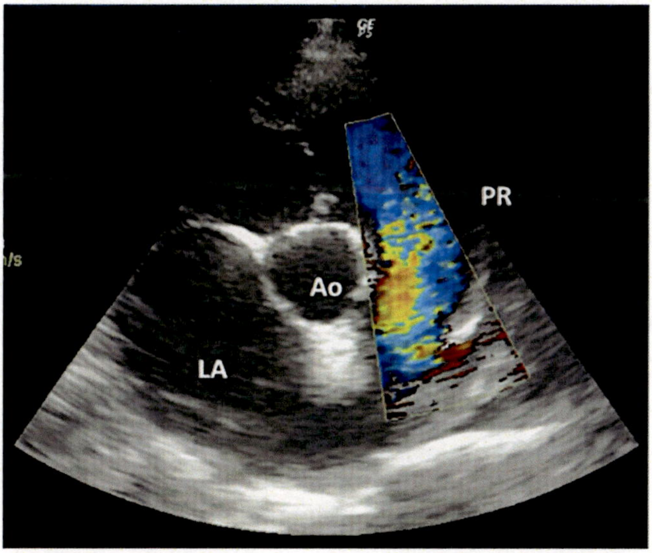

Fig. 157: 2-D echocardiogram (Right parasternal short axis view) of a dog showing pulmonic valve insufficiency (PI).

- **Aortic Stenosis**
    - Blood is unable to flow freely from left ventricle to aorta
    - Thickened left ventricular wall
    - Narrowing of left ventricular outflow tract.
    - Thickened aortic valve

- Detection of obstruction and pressure gradient by Doppler to detect severity of aortic stenosis

- **Aortic Insufficiency**
  - Dilation and hypertrophy of left ventricle
  - Almost normal thickness of septal and left ventricular free valve
  - Mild to moderate left atrial dilation
  - Thickening of aortic valve leaflets
  - Excessive systolic motion of septal and left ventricular free wall
  - Fluttering of the septal mitral valve leaflets during diastole
  - Detection of turbulence below aortic valve during ventricular diastole on Doppler echocardiography

- **Ventricular Septal Defect (VSD)**
  - Visualization of VSD in 2-D echocardiography as echolucent region in ventricular septum generally below aortic valve
  - Left atrial enlargement
  - Dilated hyperdynamic left ventricle
  - Septal dropout in M-mode echocardiography.

- **Atrial Septal Defect**
  - Visualization of ASD in 2-D echocardiography as an echo lucent space in atrial septum
  - Septal dropout in M-mode echocardiography.
  - Right to left or bidirectional blood flow across atrial septum on Doppler examination

- **Tetralogy of Fallot**
  - Overriding of aorta on the interventricular septum
  - Ventricular septal defect high on the septum just below aortic valve
  - Abnormalities in pulmonary valve and narrowing of pulmonary outflow tract
  - Thickening of right ventricular wall
  - Dextraposition of aorta in some cases

- Right to left blood flow across the VSD with the appearance of microbubbles in the ascending aorta on Doppler examination

• Chronic Mitral Valve Insufficiency (Fig.158 and 159)

The following echocardiographic changes may be detected in dogs with chronic degenerative mitral valve insufficiency.

- Functional class I heart failure may be associated with normal or increased contractility, doming /thickening of mitral valve, slight increase in chamber size with mild compensatory hypertrophy. Detection of regurgitant blood flow from left ventricle to left atrium in Doppler echocardiography.
- Functional class II heart failure may be associated with minimum ventricular hypertrophy/dilation, normal/increased ventricular contractility, slight enlargement of left atrium, LA:Ao ratio more than 1, and doming /thickening of mitral valve.
- Functional class III heart failure may be associated with dilated hypertrophied left ventricle, LA: Ao ratio is more than 2:1, thickened, domed or flailing mitral valve leaflets.
- Functional class IV heart failure may be associated with flailing mitral valve leaflets when there is ruptured chordae tendineae. Contractility may be normal or slightly reduced. Sometimes pericardial effusion is also visualized.

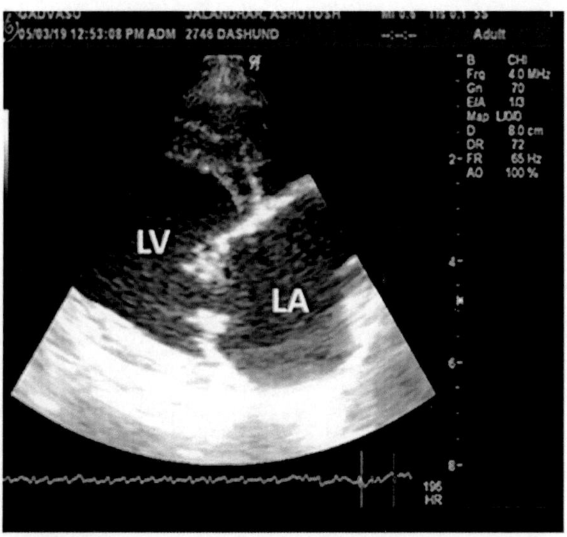

Fig. 158: 2-D echocardiogram of a Dachshund dog with chronic degenerative mitral valve insufficiency showing thickened mitral valve between LA and LV.

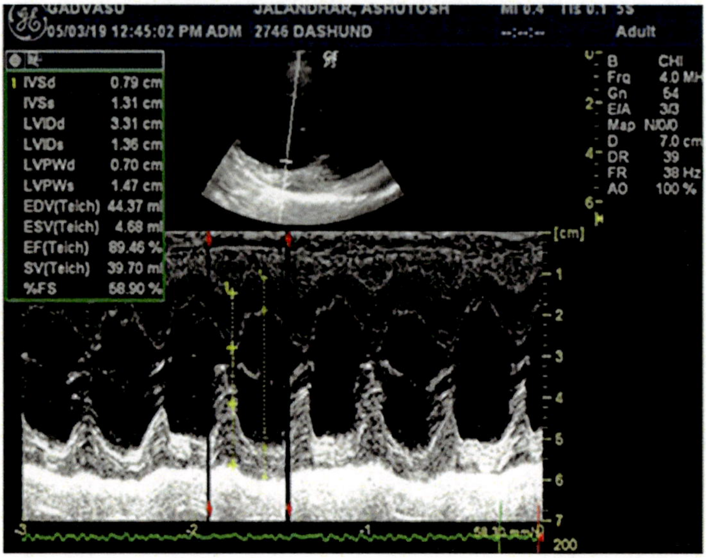

Fig. 159: M- mode echocardiogram of a dog with chronic degenerative mitral valve insufficiency showing hyperkinetic interventricular septum and left ventricular posterior wall .

- **Mitral valve dysplasia (MVD)**
  - A common congenital heart disease in cats
  - Short, thick , redundant leaflets lead to regurgitation of mitral valve
  - Left atrium and left ventricle volume overload with increased left atrial pressure
  - Enlarged left atrium and dilation of left ventricle
  - Increased shortening fraction in moderate to severe cases of MVD
  - Decreased shortening fraction in cases with myocardial failure
  - Thick valve with decreased mobility, thick short chordae and upwardly displaced papillary muscles may be visualized on 2-D echocardiography
  - Mitral regurgitation or stenosis can be confirmed on Doppler examination using left parasternal apical window.
- **Mitral Stenosis**
  - Reduced valve area
  - Enlargement of left atrium
  - Detection of turbulent flow from left atria to ventricle during diastole on Doppler examination

- **Tricuspid Insufficiency**
  - Dilation of right atrium
  - Prolapse of tricuspid valve
  - Thickening of valve leaflets
  - Flailing leaflets of the valve
  - Dilation of right ventricle with hypertrophy
  - Detection of regurgitant blood flow from right ventricle to right atrium (Fig.160) during ventricular systole on Doppler echocardiography.

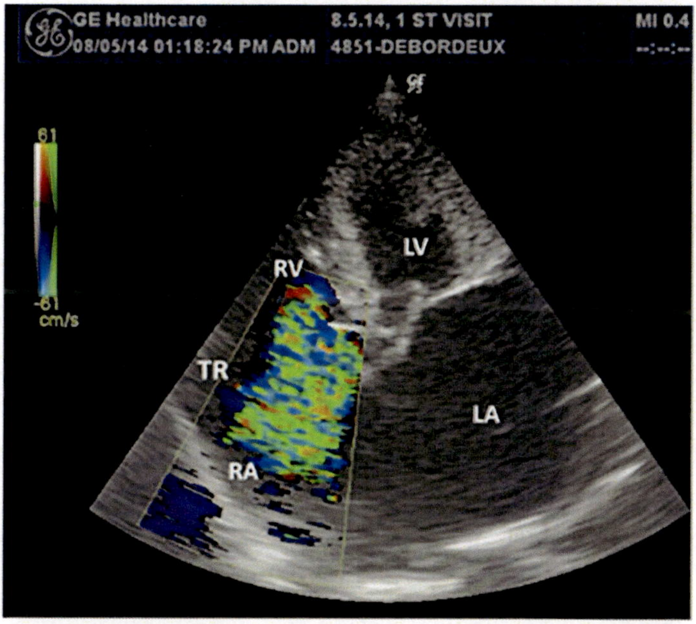

Fig. 160: Echocardiogram of a dog (left apical 4 chamber view) showing severe tricuspid regurgitation.

- **Tricuspid dysplasia**
  - Seen in cats and large breed dogs
  - Tricuspid regurgitation
  - Right atrial dilatation
  - Diastolic flattening of the ventricular septum

- **Infective Endocarditis**
  - Diffuse, localized or nodular thickening of cardiac valve (s)
  - Ruptured chordae tendineae causes swinging of AV valve leaflets
  - Mild to moderate enlargement of left atrium
  - Mild to moderate dilation of left ventricle with increased septal and free wall movement during systole
  - Detection of regurgitant or turbulent flow on Doppler echocardiography
- **Cardiomyopathy**

Canine dilated cardiomyopathy

- The following characteristic echocardiographic changes can be detected in cases of DCM (Fig. 161,162,163, 164 ,165,166,167 and 168) in right parasternal short axis view at the level of left ventricle.
- Left ventricle enlargement in both systole and diastole.
- Enlargement of left atrium and left ventricular chambers with or without enlargement of right ventricle
- Reduced contractibility of chambers as manifested by low FS% (25%) and EF %(< 40%).
- Thinning of interventricular septal wall and left ventricular posterior wall.
- Hypo kinesis.
- The following echocardiographic changes can be observed in cases of DCM in right parasternal view at the level of mitral valve.
- Increased E point to septal separation (EPSS).
- 'B bump' at the end of mitral valve diastolic motion indicates delayed closure of mitral valve and is a sign of high end diastolic LV pressure.
- The values of End diastolic volume (EDV) and End systolic volume (ESV) are calculated by using M mode Teicholz equation from LVIDd and LVIDs, respectively. There is increase in EDV and ESV in overt DCM.
- The end-diastolic and end-systolic ventricular volumes can be normalised to body surface area (BSA) to give an end diastolic volume index and an end-systolic volume index (EDVI and ESVI) in units ml / m^2. The normal value of canine ESVI has been found to be <30 ml/m^2 and the value > 80 ml/m^2 confirms systolic dysfunctions.

- Decrease in left ventricular shortening fraction suggesting decreased ventricular contractility. Left ventricular fractional shortening (LVFS) can be calculated as follows:

  LVFS = LVIDd-LVIDs/LVIDd x 100

- Thin left ventricular posterior wall and interventricular septum.
- Increased anterior mitral leaflet E-point to septal distance.

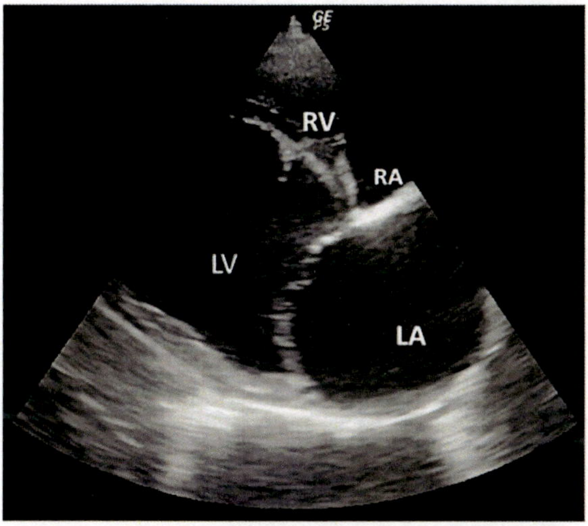

Fig. 161: 2-D echocardiogram (right parasternal long axis view) of a dog with dilated cardiomyopathy showing enlargement of left atrium and ventricle.

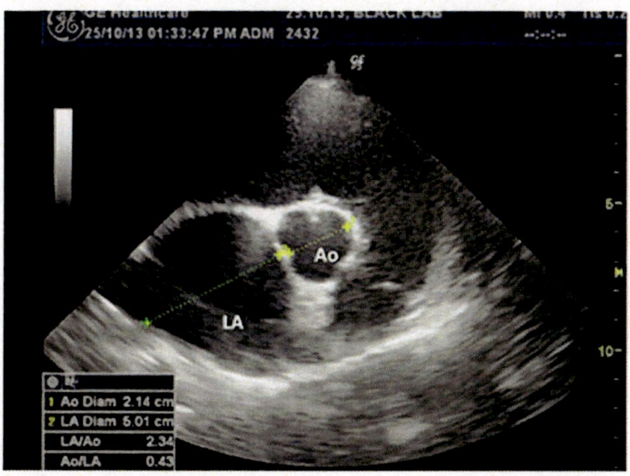

Fig. 162: 2 D echocardiogram (right parasternal short axis view) of a dog with dilated cardiomyopathy showing enlarged left atrium and increased LA: Ao ratio.

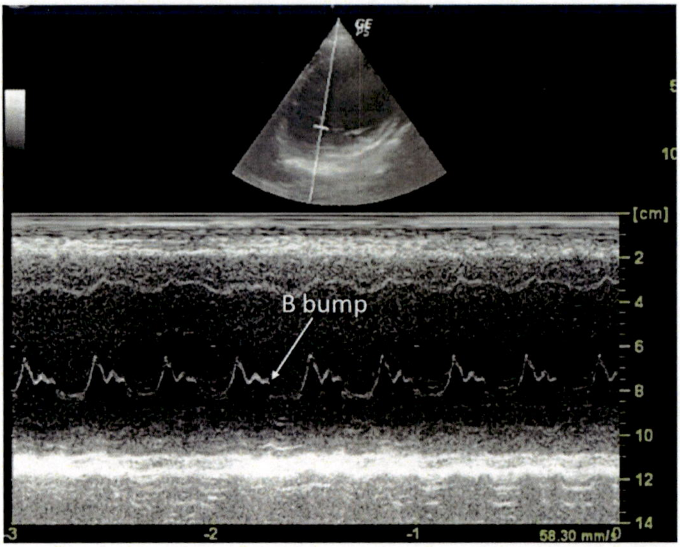

Fig. 163: M- mode echocardiogram of a dog with cardiomyopathy at the level of mitral valve showing delayed closure of mitral valve as indicated by " B bump" (white arrow).

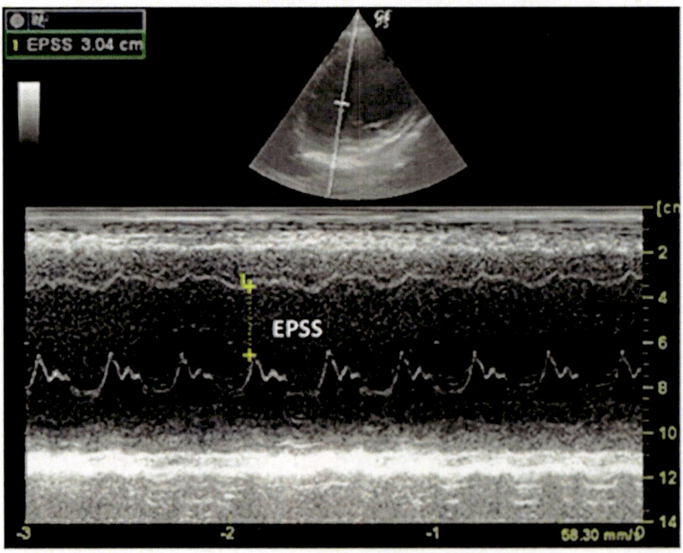

Fig. 164: M mode echocardiogram of a dog with dilated cardiomyopathy showing increased E point to septal separation (EPSS).

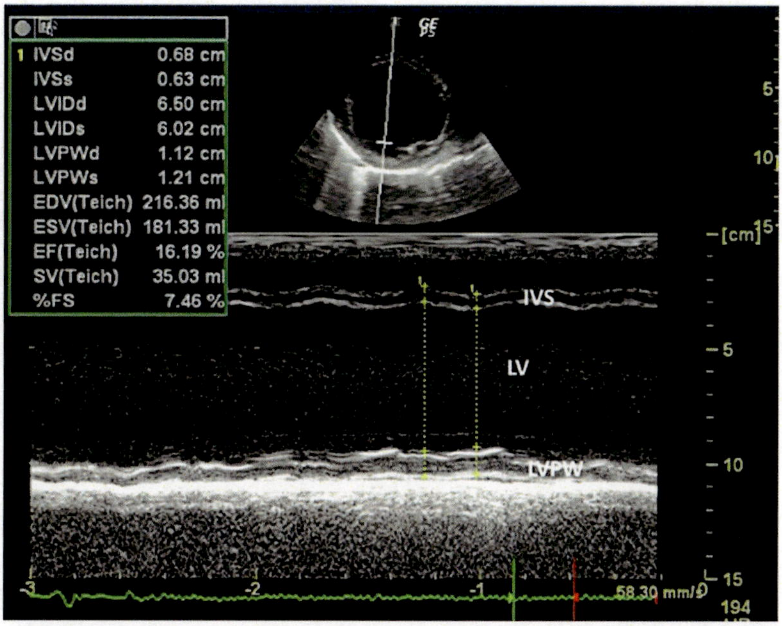

Fig. 165: M- mode echocardiogram of the left ventricle of a Dalmatian dog with dilated cardiomyopathy showing decreased systolic motion of the interventricular septum (IVS) and left ventricular (LV) posterior wall.

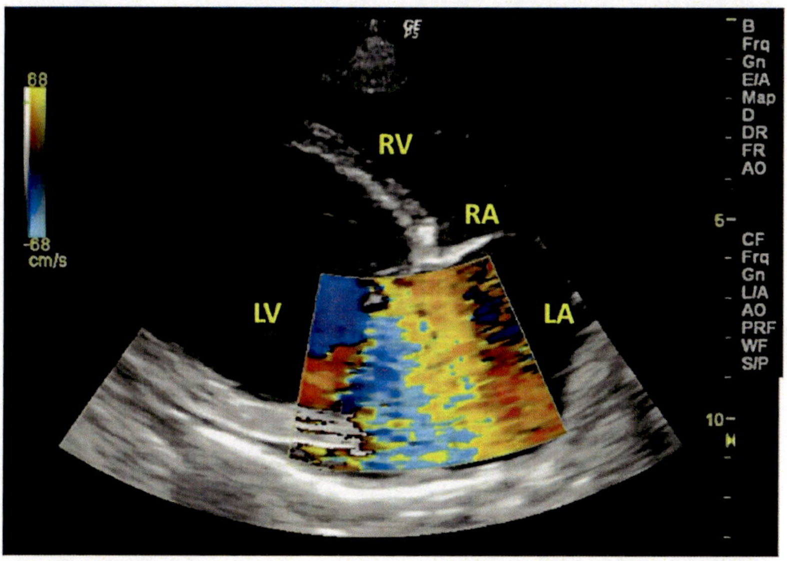

Fig.166: 2 D echocardiogram showing mitral regurgitation in a Dog with dilated cardiomyopathy.

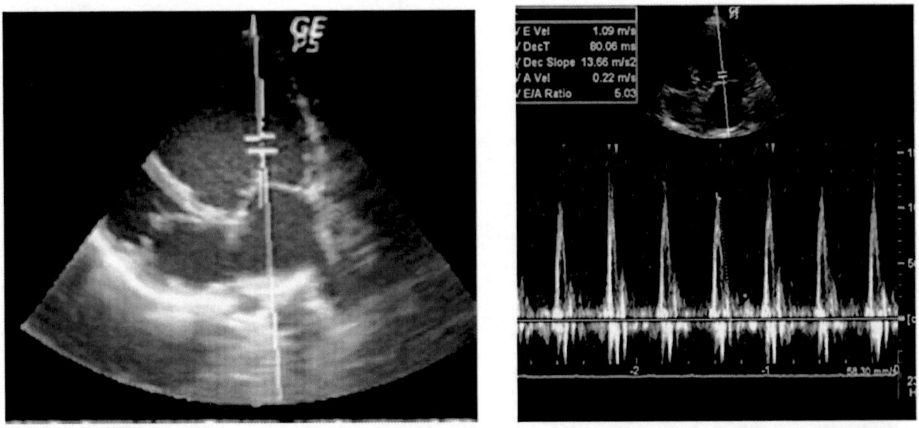

Fig. 167: Pulse wave Doppler of a dog with dilated cardiomyopathy at the level of mitral valve showing tall E wave , short A wave indicating restrictive filling pattern.

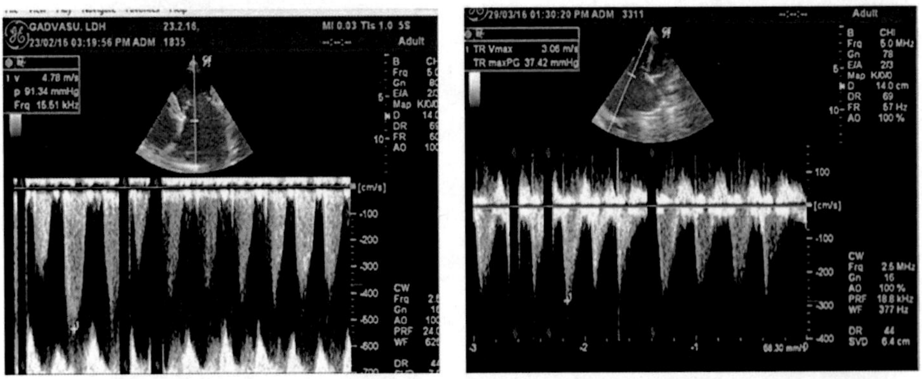

(A) **(B)**

Fig. 168: Continuous wave Doppler of dogs with dilated cardiomyopathy at mitral valve **(A)** and at tricuspid valve **(B)** showing mitral regurgitation **(A)** and tricuspid regurgitation **(B)**

Canine hypertrophic cardiomyopathy

The following echocardiographic changes can be detected in dogs with hypertrophic cardiomyopathy (Fig.169 and 170)

- Hypertrophy of left ventricle and septal wall
- Increased left ventricular free wall and septal thickness
- Diminished left ventricular lumen
- Reduced E-point-septal distance
- Hyperdynamic motion of the left ventricle

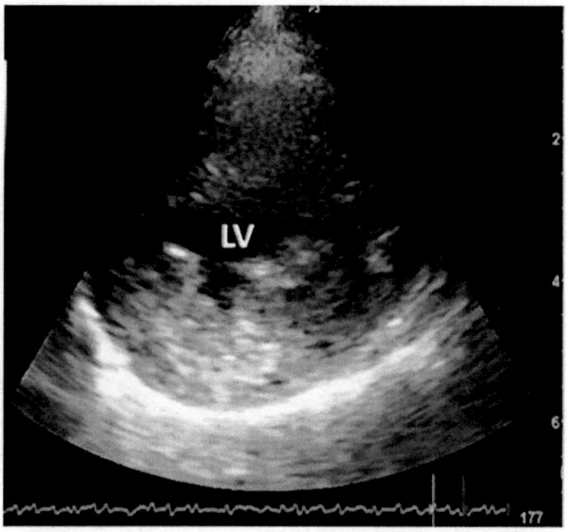

Fig. 169: 2-D echocardiogram of a dog (right parasternal short axis view) with hypertrophic cardiomyopathy showing thickened wall of the left ventricle.

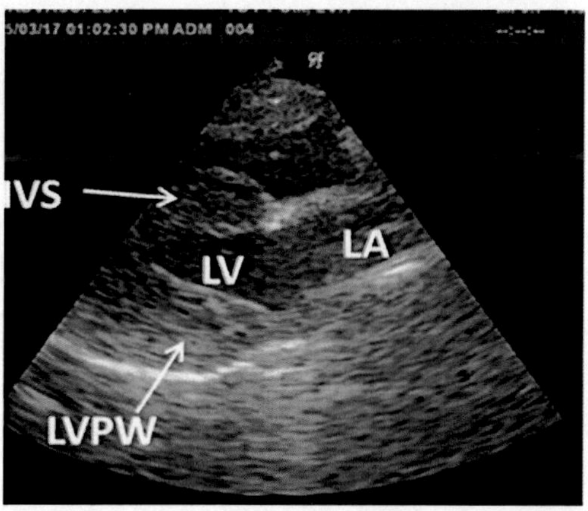

Fig. 170: 2-D echocardiogram of a dog with Hypertrophic cardiomyopathy showing thickened interventricular septum (IVS) and left ventricular posterior wall (LVPW).

Feline dilated cardiomyopathy

- Dilated lumen of left atrium and left ventricle
- Decreased thickening and wall motion of Left ventricle during systole
- Reduced fractional shortening (FS). FS may be less than 30 %.
- Increased mitral valve E-point-septal separation

Feline hypertrophic cardiomyopathy

- Reduced lumen of left ventricle
- Increased thickness of left ventricular wall
- Reduced mitral valve E-point to septal separation
- Increased Fractional shortening (FS)
- Increased left ventricular wall motion

Feline restrictive cardiomyopathy

- Lumen of left atrium is enlarged
- Slight increase in the lumen of left ventricle with almost normal wall thickness.
- No change in Fractional shortening
- Often right heart (right atrium and right ventricle) enlargement
- Pericardial Disease

- **Pericardial Effusion (Fig.171, 172 and 173)**
    - 2-D and M-mode echocardiography is of diagnostic value.
    - Heart is surrounded by anechoic pericardial fluid space.
    - Swinging of heart may be visualized in many cases

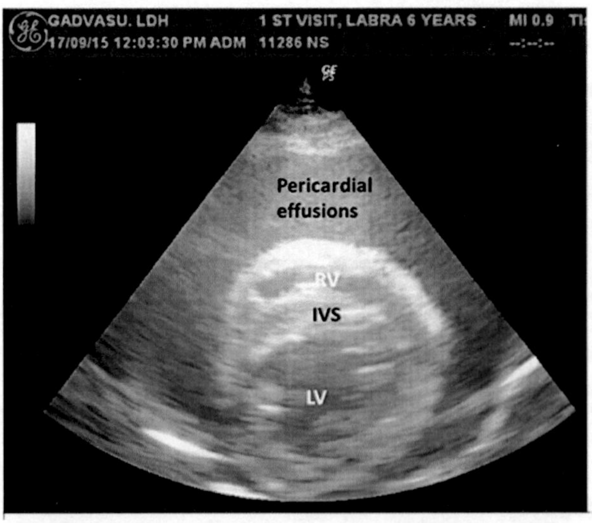

Fig.171: 2-D echocardiogram (right parasternal short axis view) of a Labrador showing severe Pericardial Effusions

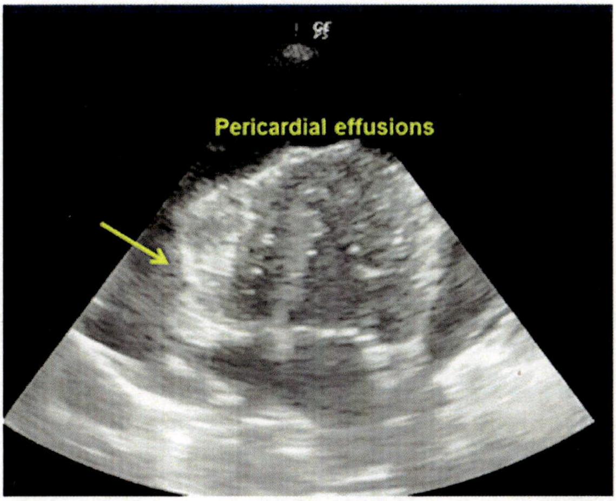

Fig. 172: 2-D echocardiogram of a Cocker Dpaniel dog with severe limb oedema, abdominal distension, coughing and exercise intolerance showing pericardial effusion due to pericardial tumour (arrow) in wall of right ventricle

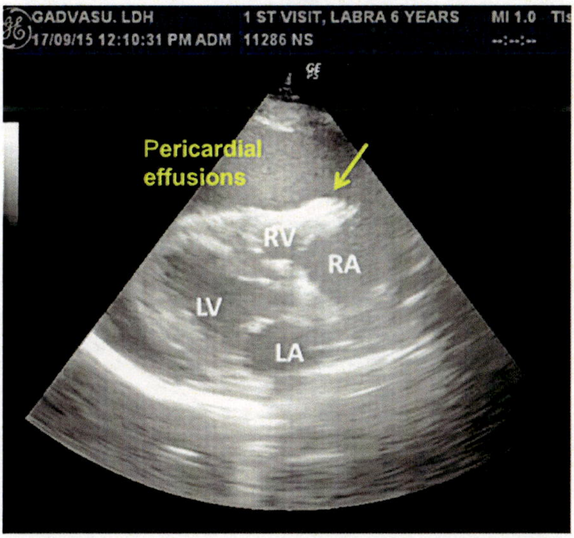

Fig. 173: 2-D echocardiogram of a Labrador with abdominal distension, exercise intolerance, dyspnoea (right parasternal long axis view) showing pericardial effusion due to pericardial tumour (increased echogenic area)

- **Constrictive pericarditis**
  - Pericardial thickening
  - Abnormal diastolic motion of the septum and left ventricular wall

• Cardiac tamponade

- Early diastolic collapse of the right atrial and ventricular walls (Fig. 174, and 175).

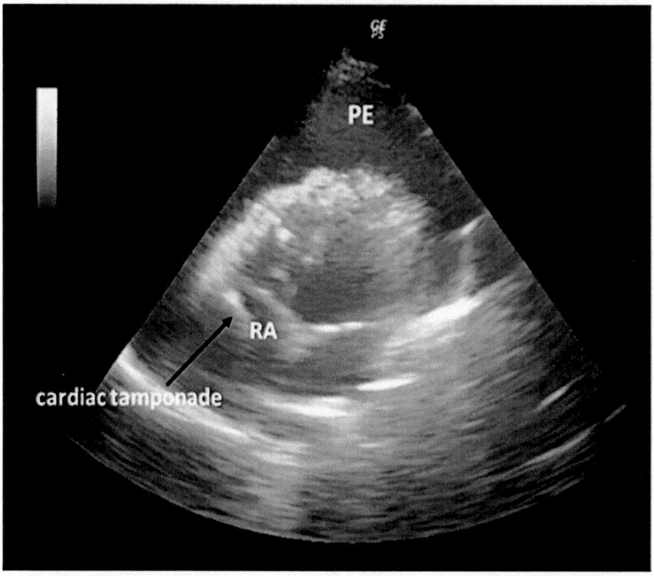

Fig. 174: 2-D echocardiogram of a dog (left apical four chamber view) showing cardiac tamponade (arrow) indicated by right atrial (RA) diastolic collapse.

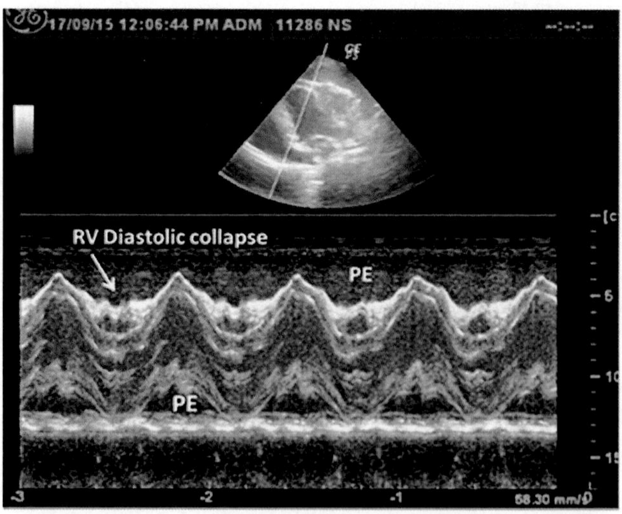

Fig. 175: M-mode echocardiogram of a dog showing right ventricular (RV) diastolic collapse (arrow) with cardiac tamponade due to pericardial effusions (PE)

- **Cardiac masses**
    - Masses can be identified in 2-D echocardiography
    - *Heartworm Disease*
    - Enlargement of right heart (right atrium and ventricle)
    - Pulmonary artery enlargement detected on 2-D echocardiography
    - Hypertrophy of the right papillary muscle
    - Hypertrophy of the right ventricular free wall
    - Paradoxical motion of the interventricular septum and septal flattening

References

Bonagura, J.D. (1983). M-mode echocardiography. Basic principles. Vet. Clin. North Am. Small Anim Pract. 13:299-319 .

Saini, N., Uppal, S.K. and Randhawa, C.S. (2017). Echocardiographic parameters and indices in healthy Labrador Retriever dogs. Israel J.Vet. Med. 72: 428-34.

Saini, N., Uppal, S.K., Tandon, R. and Kashyap, N. (2020). Doppler echocardiographic reference parameters in healthy Labrador Retriever dogs. J.Anim. Resch.10: 1-8.

Suggested Further Reading

Boon, J. A. (2011). Manual of Veterinary Echocardiography. Lippincott Williams & Wilkins, Philadelphia

Mannion, P. (2006). Diagnostic Ultrasound in Small Animal Practice. Blackwell Science Ltd. Oxford, U.K.

Tilley, L.P., Smith Jr, F.W.K., Oyama, M. A. and Sleeper, M.M. (2008). Manual of Canine and Feline Cardiology, 4th edn, Saunders.

17

Ultrasound of The Thorax (Lungs, Pleura, Mediastinum and Thoracic Wall)

J.P. Varshney and P.S. Chaudhary

Beside heart, ultrasound of the thorax facilitates the imaging of lungs, pleura, mediastinum, chest wall and diaphragm. Sonographic examination of the heart is discussed in chapter16. Because of nearly total reflection of sound waves at gas interfaces (Fig. 176) thoracic ultrasound has limitations. Pulmonary and mediastinal lesions located deep are difficult to image. Peripheral pulmonary lesions and pleural fluid can be visualized. Point of care lung ultrasound is becoming an effective tool for the diagnosis of left sided congestive heart failure in humans, dogs and cats. It can be of great help in differentiating pulmonary oedema of cardiac and non-cardiac origin. Thoracic ultrasound can assist in thoracocentesis, aspiration of lung mass or consolidated lungs. Other advantage of thoracic ultrasound is to distinguish fluid and soft tissues.

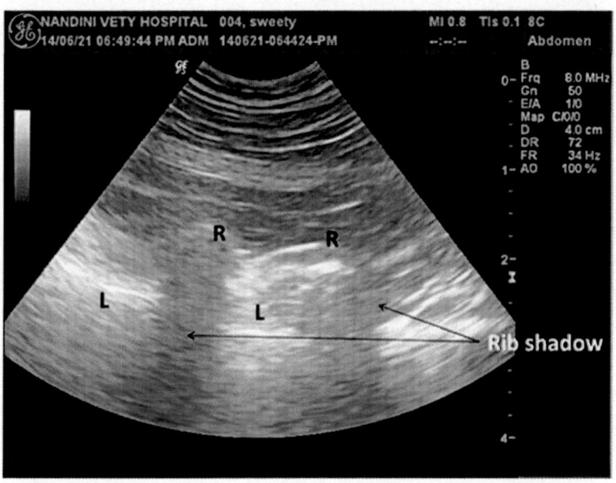

Fig. 176: Thoracic ultrasound of a dog (transducer placed in longitudinal plane on 6th and 7th ribs in upper middle thorax) showing near total reflection of sound waves at gas interface in the lung. Lung area is appearing echogenic between acoustic shadowing of the ribs. Therefore lesions deep to air filled lungs are difficult to visualize. R== Ribs, L== lung.

Techniques of Thoracic Ultrasound

- It is always advisable to conduct radiographic examination of thorax prior to ultrasound examination so that some assessment of the disease can be made and appropriate acoustic window may be decided.
- Thoracic scan of the dogs and cats can be done in sternal, lateral, or dorsal recumbency as per the condition of the patient. Dogs and cats with respiratory distress are better scanned in standing or sternal recumbency. Generally no specific preparation is needed. If sedation or anaesthesia is to be given, prior fasting is necessary.
- Dogs and cats with respiratory distress should be treated with oxygen on priority before subjecting them to ultrasound examination.
- Chemical restrain is required where ultrasound guided biopsy is to be taken.
- Pleural fluid can serve as an important acoustic window for scanning lungs and mediastinum.
- Acoustic windows for thoracic examination are parasternal (detail has been given under cardiac ultrasound), suprasternal (through thoracic inlet), sub-costal (through liver), or directly over the lesion.
- Thorax should be examined in longitudinal plane keeping the transducer perpendicular to ribs and in transverse plane keeping the transducer parallel to ribs. Visualization of caudal thorax or mediastinum can be done by adopting transhepatic approach from ventral or lateral abdominal location.
- Cranial mediastinum can be better visualized through thoracic inlet.
- Curved micro convex, curved linear array or sector transducers with small foot print can be used for ultrasound examination of the thorax. Sector or micro-convex transducers allow better penetration between ribs.
- It is better to select transducer frequency as per the size of the patient and depth of the suspected lesion. A transducer 7.5 MHz is suitable for small dogs and cats. For large breeds and deeper lesions a transducer of 5.0 MHz is appropriate. Higher frequency transducers are good for superficial lesions and low frequency transducers are good for deep lesions.

Normal Ultrasonographic Appearance of Thorax

- Thoracic wall has three layers viz. skin, subcutaneous fat and muscle. Sonographically these layers are visualized as alternating layers of hyper- and hypoechogenicity.
- Parietal pleural lining may not be visible.
- In healthy dogs and cats visceral pleura and lung surface form a continuous echogenic line.
- Normal deep lung tissue is concealed by artefacts (shadowing and reverberation). Visualization beyond most superficial layer of the lungs is not possible because about 99% of ultrasound beam is reflected at lung-soft tissue interface.
- Ribs have smooth curvilinear echogenic interface with acoustic shadowing at regular intervals.

Ultrasonographic Appearance in Diseases

- Point of care ultrasound of lung may show infinite coalescing B lines between ribs shadows within each intercostal space in cases of pulmonary oedema of cardiac origin (Murphy *et al.*, 2021). B-lines are vertical hyperechoic lines with a narrow base emerging from the surface of pleura, extending to the distal edge of the screen (Baldi *et al.*, 2012). These lines correspond to the thickening of the sub- pleural and inter-lobular septa or to the presence of extravascular fluid in the lungs (Volpicelli *et al.*, 2006).
- Sonographic image in cases of pleural effusions depends on the character and volume of the fluid present there. Transudate /modified transudate appears as anechoic with floating fine echogenic lines. With increasing cellular content of the fluid, the fluid becomes more echogenic. Localized small amount of fluid may mimic as hypoechoic mass. Pleural surface appears as thickened and irregular when the fluid is exudate or haemorrhagic.
- Roughened and thickened pleura may indicate pleuritis, neoplastic pleural disease or chronic pleural effusions.
- Decreased volume of lung lobes forming small triangular structure surrounded by fluid is seen in cases of atelectasis secondary to pleural effusions. Multifocal echogenic linear structures and foci are seen because of residual alveolar and bronchial air. Lung lobes may appear uniformly hypoechoic when there is complete collapse.

- Mediastinal masses in cranial and middle mediastinum can be visualized. There is no definite single appearance. There is a need to assess margins of the mass, its echogenicity and its relationship with mediastinal vessels. Neoplastic lesions may have well defined borders while inflammatory lesions are more irregular and vague.
- Lymphomas may appear as round, distinct and hypoechoic mass with fine echogenic capsule and a central echogenic line. In other cases there may be mixed echogenicity. Discrete hypoechoic with hyperechoic rim has been considered pathognomonic for lymphoma.
- Thymomas, mediastinal masses, may be well marginated, irregular or smooth outline. Their echogenicity may be moderate or mixed. Differentiation between lymphomas and thymomas can only be done on biopsy examination.
- Mediastinitis has varied sonographic appearances. Anechoic/hypoechoic fluid is surrounded by echogenic tissues (moderate to increased echogenicity) with poorly defined margins.
- Consolidated lung has sonographic appearance similar to liver. Small irregular hyperechoic areas in consolidated lung may be because of small pockets of remaining gas. Liver has characteristic vessels and therefore can be differentiated from lung. Mirror image artefact does not occur in the face of pleural effusion.
- Pulmonary masses are round and may have variable echogenicity (hypo, hyper or mixed echogenicity). With the development of necrosis central region may become anechoic. Homogeneous or heterogeneous lung masses have smooth deep margin while lungs have more irregular margin.
- Small diaphragm rupture may not be detected. The presence of intestines and abdominal contents on thoracic side of the diaphragm is indicative of disruption of diaphragm. Normal diaphragm is sonographically visualized as curvilinear echogenic band surrounding the cranial margin of the liver. In normal dogs mirror image artefact of liver is suggestive of intact diaphragm (Fig.177). Asymmetric cranial hepatic margin is a common finding in diaphragmatic hernia.

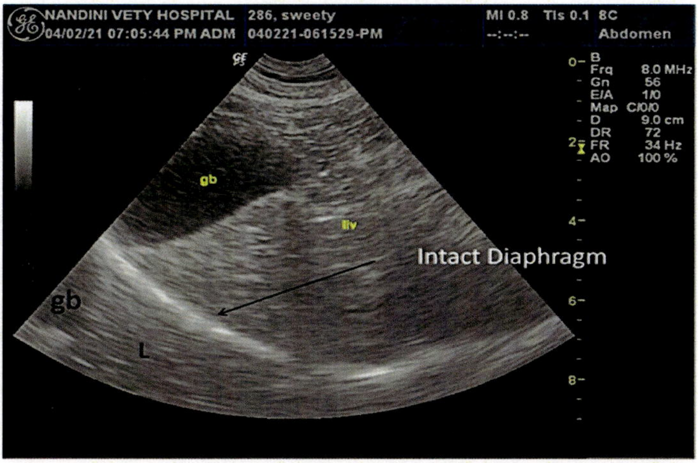

Fig. 177: Transabdominal sonogram (sagittal plane) of the liver in a normal dog. A curvilinear hyperechoic line along cranial margin of the liver (black arrow) is representing diaphragm. A mirror image artefact (gb and L) is creating the appearance of the gall bladder and liver cranial to the diaphragm. The mirror image artefact is suggesting that the diaphragm is intact.

- Thoracic wall lesions are usually neoplastic and arise from the tumours of the ribs.

References

Baldi, G., Gargani, L., Abramo, A., D'Errico, L., Caramella, D., Picano. E., Giuanta, F. and Forfori, F. (2012). Lung water assessment by lung ultrasonography in intensive care: A pilot study. Intensive Care Med. 39:74–84.

Murphy, H.D., Ward, J.L.,Viall, A.K.,Tropf, M.A.,Walton, R.L., Fowler, J.L., Ware, W.A. and DeFrancesco, T.C. (2021). Utility of point-of – care lung ultrasound for monitoring cardio-pulmonary edema in dogs. J.Vet. Internal Med. 35: 68-77.

Volpicelli, G., Mussa, A., Garofalo, G., Cardinale, L., Casoli, G., Parotto, F., Fava, C. and Frascisco, M. (2006). Bedside lung ultrasound in the assessment of alveolar-interstitial syndrome. Am.J. Emerg. Med.24:689–696.

Suggested Further Readings

Larson, M.M. (2009). Ultrasound of the Thorax (Non-cardiac). Vet. Clin. Small Anim. 39:733-745. doi:10.1016/j.cvsm.2009.04.006.

Mannion, P. (2006). Diagnostic Ultrasound in Small Animal Practice. Blackwell Science Ltd. Oxford, U.K

18

Sonographic Variations in Dogs and Cats

J.P. Varshney and P.S. Chaudhary

Abdominal organs in different species of animals have distinctive features with respect to their shape, size, location and echogenicity and echo texture. This is true for dogs and cats also. Therefore, information with respect to sonographic features of dogs cannot be taken for granted for cats in totality. It is essential for the Veterinarians engaged in sonography to have knowledge about sonographic differences in various organs in different species of animals. Major differences in sonographic features of important organs of dogs and cats are enumerated below:

Liver

- Liver of dogs is hypoechoic as compared to spleen. Portal veins have hyperechoic wall.
- Cat liver is isoechoic to falciform fat. In obese cats liver may appear hyperechoic. Portal veins are not much conspicuous.

Gall Bladder

- In dogs, cystic and bile ducts are not visualized to the level of the major duodenal papilla. Material within gall bladder is generally echogenic (Fig. 178A).
- In cats gall bladder can be bilobed. Cystic and bile ducts can be visualized to the level of major duodenal papilla. Normally gall bladder contents are not echogenic (Fig.178 B).

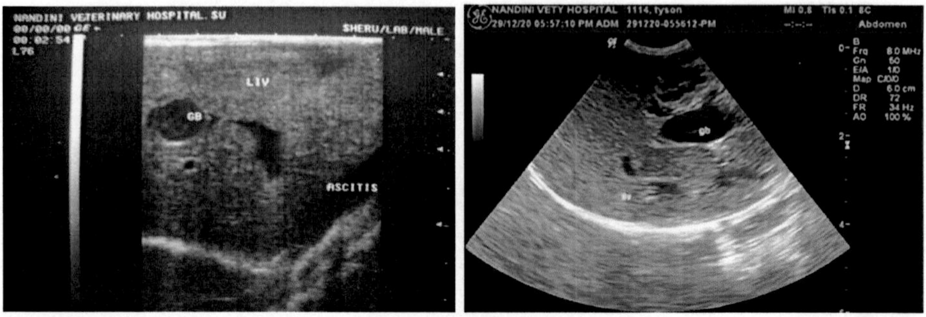

(A) **(B)**

Fig. 178: Comparative hepatic sonograms of dog**(A)** and cat **(B)**. Gall bladder content is slightly echogenic in the dog **(A)** while gall bladder contents of the cat is not echogenic **(B).**

Spleen

- Canine spleen (Fig.179 A) is variable in size. Location of craniodorsal extremity of the spleen varies depending on gastric distension. It is easy to locate spleen but difficult to trace entire spleen. The splenic portal veins are visualized along visceral surface.
- Feline spleen (Fig.179 B) is consistent in size and is lateral to the stomach. It is around 3 to 5 cm in size and about 1cm thick. Its echotexture is coarse. It is difficult to visualize as it is isoechoic to slightly hypoechoic to surrounding mesenteric fat. The splenic portal veins are less prominent but can be visualized with colour Doppler

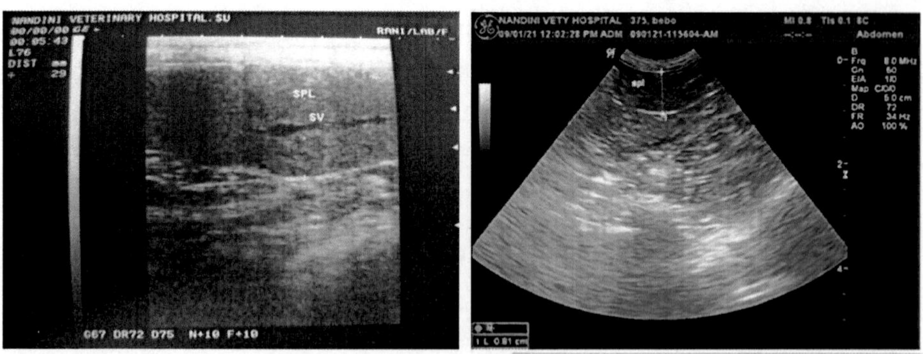

(A) **(B)**

Fig. 179: Comparative splenic sonogram of dog **(A)** and cat **(B)**. The Spleen of the dog is large, slightly hyperechoic and splenic vessel is visible (A) while spleen of the cat is small, comparatively hypoechoic and splenic vessel not prominent.

Kidneys

- Normally both kidneys are symmetrical with sharp zone of transition between cortex and medulla in dogs and cats. Cortex is relatively hyper echoic. Hyperechoic thin walled vessels are seen in renal diverticulum region.
- Kidney size in dogs depends on body conformation. An inner hyperechoic band is associated with renal cortex.
- An inner hyperechoic band associated with renal cortex is not seen in cats. Kidney size in cats is constant (approximately 3.5 to 4.5 cm). Fat deposit in renal sinus in cats is more than that of dogs. Kidneys of castrated male cats are more hyperechoic owing more fat deposition.

Urinary Bladder

- Wall layering of urinary bladder is difficult to visualize in healthy dogs and cats. The size of urinary bladder and wall thickness is variable and depends on the size of the dogs.
- Urinary bladder in felines is small in volume, consistent in size and contains suspended echogenic contents.

Prostate

- In dogs, prostate is located surrounding proximal urethra and visualized caudal to trigone area of the urinary bladder. It is uniformly hypoechoic and fusiform in neutered males and uniformly homogeneously hyperechoic and round in intact males.
- Feline prostate is not visible sonographically as it is not a discrete macroscopic structure.

Adrenals

- Adrenals of dogs are long and thin structures. Left one is peanut shaped in small dogs, and lawn chair shaped in medium and large dogs. Right one is oval shaped in small dogs, and V shaped in medium and large dogs. Mineralization of adrenals is visible in neoplastic masses.
- Adrenals of cats are oval/bean shaped, bilaterally symmetrical and hypoechoic in relation to the surrounding retroperitoneal fat. Cortex and medulla are not distinguishable. Mineralization of adrenals is an incidental finding.

Pancreas

- Normal pancreas is isoechoic to surrounding mesenteric fat in both cats and dogs.
- In dogs right lobe of pancreas is large as compared to left and is close to descending duodenum. Size of the pancreas varies depending on the size of the dogs. Normally pancreatic duct is not identifiable sonographically.
- In cats left lobe of pancreas is larger. Pancreatic duct is identifiable and is centrally located. Its diameter increases with age.

Stomach

- Gastric sub mucosal layer is thin in dogs. The presence of food material and /or gas limits evaluation of stomach in dogs. The pyloro-duodenal junction in dogs is in a more lateral position.
- Rugal folds of fundic region of the stomach in cats have hyperechoic prominent submucosal layer in cats. Gas is not common in gastrointestinal tract of cats. Pyloro-duodenal angle is narrower and more in a mid-line and dorsal in cats.

Duodenum

- Duodenum of dogs has a thicker mucosal layer than that of jejunum and its thickness varies according to weight of the dog.
- Mucosal layer of duodenum of cats is thin and similar to that of jejunum.

Ileum

- The muscular is, submucosal and mucosal layers of the ileum wall are more equal in thickness in dogs.
- The muscularis and submucosal layers of the ileum wall in cats are thicker than that of mucosal layer.

Cecum

- Cecum of the dogs is usually gas filled and its differentiation from ascending colon is difficult.
- Cecum of cats is not gas filled and can be differentiated from ascending colon.

Colon

- Colon is thinnest segment of gastrointestinal of dogs identifiable from pelvic inlet to the ileum.
- In cats colon is also thinnest segment of gastrointestinal tract identifiable from pelvic inlet to the ileum.

Anal Sacs

- Anal sacs are located on the both side of the rectum on dorsal image. Most surfaces of the anal sac tissue are surrounded by the hypoechoic external sphincter muscle.
- The anal sac tissue may occasionally appear as hyperechoic thin line.
- In dogs anal sacs are ellipsoidal
- In cats anal sacs are rounder.
- The normal anal sac contents of dogs appear as hypoechoic with diffuse point like hyperechoic debris.
- The normal anal sac contents of cats appear as more hyperechoic.

Abdominal Lymph Nodes

- In dogs medial iliac lymph nodes are fusiform and are sonographically identifiable.
- In cats normal medial iliac lymph nodes are sonographically not identifiable.
- The jejunal lymph nodes in dogs are oval /elongated and hypoechoic as compared to surrounding mesenteric fat. These nodes are much larger in puppies.
- The jejunal lymph nodes in cats are oval/bean shaped and hypoechoic as compared to surrounding mesentery. These glands are located on the right of the umbilicus, medial to the ileocecocolic junction and adjacent to the cranial mesenteric portal veins. The ileocolic lymph nodes in the cat are located near to the ileocecocolic junction.

19

Focused Assessment with Sonography for Trauma (FAST)

J.P. Varshney and P.S. Chaudhary

Focused assessment with sonography for trauma (abdominal and thoracic) refers to the limited ultrasound examination with the main focus on quick identification of the presence of free fluid within peritoneal, pleural and pericardial spaces in trauma cases in intensive care units. Despite limitations, findings of FAST are helpful in stabilizing the emergency patients.

- Focused assessment with sonography for trauma (FAST) came into being for the first time in human medicine as an extension of the physical examination by trauma surgeons in1990s.
- Use of focused assessment with sonography for trauma (FAST) in emergency cases in animals to detect free fluid in abdomen and thorax dates back to early 2000s (Boysen *et al.,* 2004, Lisciandro *et al*., 2008 and 2009, and Lisciandro, 2011). Now it is known as AFAST (Abdominal Focused Assessment with Sonography for Trauma) and TFAST (Thoracic Focused Assessment with Sonography for Trauma).
- Since then AFAST is being used as a tool to evaluate soft tissue abnormalities and ascites in abdomen in emergency trauma patients.
- AFAST is a screening tool that is being performed to assess free fluid and soft tissue abnormalities in all trauma patients to capture important problems that may otherwise be missed on physical examination.
- TFAST is used to identify the presence of fluid within pleural and pericardial spaces.
- AFAST and TFAST have also been used in non-traumatized cardiovascularly unstable and dyspnoeic dogs and cats in emergency and critical care settings to detect free fluid (McMurray *et al*., 2016).

- In emergency settings, use of AFAST and TFAST is being recommended as an extension of physical examination.

Scanning Protocol

- Emergency patients need not be shaved. Images can be obtained by parting fur and applying gel/alcohol on skin.
- Scanning can be done in standing, sternal or lateral recumbency position. Right lateral recumbency is a preferred position as echo and electrocardiography can also be performed, gall bladder and caudal vena cava can be visualized, and it is safe to perform abdominocentesis also.
- The transducer is placed in longitudinal scanning plane throughout AFAST scanning with marker towards head and screen marker to the left of screen. The transducer is moved and fanned at each FAST site to increase the sensitivity so that even small pockets of the free fluid can be detected.
- TFAST examination is performed in dogs and cats placed in alternating left and right lateral recumbency or sternal recumbency. Dyspnoeic animals should be given oxygen supplementation first and then scanned in sternal recumbency.
- Serial FAST examinations are helpful in detecting delayed fluid accumulation and also the progress of resolution of free fluid.

AFAST Windows to Evaluate Target Organs

- AFAST scanning is done through five windows (DH, SR, CC, HRU and FS) as shown in the Fig.180.
- Diaphragmatico-hepatic (DH) view- Transducer is placed just caudal to xiphoid. By fanning and rocking, liver, gall bladder, heart, lung, pleural cavity and caudal vena cava is examined.
- Spleno-renal (SR) and hepato-renal (HR) views- Transducer is placed just caudal to costal arch. By fanning and rocking, spleen and left kidney are examined.
- Cystocolic (CC) View – Transducer is placed just lateral to midline over caudal abdomen. By fanning and rocking urinary bladder and genitals are examined.
- Hepato-renal umbilical (HRU) and spleno-renal umbilical Views- Transducer is placed at the level of umbilicus. By fanning and rocking abdominal masses, small intestine and ileum are examined..

- Focused spleen (FS)- Transducer is used by sliding and fanning following the spleen cranially to caudally. Spleen extends from mid line to the left kidney. This window is used to visualize splenic parenchymal abnormalities, infarcts, masses and echogenicity (Dark Swiss cheese heterogeneous echogenicity rules out splenic torsion; Bright Swiss cheese heterogeneous echogenicity rules out lymphoma).

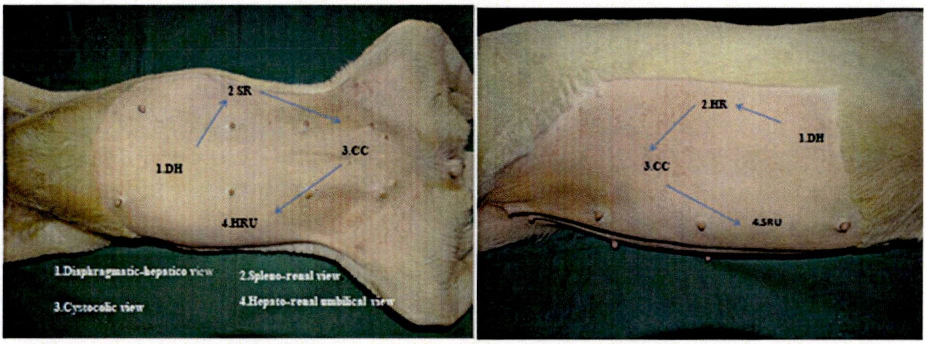

Fig. 180: Showing acoustic windows for scanning in right and left lateral recumbency.

Recording of AFAST Observations

- It has been suggested that the observations of AFAST scanning are better recorded as "suspect abnormalities" so that they are not assumed as diagnostic (for example as suspected mucocele, suspected renal pelvis dilation or suspected cystic calculi) and can be further assessed employing radiography, complete ultrasonography and other tests as needed.

Abdominal Fluid Scoring

- Abdominal fluid scoring is best done in lateral recumbency. However, it may be done in standing or sternal positions. If fluid is detected in sternal or standing position, then the dog/cat is placed in either right or left lateral recumbency. A cooling period of 3-4 minute is given before scoring so that free fluid is redistributed for valid score.
- Fluid is assessed in DH, SR, CC and HRU views and score is given as 0 (no fluid). ½ (weak positive, maximum dimension < 5 mm in cats, < 10 mm in dogs)) or 1 (strong positive, maximum dimension > 5 mm in cats, 10 mm in dogs). Add these score numbers together for a final score with a maximum of 4 (Lisciandro, 2020; Lisciandro *et al.*, 2020).
- Total score of<3 mm and > 3 mm are considered as small - volume haemorrhages and large- volume haemorrhage (effusion) respectively (Lisciandro, 2020).

Indications of Positive AFAST Findings

- AFAST scan in trauma cases is suggestive of blood. Nevertheless, ascites, urine, bile or other forms of peritonitis cannot be ruled out.

TFAST

- Focused echocardiography is done to assess pericardial space.
- Primary aim of TFAST is to detect the presence of gas within left/right pleural spaces.
- For identifying gas, the probe is placed dorso-lateral along the thoracic wall with probe notch pointing cranially within 7 to 9 intercostal spaces on both side. Pneumothorax can be detected only when pleural air is located directly beneath the transducer.
- Thoracic effusion (pleural and pericardial) has ultrasonographic features similar to peritoneal effusion.

References

Boysen, S.R., Rozanski, E.A., Tidwell, A.S., Holm, J.L. Shaw, S.P. and Rush, J.E. (2004). Evaluation of focused assessment with sonography for trauma protocol to detect abdominal fluid in dogs involved in motor vehicle accidents. J. Am. Vet. Med. Assoc. 225:1198-1204.

Lisciandro, G.R.(2011). Abdominal and thoracic focused assessment with sonography for trauma, triage, and monitoring in small animals. J.Vet. Emerg. Crit. Care. 21:104-122. doi:10.1111/j. 1476- 4431.2011.00626.x

Lisciandro, G.R. (2020). Cageside ultrasound in the emergency room and intensive care unit. Vet. Clin. North Am. Small. Anim. Pract. 50:1445-1467. doi:10.1016/j.cvsm.2020.07.013.

Lisciandro, G.R., Lagutchik. M,S., Mann, K.A., Voges, A.K. and Fosgate, G.T. (2008). Evaluation of a thoracic focused assessment with sonography for trauma (TFAST) protocol to detect pneumothorax and concurrent thoracic injury in 145 traumatized dogs. J. Vet. Emerg.Crit. Care. 18:258-269. doi:10.1111/j.1476-4431.2008.00312.x

Lisciandro, G.R., Lagutchik, M.S., Mann, K.A., Fosgate, G.T., Tiller, E.G., Cabano, N.R., Baur, L.D., Book, B.P. and Howard, P.K..(2009).

Evaluation of an abdominal fluid scoring system determined using abdominal focused assessment with sonography for trauma in 101 dogs with motor vehicle trauma. J. Vet. Emerg. Crit. Care. 19: 426-437. doi: 10.1111/j.1476-4431.2009.00459.x

Lisciandro, G.R., Fosgate, G.T., Romero, L.A., Hauke, S.M., and Bridgeman, C.H..(2020). The expected frequency and amount of free peritoneal fluid estimated using the abdominal FAST-applied abdominal fluid scores in healthy adult and juvenile dogs [published online ahead of print, November 11, 2020]. J. Vet. Emerg.Crit. Care. doi:10.1111/vec.13029 .

McMurray, J., Boysen, S. and Chalhaub, S. (2016). Focused assessment with sonography in nontraumatized dogs and cats in the emergency and critical care setting. J. Vet. Emerg. Crit. Care (San Antonio) 26:64-73. doi: 10.1111/vec.12376. Epub 2015 Oct 7.

Further Reading

Gillman, L. M., Ball, C.G., Panebianco, N., Al-Kadi, A. and Kirkpatrick, A.W. (2009). Clinician performed resuscitative ultrasonography for the initial evaluation and resuscitation of trauma. Scand. J. Trauma Resuscitation Emerg. Med. 17: 34. doi: 10.1186/1757-7241-17-34. PMC 2734531. PMID 19660123.

20

Sonographic Findings in Diseases: At A Glance

J.P. Varshney

Architecture of the organ is affected in the primary or secondary diseases of the organs. Ultrasonography plays a significant role in detecting the changes in the organs in various diseases. Significant sonographic variations from that of normal sonographic features in different organs in diseases are given below:

Diseases	Sonographic Findings
Ascites (Peritoneal Effusions)	Increased amount of anechoic fluid in peritoneum.
Liver Diseases	
Hepatitis/Liver congestion	Diffuse hypoechoic liver
Hepatic nodular hyperplasia	Hyperechoic/hypoechoic/mixed focal/multiple lesions in liver.
Hepatic cyst/abscess/	Focal/multiple hypoechoic lesion in liver.
haematoma	Abscess and haematomas may have mixed echoes also.
Hepatic lymphosarcoma	Focal/multiple or diffuse hypoechoic/hyper echoic lesion in the liver.
Hepatocellular carcinoma	Focal/multifocal hyperechoic lesions in liver.
Steroid hepatopathy	Hyperechoic lesion(s) in liver.
Fat deposits	Focal/multifocal hyperechoic lesions in liver.
Histoplasmosis	Diffuse hypoechoic liver.
Cirrhosis/fibrosis or lipidosis	Diffuse hyperechoic liver.

Intra hepatic porto-systemic	Patchy hyperechoic small areas.
Shunt	Small liver with detectable veins. Inhtrahepatic shunts between portal and hepatic vasculature.
Arterio-venous fistula	Dilated and tortuous vessels
Gall Bladder	
Sludge	Echogenic material gravitates to the dependent part of the gall bladder.
Tumours/Polyps	Pedunculated hyperechoic mass within gall bladder lumen and thickened G.B.wall.
Calculi /stone	Hyperechoic solitary structure with acoustic shadowing.
Cholecystitis	Odematous, thickened gall bladder wall giving double wall appearance.
Extra-hepatic billiary Obstruction	Dilation of common bile duct.
Mucocele	Linear echogenic striations (stellate or kiwi like) and distended gall bladder
Spleen	
Haemangiosarcoma and haematoma	Hypoechoic or mixed echoic lesion.
Acute haemorrhage	Echogenic owing to acoustic interfaces by aggregated erythrocytes.
Focal splenic infarcts	Marginated round or wedged shaped nodules around splenic periphery. Initially lesion is hypoechoic.
Venous congestion	Diffusely hypoechoic spleen.
Abscess	Encapsulated lesion with hypoechoic or mixed echotexture.
Nodular Hyperplasia	Hypoechoic to isoechoic nodular lesions/mass.
Myelolipomas	Rounded or irregularly shaped hyperechoic foci of variable sizes.
Dystrophic mineralization	Focal hyperechoic speckles and thin lines throughout splenic parenchyma.
Splenic torsion	Coarse, diffuse, lacy hypoechoic to anechoic parenchymal pattern with interspersed linear echoes or hypoechoic pattern with small hyperechoic speckles.
Lymphoma	Multiple hypoechoic nodules of different size (honeycomb pattern, moth eaten appearance, spotted spleen or leopard spots), or diffused increased/decreased echogenicity with coars echotexture.

Stomach

Stomach Dilatation	Thin wall, loss of layering and less distinct rugal folds.
	Gaseous dilatation show reverberation artefact.
Congenital hypertrophic pyloric stenosis	Circumferential thickening of pylorus, and thickening of muscularis layer.
Foreign Bodies (pyloric region)	Irregular shape bodies with strong acoustic shadowing.
Chronic hypertrophic pyloric gastropathy	Increased thickness of muscular layer and pyloric wall.
Gastritis	Diffuse mild to moderate gastric wall thickening without loss of wall layering.
Neoplasm	Focal loss of gastric wall layering with wall thickening.
Eosinophilic sclerosing fibroplasia in cat	Focal mass lesion with mural thickening at pyloric antrum and loss of wall layering.
Uremic Gastritis	Thickened gastric wall with a hyperechoic line in mucosal and submucosal layer.

Intestines

Lymphoma in cats	Focal or multiple masses with thickened wall and loss of layering.
Adenocarcinoma in cats	Circumferential transmural thickening and loss of layering.
Intussusception	Multi-layered appearance in longitudinal plane. Concentric ring appearance in transverse plane.
Adenocarcinoma (Large intestine)	Nodular pedunculated mass. Circumferential transmural thickening with loss of wall layering pattern.
Mast cell tumour (Colon of cats)	Focal or diffuse wall thickening.
Fungal colitis	Focal wall thickening or masses.
Inflammatory bowel disease	Mild to moderate symmetrical wall thickening, diffuse echogenic mucosa or presence of bright mucosal speckles.
Anal sac tumour	Circumscribed or infiltrative masses of increased echogenicity.

Pancreas

Acute pancreatitis	Enlarged hypoechoic structure is seen ventral to the portal

	vein, medial to the right kidney and adjacent to duodenum.
Chronic pancreatitis	Thickened hyperechoic/ heterogeneous pancreas
Necrotizing pancreatitis	Hypo to anechoic regions in pancreas due to haemorrahge or necrosis.
Insulinomas	Small solitary or multiple hypoechoic nodules within pancreas.
Pancreatic cysts	Round anechoic structures with distal enhancement.
Pancreatic abscess	Thick irregular wall structures with distal acoustic shadowing and reverberation artefacts.
Pancreatic oedema	Tiger stripe appearance of pancreas (multiple anechoic areas).
Urinary Tract	
Cystic kidney	Rounded anechoic smooth sharply demarcated thin walled structures in kidney.
Haematomas	Structures with mixed echoic contents within renal cortex or medulla.
Abscess in kidney	Poorly demarcated cavity having irregular contours, sedimentation, echoes and variable degree of distal acoustic enhancement .
Renal infarcts	Well defined wedge shaped cortical lesions. Chronic infarcts are hyperechoic with focal cortical depression.
Nephrocalcinosis	Hyper attenuating foci with distal acoustic shadowing.
Renal Tumours	Homogeneous/heterogeneous; hypoechoic/ isoechoic /hyperechoic; regular/irregular margin; hypoechoic halo at the periphery of the cortex; hyperechoic foci or striations throughout the medulla; hypoechoic medullary or cortical nodules or masses.
Chronic interstitial	Small, irregular and diffusely hyperechoic kidney nephritis having no cortico-medullary demarcation.
Hydronephrosis	Renal diverticuli appear as anechoic finger like projections extending from anechoic renal pelvis.
Ureterocele	Thin walled round structure containing an anechoic fluid within the neck of urinary bladder.
Cystic calculi	Variable sized spheric and hyperechoic curvilinear interface with distal acoustic shadowing and sedimenting in the dependent portion of the bladder.
Blood clot	Irregular shaped hyperechoic material without distal acoustic shadowing in the urinary bladder.

Chronic cystitis	Thickened bladder wall with irregular mucosal surface.
Transitional cell carcinoma	Heterogeneously hyperechoic/isoechoic/ hypoechoic irregular mass with broad based attachment projecting into bladder lumen.
Urethral calculi	Small curvilinear hyperechoic foci with distal acoustic shadowing.
Prostatitis	
i.Acute	Loss of homogenous echo pattern. Symmetrical /asymmetrical enlargement. Hypoechoic appearance of the parenchyma.
ii. Chronic	Parenchyma shows patchy increased echogenicity with focal echogenic regions. In unresolved chronic cases, patchy hypoechoic areas may appear and with time coalesce as small fluid filled irregularly marginated areas suggesting micro abscesses.
Benign Hyperplasia of prostate (BHP)	Loss of homogenous echo pattern. Early cases may show symmetrical enlargement with an overall increased echogenicity. It may be patchy. If gland is significantly enlarged, it bulges outside and may lose its bi-lobed appearance.
Prostatic cysts	Rounded thin walled anechoic areas. Small intra -prostatic cysts are seen in early cases of BHP. In long standing cases these cysts become large and may protrude from the margin of the gland. Large para-prostatic cysts are attached by a thin stalk like structure having anechoic fluid that may become more echogenic with sediment.
Prostatic abscess	Rounded thick walled anechoic/hypoechoic areas with moderate posterior acoustic enhancement.
Prostate neoplasia	Loss of homogenous echo pattern. Early cases may have focal hypoechoic lesions which are difficult to differentiate from other prostatic pathology. In later stage, the gland becomes asymmetrical with irregular margins and markedly hyperechoic heterogeneous parenchyma with irregular anechoic regions and zone of calcification creating acoustic shadowing.

Uterus	
Hydrometra/mucometra	Anechoic fluid in uterine lumen.
Pyometra	Thickened uterine wall with anechoic contents in uterine lumen.
Tumour	Different echogenic mass projecting in the uterine lumen.
Ovaries	
Cystic ovaries	Thin walled anechoic fluid filled structures within ovaries with distal acoustic enhancement.
Ovarian tumour	Variable size mass with complex internal architecture.
Vagina	
Tumour	Hyperechoic mass in vaginal passage.
Testicles	
Orchitis	Hypoechoic echogenicity of testicles.
Cysts	Anechoic fluid filled structures with posterior acoustic enhancement.
Hydrocele	Testicles having typical anechoic area.
Torsion of spermatic cord	Also known as testicular torsion. Early changes spermatic chord are associated with enlargement of epididymis and presence of hydrocele.
	Testicular and spermatic chord enlargement with decreased parenchymal echogenicity may be observed.
Thyroid Glands	
Primary hypothyroidism	An irregular outline of the gland with hypoechoic parenchyma and decreased size and volume.
	Round to oval shape thyroid lobes in transverse plane.
Muscle, Tendon, Joints and Subcutaneous Tissue	
Subcutaneous oedema	Cobble stone appearance layering with hypoechoic fluid.
Acute Tendon Injury	Hypoechoic changes within tendon.
Chronic Tendon injury	Hyperechoic changes within tendon.
Nervous System	
Hydrocephalus	Enlargement of ventricular system and atrophy or hypoplasia of surrounding nervous tissue.
Brain tumour	Hyperechoic lesion.
Spinal cord Trauma	Hyperechoic changes

Ophthalamic Diseases	
Hyphema	Echogenic change in anechoic anterior chamber.
Cataract	Thickening of anterior and posterior surfaces of the lens. During an early stage hyperechoic line within lens and echogenic anterior or posterior cortices.
Clot in Vitreous chamber	Amorphous echogenic heterogeneous mass.

Section 3: Other Animals

21

Ultrasound In Ruminants

J.P. Varshney and P.S. Chaudhary

For the sake of convenience ruminants are broadly divided into two categories as large ruminants and small ruminants. Large ruminants consist of cattle and buffaloes and small ruminants consist of goats and sheep. Sonography is becoming an important part of diagnostic modalities in ruminants also. Its major use in ruminants is in reproduction and lameness.

Large Ruminants

- Sonography in cattle and buffaloes is mainly used in the field of reproduction and lameness.
- Its transabdominal use to visualize gastrointestinal tract is very much limited. Efforts have been made to use transabdominal ultrasound in the diagnosis of peritonitis, abomasal displacement (left and right), abscesses, paralytic ileus and intussusception etc.
- Ultrasound can also be used in variety of non-reproductive imaging such as thoracic ultrasound can be used to investigate respiratory disease, teat ultrasound to investigate difficult milkers or reticulum ultrasound to investigate suspected hardware disease or motility disturbances, or top line ultrasound for a more objective measure of body condition score (Pothmann *et al.,* 2015).
- Ultrasound examination at the base of the ear (Fig.181), using a 7.5MHz linear probe, can detect subclinical otitis in calves and is quite specific for diagnosing clinical cases of otitis (Bernier Gosselin *et al*., 2014).

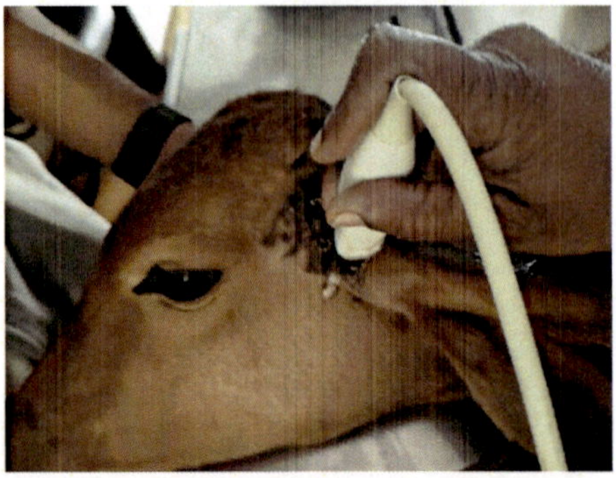

Fig. 181: Showing sonographic examination of ear canal of a calf. The transducer is placed caudal to the vertical mandibular ramus, and ventral to the base of ear.

- A rectal probe can be used to diagnose lung disease before the onset of clinical signs in neonatal calves with 94% sensitivity and 100% specificity (Ollivett *et al.*, 2015).
- The musculoskeletal system can also be examined with a rectal probe. It can be used to image gross evidence of extension of deep digital sepsis up to a flexor tendon sheath, or for differentiation between causes of swellings associated with lameness (Kofler *et al.,* 2014).

Ultrasound Technique and Windows

Trans abdominal Ultrasound

- Trans abdominal ultrasonographic imaging in cattle and buffaloes can be done in standing position without any sedation.
- A 3.5 to 5.0 MHz convex transducer is appropriate to examine peritoneum, abomasum, duodenum, jejunum and colon.
- The abdominal area is marked into six ultrasonographic windows (Zone 1 to zone 6) based on anatomy in healthy animals (Fig.182 and183) as described by Munday and Mudron (2016).
- Zone-1 is on the left side extending from tuber coxae to the 6th to 8^{th}intercostal space containing rumen and reticulum.
- Zone-2 is on the left (2L) and right (2R) side of the sternum, in the ventral third of the abdomen extending from 6th to 9th intercostal space, with dorsal border at the level of 10 cm above the olecranon and ventral border at the level of olecranon.

- The omasum is in the zone -3 that extends from the 7th to 10^{th}intercostals space on the right side.
- Zone -4 has abomasum, pylorus and part of cranial duodenum. It extends approximately from 10 cm caudal to the xyphoid process of the sternum and to the right paramedian region of the ventral midline to the level of the umbilicus.
- Zone -5, containing liver and cranial duodenum, is in the dorsal half of the abdomen, extends from transverse process of the thoracic vertebrae dorsally to the level of the articulation humeri ventrally from the 10th - 12^{th}intercostals space.
- Zone -6 extends from the 10th inter costal space to the tuber coxae and is divided in to A, B and C subzones.

  Zone 6A extends from transverse process of the lumbar vertebrae dorsally to at the level of the articulation humeri ventrally and contains the colon.

  Zone 6B extends from at the level of the articulation humeri dorsally to the level of the articulation cubiti ventrally and contains jejunum and parts of the colon.

  Zone 6C extends from the level of the articulation cubiti dorsally to the linea alba ventrally and contains loops of the jejunum.
- Area for scanning is prepared by cleaning, shaving and applying acoustic gel as described earlier.

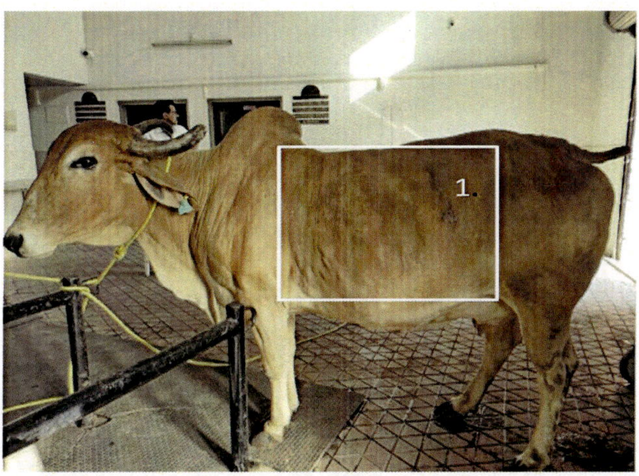

Fig. 182: Left side of the cow showing zone **1. Zone 1** is accoustic window for screening rumen and reticulum.

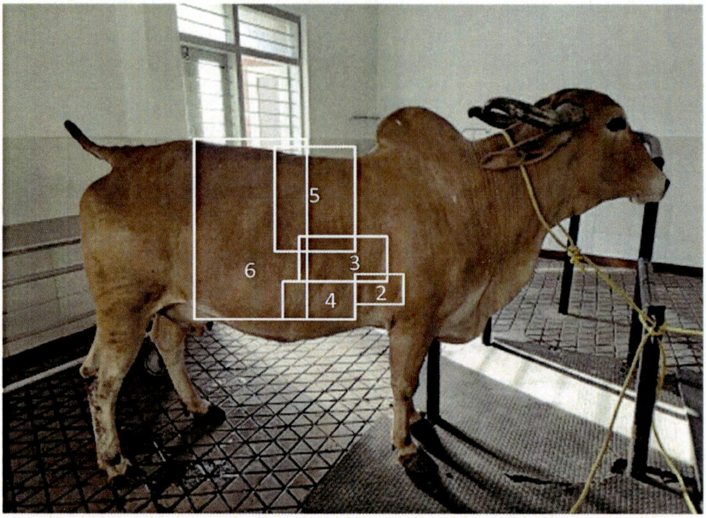

Fig. 183: Right side of the cow showing zone **2, 3, 4, 5 and 6.** The **Zone 2** is accoustic window for screening reticulum. **Zone 3** is accoustic window for screeing omasum. **Zone 4** is accoustic window for screening abomasum, pylorus and some part of cranial duodenum. **Zone 5** is accoustic window for screening liver and cran ial duodenum. **Zone 6** is accoustic window for screening. **Zone 6** is accoustic window for screening jejunum and colon.

Umbilicus Ultrasound

- This is a simple, valuable, technique for imaging the contents of an umbilical or inguinal hernia.
- Umbilicus ultrasound is performed in calves in standing position.
- The site is prepared by clipping/shaving and soaking the site with gel or alcohol.
- The transducer is pressed perpendicular to the long axis of the body, against the extra abdominal portion of the umbilical defect. Examination is done by slowly sliding the transducer cranially and caudally.
- Umbilical remnant infections, appear as a tube or cord
- Infected umbilical vein remnants travel cranially toward the liver.
- Urachal remnants travel caudally toward the apex of the urinary bladder.
- Infected umbilical artery remnants are traced caudally and may continue around the urinary bladder toward the aorta.

Thoracic Ultrasound

- It can be used to screen calves at risk for pneumonia before anaesthesia for surgical procedures.
- The calf is restrained appropriately. Hair clipping/ shaving of the site is done to improve the quality of images.
- The lung field can be visualized from 10th to 1^{st}intercostal space on the right, and from 10th to 2 ndintercostal space on the left.
- The probe is pressed between and parallel to the ribs, starting at the caudo-dorsal margin of the lung field.
- The footprint of the probe can be angled slightly cranially or caudally to keep the image between the ribs.
- The aerated lung surface creates a hyperechoic line, and reverberation artefact beyond the line. The line slide back and forth with inspiration and expiration and referred as the, "glide sign". Echogenic line produced by ribs needs to be differentiated from that produced by lung surface by slight repositioning or fanning of the probe
- Each rib space is scanned from the dorsal lung margin, just below the epaxial musculature to the ventral margin of the lung.
- Positioning the probe between elbow and thorax facilitate examination of cranial lung.
- In cranial lung the thymus needs to be differentiated from consolidated lung. The thymus is not continuous with the lung surface and does not move with the lung.
- Normal lung surface appears as the smooth echogenic gliding hyperechoic line.
- Fluid in the thorax appears as anechoic space between the thoracic wall and the lung surface.
- Roughened pleura are visualized as an irregular echogenic line with irregular reverberations (comet tails).
- Abscess or consolidation in lungs is visualized as less echogenic lesion in the lung surface. Large consolidated areas are visualized similar to liver.

Per Rectal Ultrasound

- This window is commonly used to examine reproductive tract of the bovine.
- Bovine rectal probes are linear of 4.5 to 10 MHz frequency. Low frequency curvilinear rectal probes have greater penetration.
- Acoustic gel is applied on the transducer and it is covered with plastic sleeve (Fig.184) and then inserted into the rectum with the help of the hand (Fig, 185) to scan the organs.

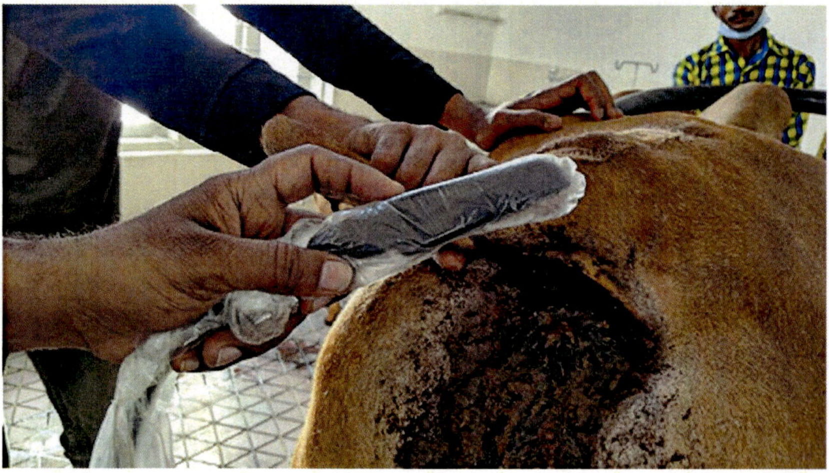

Fig. 184: Rectal probe is placed in a plastic sleeve

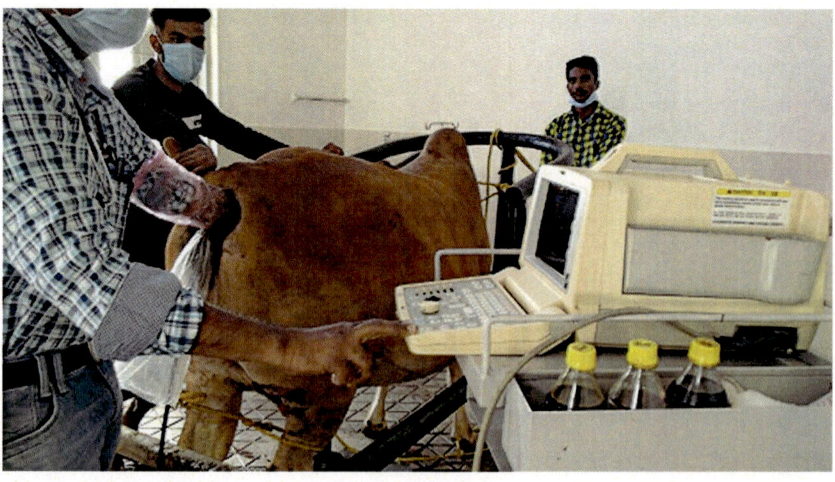

Fig. 185: Showing transrectal sonography in a cow

- In addition to reproductive tract examination, the urinary tract ,bony pelvis , portions of the small and large intestines, or even abdominal fat necrosis (Tharwat *et al.*, 2012), can also be examined during a rectal ultrasound.

Sonographic Features of the Organs in Ruminants

- Rumen wall appears as a thick echogenic line adjacent to left abdominal wall .Rumen wall (Fig.186) is generally 5 to 6 mm thick except at ruminal groove. Wall layering of rumen is not distinct. Ruminal ingesta appears as anechoic to hypoechoic interspersed with gas and fluid Fig.186). Internal reverberation artefacts (Fig.189) suggests gaseous zone in dorsal rumen sac.

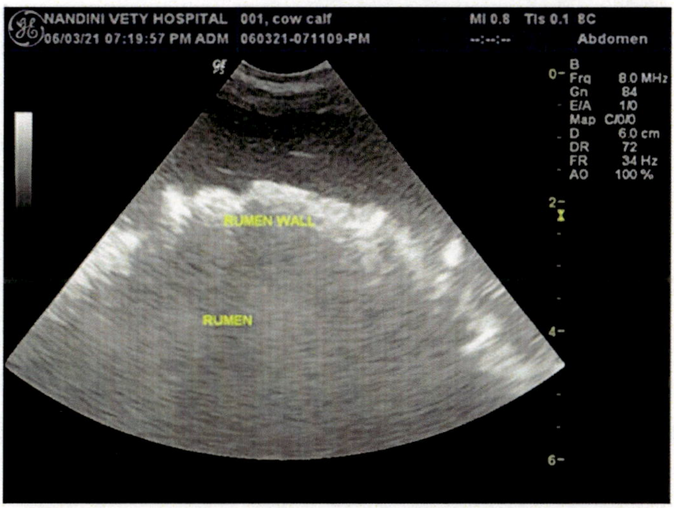

Fig. 186: Trans abdominal sonogram of the rumen of a cow calf showing wall of the rumen and ingesta

- Reticular wall (Fig.187) is slightly less thick (4 to 5 mm) than that of rumen.

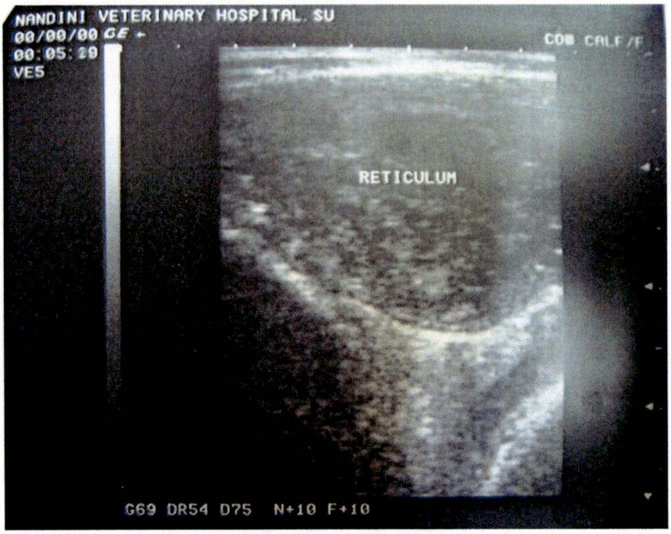

Fig. 187: Trans abdominal sonogram of reticulum of a cow showing reticulum, it's wall and ingesta.

- Omasal wall is slightly less thick (3 to 4.5 mm) than that of reticulum.
- Abomasal wall (Fig.188) is slightly less thick (2 to 2.5 mm) than that of omasum.

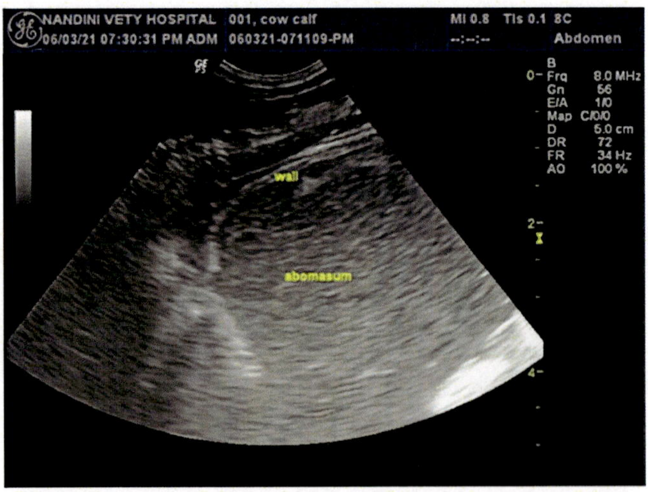

Fig. 188: Transabdominal sonogram of abomasum of a cow.

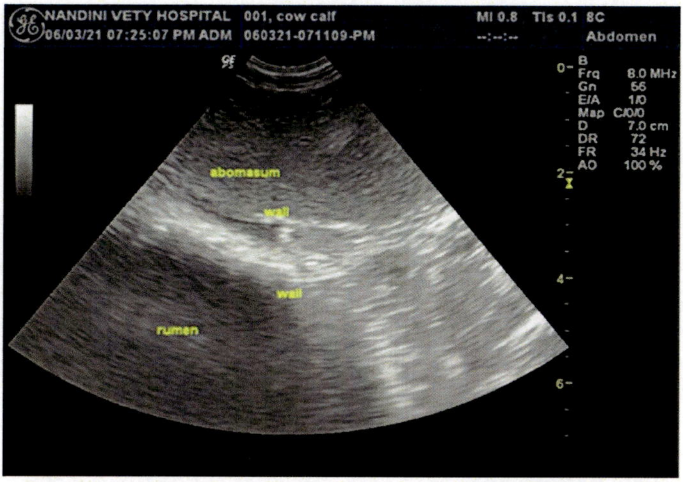

Fig. 189: Transabdominal sonogram of a cow showing rumen and abomasum. Difference in the thickness of the wall of the rumen and abomasum can easily be appreciated. Internal reverberation artefacts in the rumen suggests the gaseous zone.

- The spleen (Fig. 190) is homogeneous in echo texture and contains small regular anechoic blood vessels.

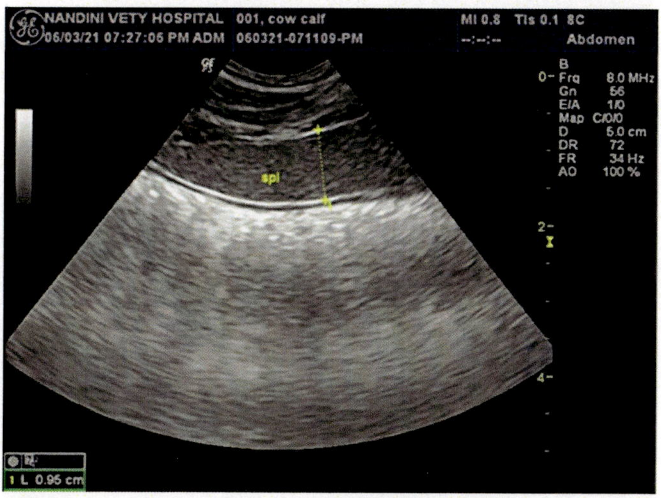

Fig. 190: Transabdominal sonogram of the spleen of the cow calf. The spleen appears as homogeneously echogenic structure.

- The liver in large ruminants is less homogeneous and more hypo echoic than the spleen. Portal vein has echogenic wall (Fig.191 A). Gall bladder appears anechoic fluid filled structure (Fig.191 B).

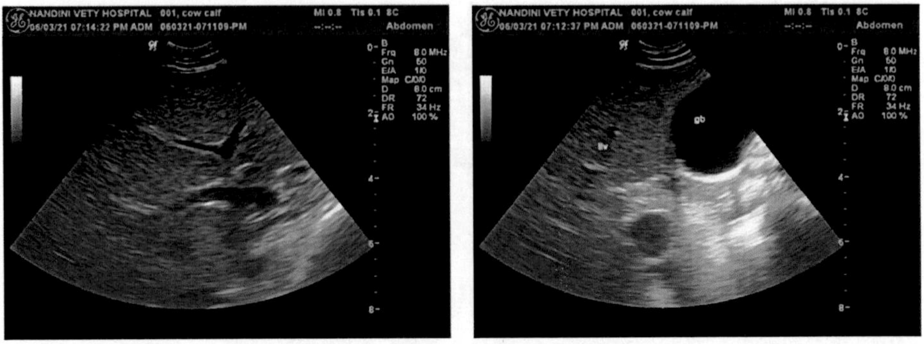

(A) **(B)**

Fig. 191: Transabdominal sonograms of a cow showing liver **(A)** and gall bladder **(B)**.

- In cows renal parenchyma is hypoechoic (Fig.192) and is less echogenic than that of liver. Renal sinus is hyperechogenic. Renal pyramids are hypoechoic areas in renal parenchyma. Kidneys are approximately of 10 x 5 cm size.

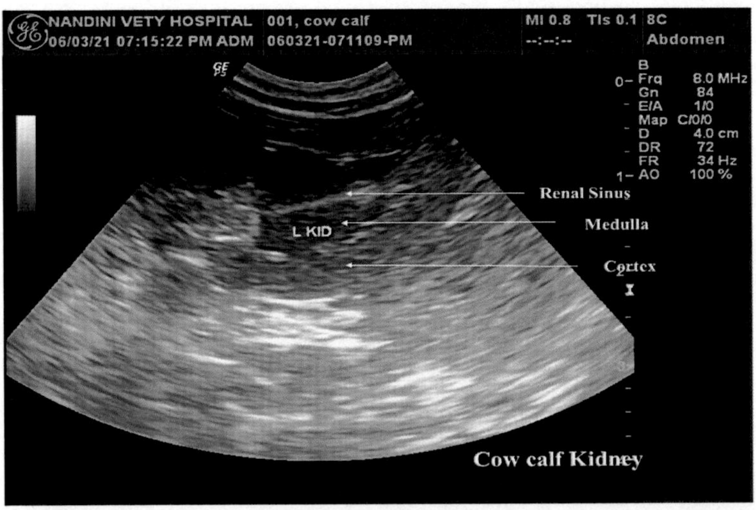

Fig. 192: Sonogram of the left kidney of a cow calf imaged through right paralumbar fossa keeping the transducer parallel to the longitudinal axis .Renal pelvis appears echogenic. Medulla is hypoechoic and cortex is more echogenic than medulla. The echogenic appearance of ruminants kidney is almost similar to that of canines.

Sonographic Features of Gastro intestinal Diseases

- Left side displacement of abomasum leads to displacement of intestines and liver cranially and ventrally in the right abdomen.

- In cattle with paratuberculosis, jejunum is displaced in zone 3 from zone 6B and 6C and wall thickness increases 3 to 4 times.
- For vagus indigestion reticulum is imaged at the cranial most portion of the abdomen. Its caudal border creates a cleft as it lies against the rumen. Luminal contents are not imaged due to gas produced by bacteria along the wall.
- Ventral abdominal approach just behind xiphoid is not appropriate to scan liver in caprine because of gas in rumen and intestines.
- Visualizing through last intercostal approach (lateral abdominal wall) facilitates scanning of major portion of the liver in caprine.
- Sonographic features of hepatic parenchyma, vasculature and biliary system of caprine are similar to canines. But images are of a little inferior quality.
- Sonography is generally recommended to identify *Echinococcus granulosis* cysts in the liver of sheep. The cysts appear as anechoic, rounded, unilocular structure with ellipse circumference of about 2 to 5 cm diameter and well defined borders. The contents of the cysts are hypoechoic. The interior of the cysts may contain echogenic particulate material.
- In large ruminants (cows and buffaloes) hepatic sonography may facilitate the diagnosis of hepatic abscesses, fatty degeneration and obstructive cholestasis.
- In goats the kidneys are imaged in standing position from lateral abdomen at paralumbar fossa by placing transducer cranio-dorsally. Left kidney is easily visualized. Sonographically kidney is visualized as having hyperechoic central zone, hypoechoic medulla and intermediate cortex. Kidneys are located easily in transverse plane.
- Per rectal approach is taken to image kidneys and urinary bladder in large ruminants. A 6 to 8 MHz rectal transducer is appropriate.
- In cases of traumatic reticulitis, reticulum wall becomes thick and reticular echogenicity increases.
- In acute omphalitis, umbilical cord is homogeneous and hypoechoic. While in purulent cases it is hyperechoic.
- An anechoic area touching umbilical area in the abdomen is seen in urachal fistula. Bladder wall becomes thick and anechoic fluid is seen in urachus lumen .

Bovine Reproductive Tract

- Per rectal approach is more appropriate.
- Ultrasonography is useful in diagnosing cystic ovaries (Fig.193). Follicular cysts are large (> 25 mm), non-echogenic with very thin wall. While luteal cysts appear as nonechogenic areas (Fig.194) surrounded by echogenic tissues of varying thickness.

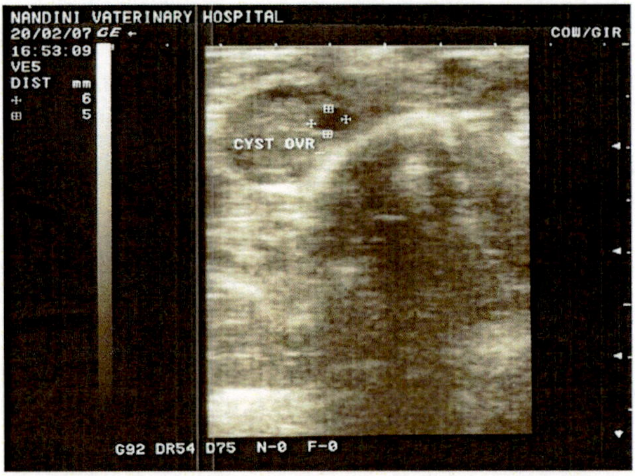

Fig. 193: Transrectal sonogram of a Gir cow showing anechoic rounded structure in the ovary suggesting ovarian cyst.

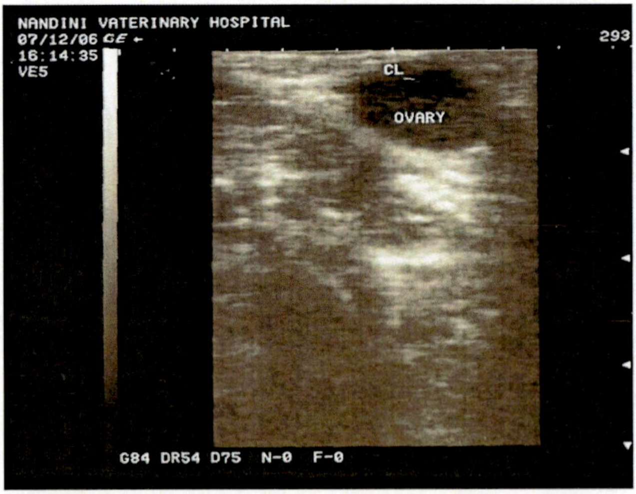

Fig. 194: Transrectal sonogram of a cow showing ovary with corpus luteum.

- Sonography is being commonly used to detect pregnancy in ruminants (Fig, 195).

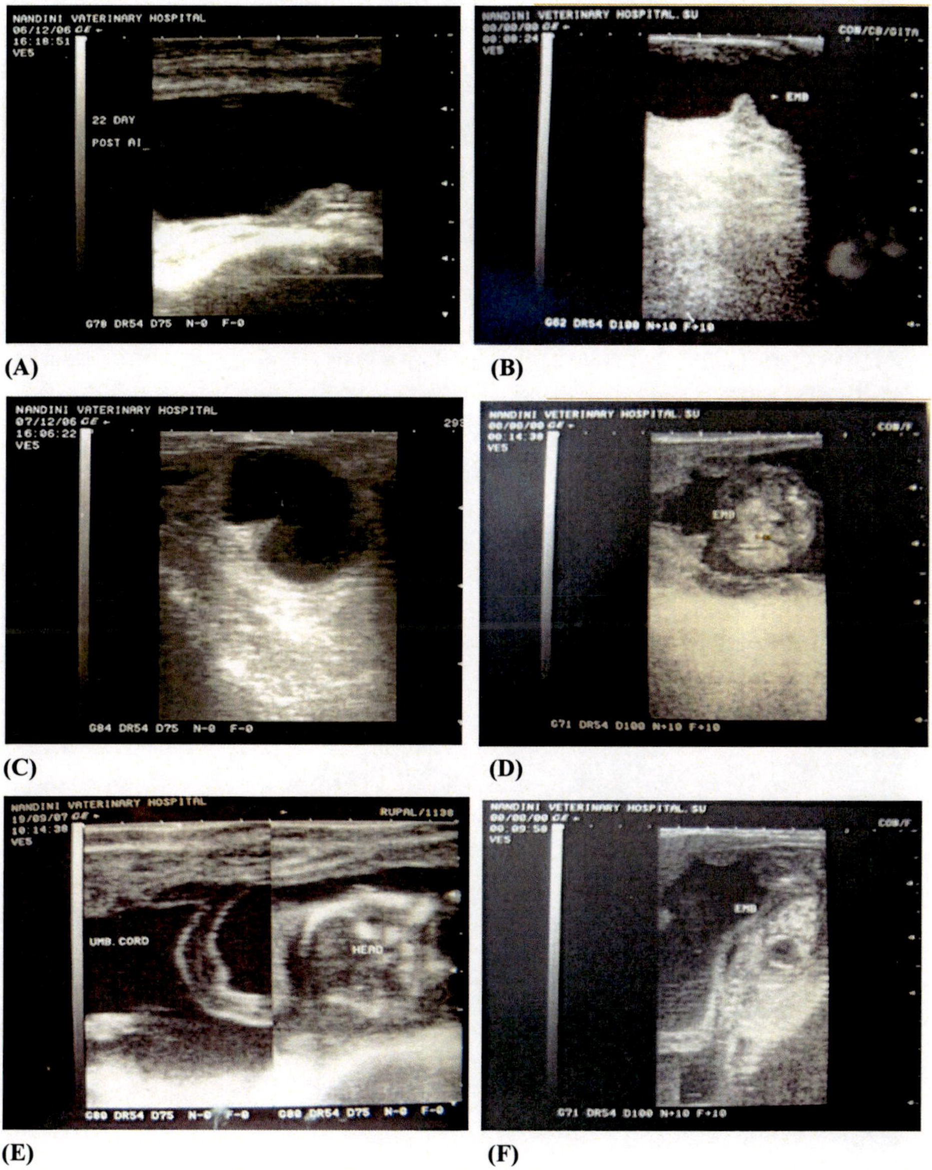

(A) (B) (C) (D) (E) (F)

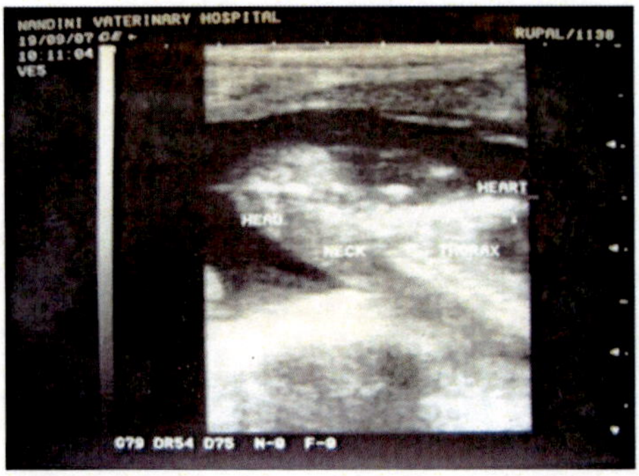

(G)

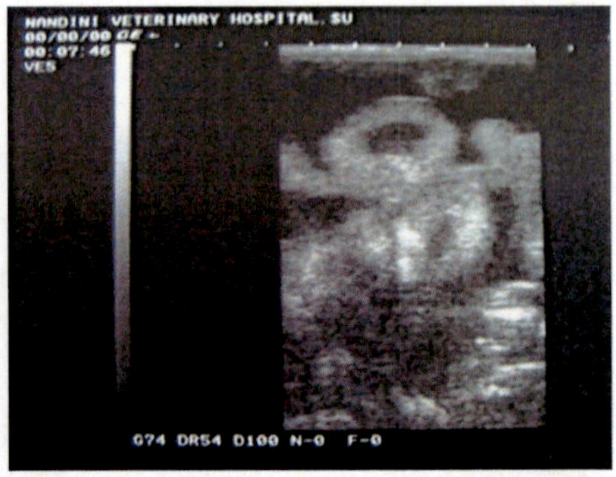

(H)

Fig. 195: Transrectal sonogram of cows showing approximately different stages of pregnancy post artificial insemination (A.I.). A = 22 days post A.I., B = 25 days post A.I., C = 27 days post A.I., D= 30 days post A.I., E = 40 days post A.I., F= 45 days post A.I., G = 56 days post A.I., and H= cotyledons

- Sonography can be used in bovines to diagnose endometritis, pyometra (Fig.196), mucometra, cervicitis (Fig.197), an early embryonic mortality (Fig.198) and mummified and macerated fetuses. The uterus is distended and lumen is filled (varying grades) with partially echogenic snowy patches in inflammatory conditions of uterus. Visualization of fragments in uterine lumen indicates foetal remnants. Macerated foetal conditions can be identified by suspended echogenic particles in foetal fluid and thickened uterine wall. Uterine fluid is absent and foetal mummy appears as poorly defined echogenic mass in cases of mummified fetuses.

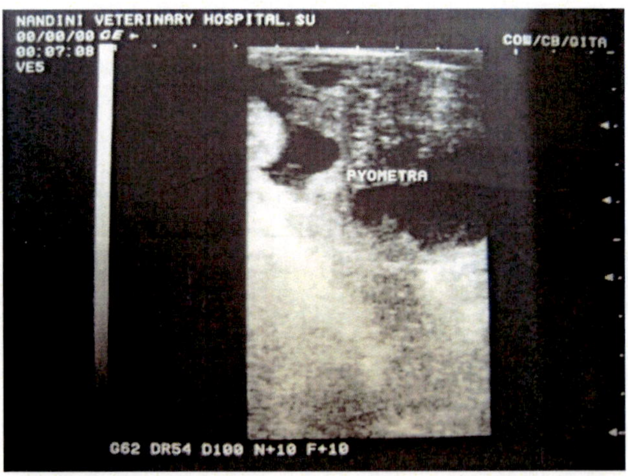

Fig. 196: Transrectal sonogram of a cow showing anechoic/hypoechoic fluid filled pockets in the uterine lumen with hyperechoic thickened uterine wall suggesting pyometra.

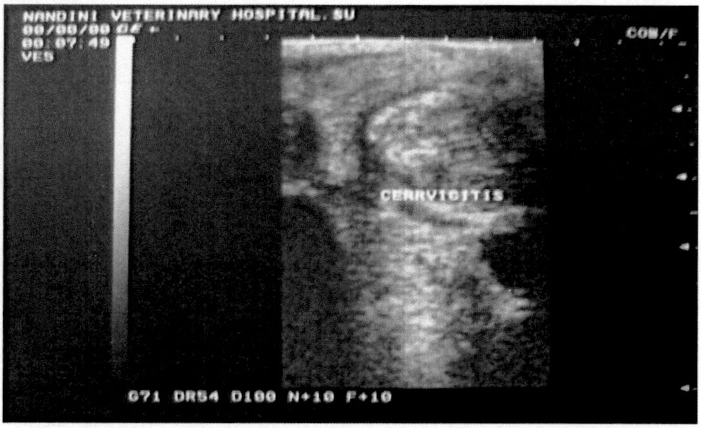

Fig. 197: Trans rectal sonogram of a cow showing hyperechoic thickened cervix suggesting chronic cervicitis

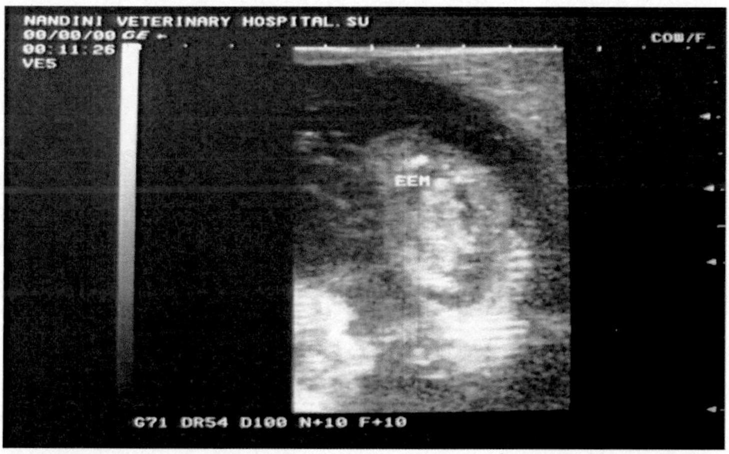

Fig. 198: Transrectal sonogram of a cow at 40 day pregnancy showing an embryo without heart beat suggesting an early embryonic mortality.

- Testis and scrotum can be imaged in domestic animals using sector transducer of 6 MHz in standing position.
- Parenchyma of normal testis is homogeneous with coarse medium echo texture.
- The epididymis is less echogenic than testicular parenchyma.
- The mediastinum testis is visualized as central linear hyperechoic structure of varying echogenicity.

- The scrotal septum can be visualized as highly echogenic line between testicles.
- The scrotal skin is visualized as a thick hyperechoic structure encircling the testicles.

Ovum or Oocyte Pick-up Technology

- An ultrasonic guided aspiration of bovine follicular oocytes was first proposed in Denmark in 1987 (Callesen *et al.*, 1987) and real OPU was first established in cattle in 1988 by a Dutch team (Pieterse *et al.*, 1991).
- *In vitro* fertilization, production of cloned or transgenic animals and creation of oocyte banks have increased the scope of sonography.
- Ultrasound guided transvaginal ovum pick up (USG-TV-OPU) technique has revolutionized the embryo transfer industry.
- Oocyte pick up (OPU) is an ultrasound guided technique in which oocytes are aspirated using a needle connected to a suction pump.
- An OPU device consists of a scanner, transducer, needle guidance system and suction apparatus. A 19-g disposable long needle is connected to silicone tubing by means of a stainless steel connector. The system is inserted into a stainless tube. The needle guidance system is incorporated into OPU device together with transducer (transvaginal convex transducer of 5 to 7.5 MHz) of an ultrasonographic scanner (real time B- mode scanner) with a unilateral scanning field.
- The animal is controlled in a standing position in cattle crate. Faeces are removed by back racking. Perineal area and vulva are washed and clean thoroughly. An epidural analgesia is given using 2% xylocaine hydrochloride. A transducer covered with latex sleeve is inserted into vagina and each ovary is scanned to visualize the number and size of the follicles. By one hand left ovary is hold through per rectal palpation and by another hand transducer is taken forward and ovary is positioned against the head of the transducer. By manipulation follicle is positioned on puncture line. A small quantity of flushing medium is sucked into the needle before placing it into needle guiding system. The needle is pushed through vaginal wall into the follicle. A constant vacuum pressure (50 mm Hg) is applied till follicle is disappeared from the monitor. The procedure is repeated for the adjacent follicles and for other ovary.

Bovine Mammary Glands

- Imaging of udder and teats is another important area of the application of sonography in bovine medicine.
- Use of ultrasonography as teat and udder diagnostic modality is comparatively of recent origin.
- Sonographic examination of mammary gland as a whole was first carried out by Caruolo and Mochrie (1967) as an A –mode sonography using 1MHz transducer. In 1986 Cartee and his associates tested B-mode sonography to diagnose milk flow disturbances (Klein *et al.*, 2005). Later teat examination were made using 3.5 to 5 MHZ transducers (Seeh *et al.*,1996).
- Diagnosis of many pathological conditions of mammary system is facilitated by sonography which is otherwise difficult.
- Ultrasonography is a helpful in detecting pathological alterations of the udder such as inflammation, mucosal lesions, tissue proliferation, foreign bodies, milk stones, congenital changes, hematoma, and abscess.
- Ultrasonography of the teat allows localization and demarcation of the extent of pathological changes.
- Udder and teat sonography is performed in standing position. Surface is prepared by shaving, cleaning, disinfecting and applying gel.
- Linear or sector transducers of 5 to 10 MHz are appropriate for udder and teat sonography.A high frequency probe (7.5-10.0 MHz) yields better result in visualizing the teat structures (teat canal, rosette of Fuerstenberg, teat cistern, gland cistern). A 5.0 MHz probe yields better result in visualizing the glandular parenchyma.
- Saline infusion or water bath technique improves the visualization of teats.
- The probe is placed on the caudal and lateral surface directly on the teat (Fig.199) and udder skin. Scanning is done by placing transducer transversely and longitudinally to the udder.

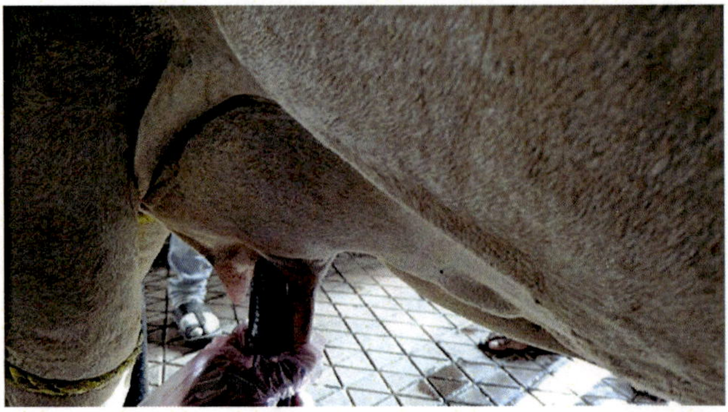

Fig. 199: Scanning of teat and udder by direct placement of transducer

- Teat is better examined using water bath technique (Fig. 200). It is done by immersing the teat into a plastic bag or cup filled with hot water (30-37 °C). The probe is placed on the cup, or build into the cup. The teat is examined horizontally by placing the probe at a right angle to the axis of the teat, or in a vertical position with the probe parallel to the teat.

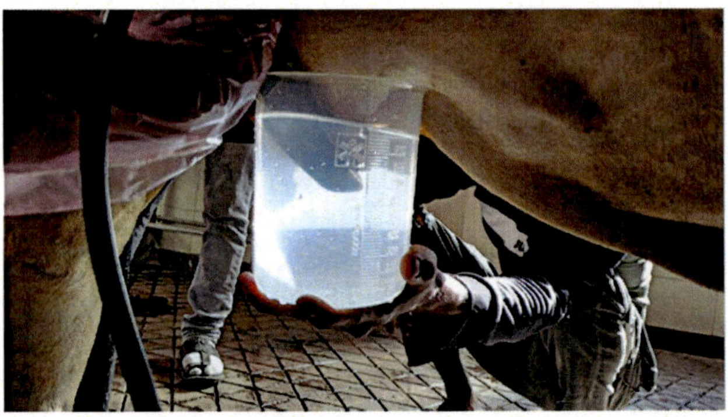

Fig. 200: Showing scanning of teat using water bath technique

- The glandular parenchyma of the udder is sonographically homogeneous and hyperechoic with anechoic alveoli.
- The gland sinus is visualized as anechoic area continuous with teat sinus.
- The lining of the wall of gland sinus may appear as mixed hyper-hypothetic folds.
- The lactiferous ducts may be visualized as anechoic areas within the hypothetic matrix of the fold.
- Normal teat wall sonographically appears as three fold layer structure (Fig. 201). Teat skin is visualized as thin bright echoic line followed

by thicker homogeneous less echoic layer with inclusion of anechoic cavities (muscular /connective tissue layer having blood vessels) and a thin bright line mucus membrane.

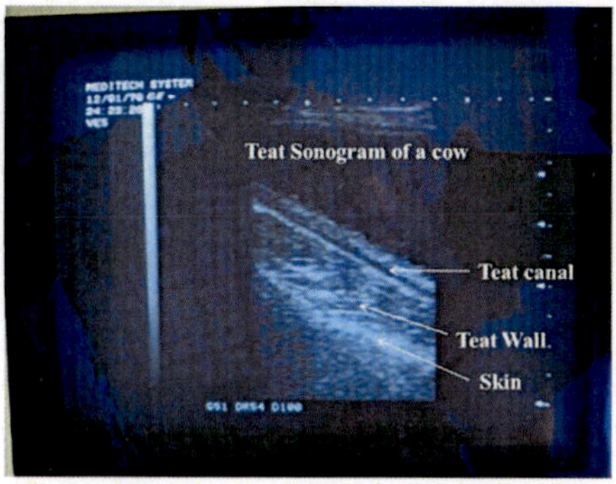

(A)

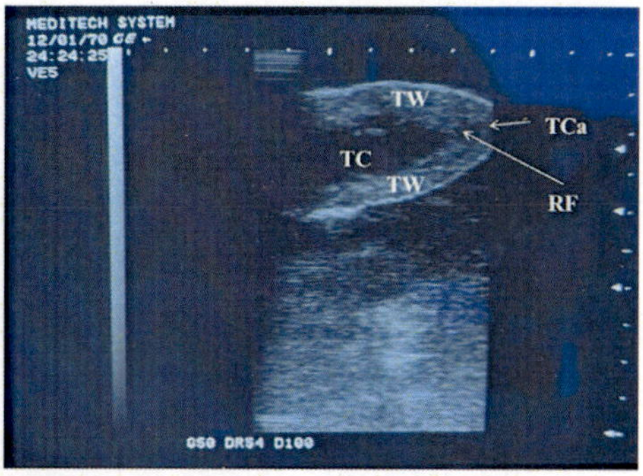

(B)

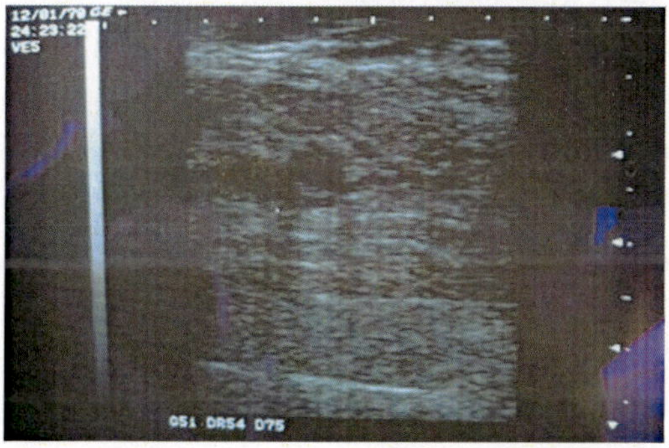

(C)

Fig. 201: Teat Sonogram **(A and B)** of a healthy cow showing skin, teat wall and teat canal. From outside to inside skin appears as bright echogenic line. Muscularis /connective tissue layer appears as thickest homogeneous less echogenic with anechoic cavities. Internal boundary as mucus membrane appears as thin bright line circumscribed on each side by parallel hypoechoic bands. Tca= teat canal, TW= Teat wall, TC= Teat cistern, RF= Rosette of Fustenberg. RF is actually transition between teat canal and teat cistern. Sonogram of the glandular parenchyma **(C)** is showing homogeneously hyperechoic echo texture with anechoic alveoli.

- Normal teat canal is visualized as a thin, white, hyperechoic line (Fig.201) circumscribed on each side by parallel thick, dark hypo- to anechoic bands.
- The boundary between mammary gland and teat cistern may appear as round anechoic structure.
- Intraluminal teat obstruction is sonographically visualized as hyperechoic shadow located near to the teat mucosa.

- In cases of thelitis central hypoechoic image of teat canal is replaced by thick hyperechoic teat lining.
- Sonographic changes in cases of subclinical mastitis have been reported as homogeneous hypoechoic parenchyma, hypoechoic contents of the gland cistern, irregular contour lining of teat canal, thickened teat wall and loss of three layered characteristic of teat wall.
- Teat fistula tract may appear as hypoechoic tubular structure.
- Udder and teat fibrosis/atresia shows hyperechoic appearance with a loss of normal typical echo pattern.
- Udder abscess/necrosis/gangrene are visualized as hypoechoic space occupying images within homogeneous hyperechoic udder parenchyma.
- Udder haematoma appears as hypoechoic space occupying image within homogeneous hyperechoic udder parenchyma.
- Varicosity of udder is sonographically characterized as an anechoic elongated vein with homogeneous hyperechoic udder parenchyma on sagittal plane and as numerous anechoic spaces within the homogenous hyperechoic udder parenchyma on transverse plane.
- Other use of ultrasonography of the udder is for detailed measurements of the length and diameter of the teat canal, cistern, and the thickness of the teat wall (Gleeson *et al.*, 2002; Ślosarz *et al.*, 2010, Stándík *et al.*, 2010).

Pregnancy Diagnosis

- Transrectal approach is suitable for determining pregnancy in cows and buffaloes.
- Transducer of 5.0 to 7.5 MHz is preferred for an early pregnancy diagnosis.
- Transducer of 3.0 or 3.5 MHz is suitable for visualizing internal organs of the foetus.
- Early conceptus is irregular in shape and anechoic vesicular structure within uterus.
- Until day 26, embryonic vesicle increases in length.
- Heart beat can be visualized between day 26 and 29.
- Fore limb buds can be visualized between 28 to 31 days.

- Hind limb buds can be visualized between 30 to 33 days.
- Embryonic vesicle occupies both the horns by day 32.
- Split hooves can be visualized between 42 to 49 days.
- Foetal movements can be seen between 42 to 50 days.
- Ribs can be visualized between 51 to 55 days.
- Head, thorax, abdomen and pelvis are visible during first four months.
- Fluid filled structures are easily recognized owing to their anechoic contents.
- Under field conditions pregnancy can be detected as early as day 30 post breeding by using an ultrasound.
- Sex determination can be done by employing transrectal real time ultrasonography between 50 to 100 days pregnancy.
- Genital tubercle migrates from initial position between hind limbs towards umbilical cord in males and towards tail in female foetuses.
- Optimal age for gender identification is between 59 to 68 days post ovulation.
- After day 60, scrotal swelling in male and mammary glands in female foetuses can be visualized.
- Identifying a male foetus is comparatively easy.

Small Ruminants

- Use of ultrasound in reproductive management of small ruminants (goats and sheep) dates back to 1960.
- It is being increasingly attempted for pregnancy diagnosis in goat and sheep also during last few decades.
- Recent advances in ultrasound technology such as its portability, ease of contact lubrication, and wireless streaming have increased the speed and convenience of ultrasound scanning.
- With real time B scan pregnancy can be diagnosed as early as 25 days of gestation. It is also being used to determine foetal number, their viability and some reproductive disorders.
- Transrectal approach for ultrasonographic examination is not feasible in caprine and ovine patients.

- Trans abdominal approach (Fig.202) for ultrasonographic examination yields poor sonographic images owing to excessive gas and ingesta in the gastrointestinal tract. Nevertheless, cystic ovaries and uterine pathology can be identified. Their sonographic features are almost similar as described in other species.

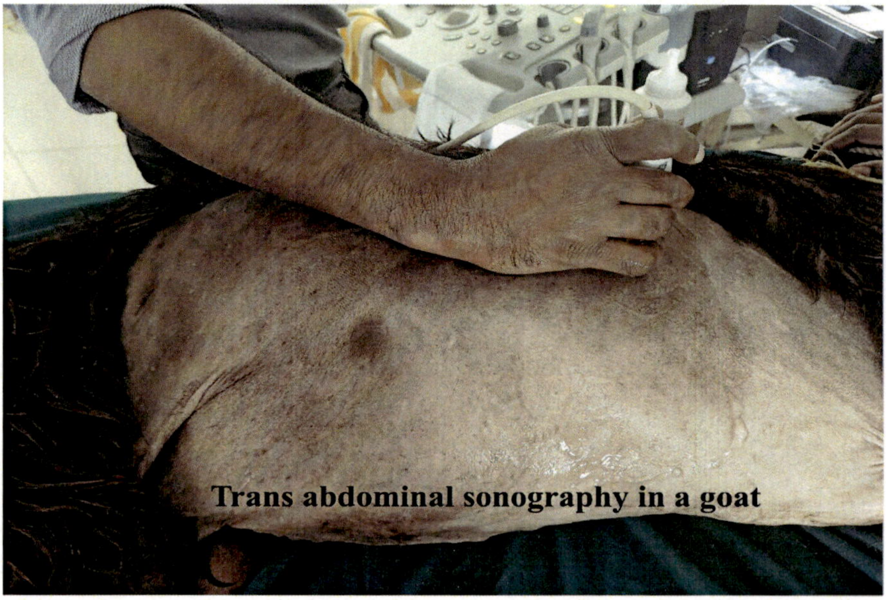

Fig. 202: Showing trans abdominal sonography in a goat

Pregnancy Diagnosis

- Ultrasound has been used in reproductive management of sheep and goats since 1960s.
- A transducer of 5 MHz is suitable for pregnancy diagnosis at early stage.
- A transducer of 3 MHz is suitable for pregnancy diagnosis at late stage and foetal monitoring.
- Transabdominal approach can be done from ventral abdomen in standing position. It is very accurate and efficient means of pregnancy diagnosis in sheep and goat.
- Prepare the inguinal area across the abdomen cranial to pelvic brim.
- Acoustic gel is applied.
- The ideal window of pregnancy for transabdominal scanning is between 40 to 70 days of gestation.

- Trans rectal approach using high frequency transducers (5-10 MHz) can be done at day 30 to 40. It is better to avoid rectal approach.
- With real time B- scan ultrasound pregnancy can be detected as early as 25 days of gestation.
- Presence of fluid in uterine lumen, evidence of placentome (Fig. 203) or detection of foetus (es) is the sonographic features of pregnancy in small ruminants.

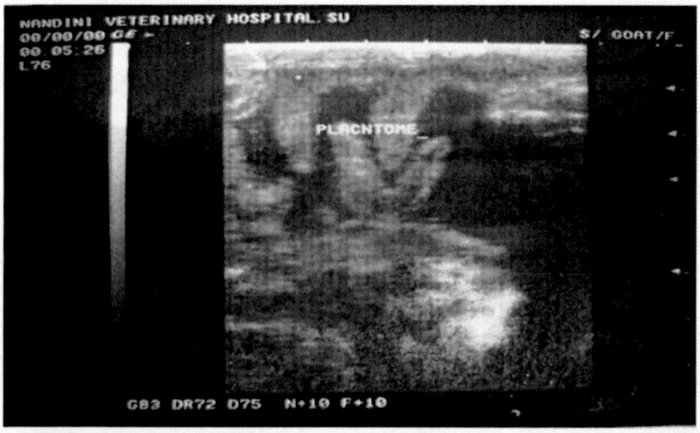

Fig. 203: Trans abdominal sonogram of a goat showing the presence of placentome (echogenic densities in the uterine wall) in the uterus suggesting pregnancy.

- Foetal heart beat can be detected after 25 days.
- Foetal movement or foetal heart beat (Fig. 204) are the indication of viable foetus.

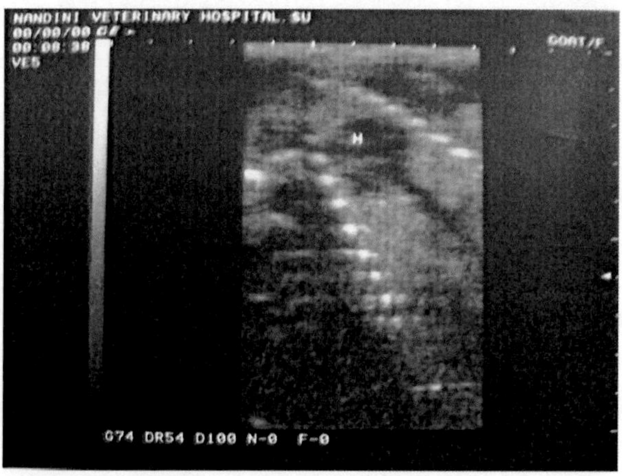

Fig. 204: Trans abdominal sonogram of a goat showing heart. Its beat is the indication of live foetus.

- Echogenic densities in the uterine wall by 26 to 28th day post breeding indicate placentomes.
- Number of foetuses can be counted in standing position, about 20 cm above the udder, between 45 to 90 days of gestation.
- It is difficult to count number of foetuses in late gestation because of large size of foetus (es).
- Foetal age can be determined by measuring width of foetal skull (Fig. 205) during 40 to 100 days of gestation.

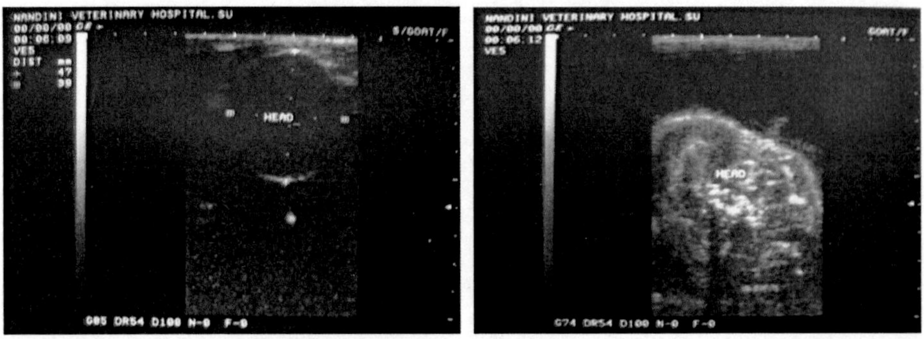

Fig. 205: Trans abdominal sonograms of a goat showing foetal skull. Foetal age can be determined by measuring width of foetal skull.

- Pregnancy can also be detected with higher frequency probes (5-10 MHz) inserted in the rectum .With per rectal approach the probe is closer to the gravid uterus and visualization of pregnancy is possible as early as day 18 in special circumstances. Generally per rectal visualization is not used in sheep and goat.
- Pregnancy is determined by visualization of the amniotic vesicle, the fetus, or the characteristic "C" shaped concave placentome.
- Detection of the amniotic vesicle (the fetus surrounded by anechoic fluid and bordered by a hyperechoic circular membrane), is the diagnostic feature of pregnancy from day 35 to 45.
- After 40 to 45 days, the densely echogenic placentomes and echogenic recognizable structures of foetus are the most prominent features of pregnancy
- After 100 to 120 days, the size of the foetus (es) is large in relation to the fluid.

Determination of stage of pregnancy

- Stage of pregnancy can be determined with accuracy of ±4 days with transabdominal scanning approach.
- The relative proportions of placentome size (component of the sheep/goat placenta) to fluid space volume to fetal size along with changes in density of fetal bones are also used to predict stage of pregnancy with a high degree of accuracy.
- Measurements of the size of the embryonic vesicle in early stage or of various anatomical features of the fetus (biparietal diameter, crown to rump length, length of fused metacarpal bone) in late stage are valuable in predicting foetal age with accuracy.
- The predictive value of these measurements have been reported as: embryonic vesicle day 28-40, crown to rump length day 40-70, biparietal diameter day 40-100. Taking measurements becomes difficult when gestation is more than 70 days.

Foetal Viability

- After 35 days gestation foetal heart beat can be detected in trans abdominal ultrasonography. Heart (Fig. 206) beat of foetus confirms viability of the foetus.

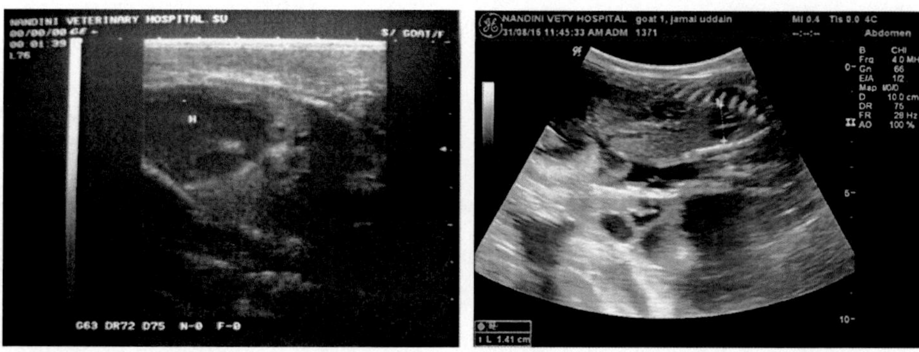

Fig. 206: Trans abdominal sonograms of a female goat showing beating heart (H) of the foetus suggesting viable foetus.

- Health and viability of the foetus (es) is indicated by lack of echogenicity of amniotic fluid, normal amount of fluid as per gestational stage, normal fetal posture and movement, and crisp placentome margins.
- Increased fluid echogenicity, floating membranes, collapsed fetal posture, no detectable heart beat or fetal movement is suggestive of dead foetus.

- Hyperechogenic placentome (Fig. 207) is also suggestive of nonviable pregnancy.

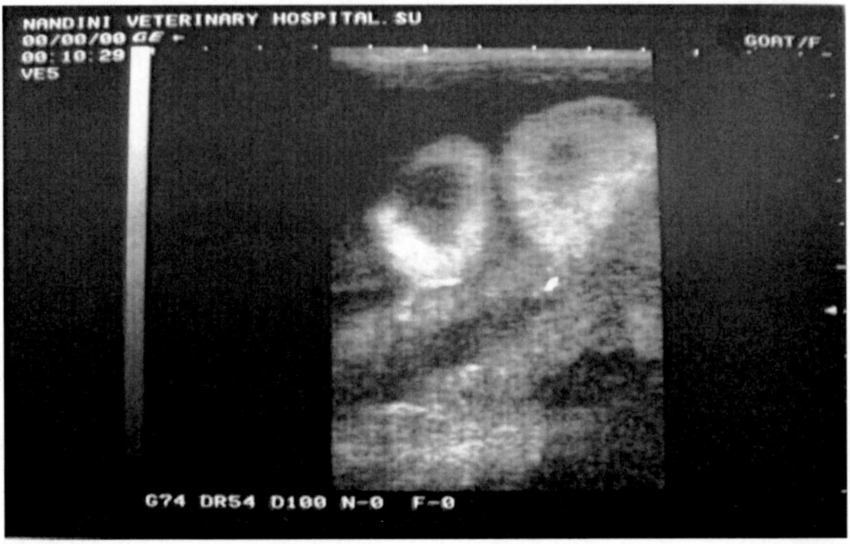

Fig. 207: Trans abdominal sonography of a female goat showing hyperechoic placentome suggestive of non-viable foetus.

Determination of foetal number

- Number of foetus can be determined with reasonable accuracy between 40 to 70 days of gestation.
- When fetuses are more in number the chances of error are increased in predicting the number of fetuses correctly.

Detection of Other Abnormalities

- The observable margins of the enlarged uterus, and visible caruncles without foetus and fluid is suggestive of recent abortion in does.
- Hydrometra is visualized as an anechoic fluid-filled uterus, and membranous strands in the lumen of the uterus.
- Pyometra is visualized as an echo dense fluid having a swirling appearance in the uterus.
- Retained fetal mummy or macerated fetus is identified by the presence of hyperechoic bone shadows and absence of fluid.

- Hydrometra in goats (pseudo pregnancy), is visualized as the accumulation of anechoic/hypoechoic fluid with membranous strands in the lumen of uterus causing variable degree of distension in the presence of a corpus luteum. Does intended for synchronized breeding programs should be screened by ultrasonography for hydrometra.
- Recently aborted does shows observable margins of the enlarged uterus, with caruncles without fetus or fluid.
- In case of pyometra (Fig. 208), echo dense fluid having swirling appearance is visualized sonographically.

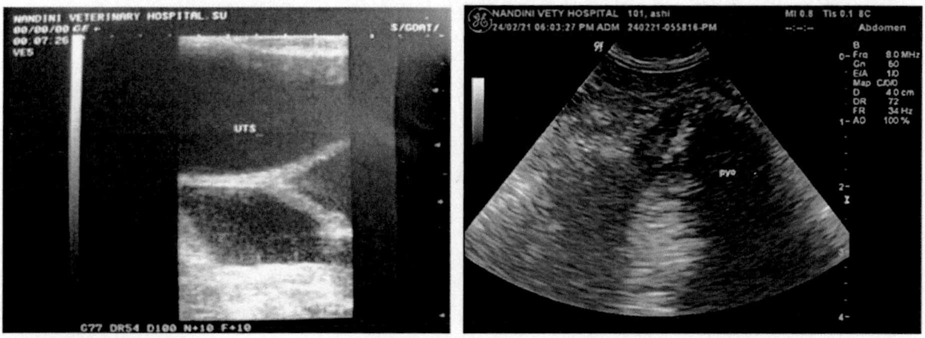

Fig. 208: Trans abdominal uterine sonogram of a goat showing anechoic and echodense fluid and thickened uterine wall suggesting pyometra.

- In the case of a retained fetal mummy or macerated fetus, hyperechoic bone shadows are visualized in the absence of fluid contrast, either in an organized (mummy) or disorganized (macerated fetus) pattern.

Scanning of Urinary system

- Ultrasonography is also being used to detect uroliths in urinary tract (Fig. 209) of small ruminants. The uroliths at the level of the urethral process and /or at the level of penile sigmoid flexure are common and can be easily detected by transabdominal ultrasonography. Transducer is placed high in the inguinal region at the junction of the medial aspect of the hind limb and abdominal wall. The probe is tilted towards the left tubercoxae and the directed slowly cranially and ventrally to scan caudal abdomen near the pelvic brim. Calculi and fine sediments are sonographically appears as multiple small echogenic structures in the ventral aspect of the bladder. Calculi are hyperechoic with acoustic shadow. Blood and fibrin are less echogenic than calculi.

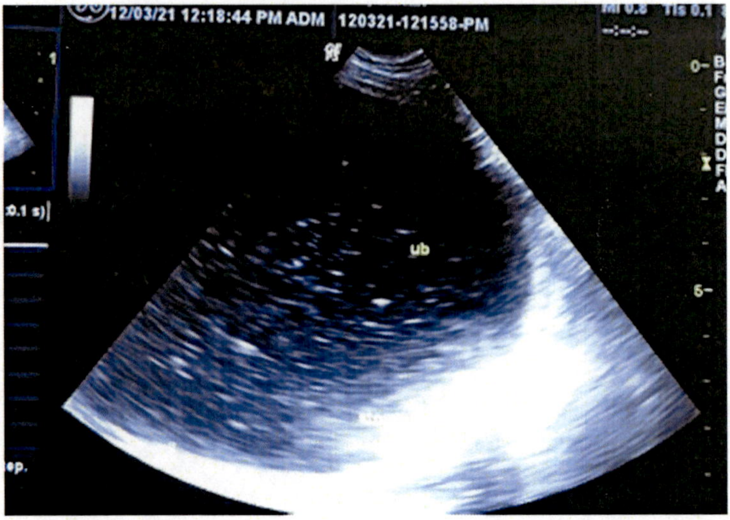

Fig. 209: Trans abdominal sonogram of a male goat (64 kg.) with urinary dribbling for a month showing hyperechoic crystals/calculi in the urinary bladder with thickened urinary wall suggesting crystalluria

- Risk of hydronephrosis increases when urethral obstruction stands for >48 hours. Both kidneys can be scanned by transabdominal approach through right paralumbar fossa. Kidneys with hydronephrosis show dilatation of renal pelvises with echo lucent fluid. Severe cases of hydronephrosis show absence of cortical tissue; dilated pelvis and medullary pyramids surrounded by echo lucent fluid.
- Urinary bladder rupture leading to uroperitoneum is sonographically characterized by a large accumulation of anechoic fluid exterior to the margins of urinary bladder. Many times ruptured bladder is not visible. In this circumstance, detection of anechoic fluid at the place of bladder in the abdomen suggests uroperitoneum.
- Urethral rupture results in accumulation of urine in subcutaneous space, muscle and fascia in ventral abdomen and inguinal region. Ultrasonographically multiple anechoic fluid pockets within swollen tissues may be visualized,

Scanning of Liver

- Scanning for liver from ventral abdomen approach just behind xiphoid cartilage does not yield quality images because of gas in rumen and intestines.

- A major portion of the liver parenchyma can be visualized from lateral abdominal wall approach (including last intercostal space).
- Sonographic features (Fig.210) of liver, gall bladder, hepatic vasculature of caprine are comparable with canine. But images are of little inferior quality. Liver in small ruminants is less homogeneous and more hypo echoic than the spleen. Hepatic vein has no echogenic wall. Gall bladder appears anechoic fluid filled structure (Fig. 210).

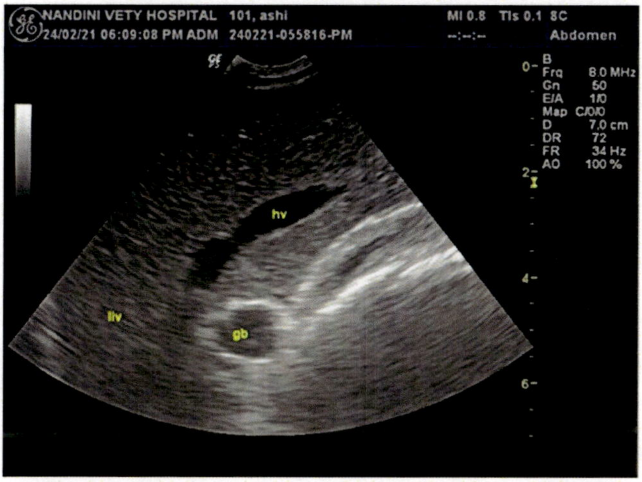

Fig. 210: Trans abdominal sonogram of a goat showing liver, gall blader and hepatic vein.

- In sheep, liver scanning is being used to detect cysts of *Echinococcus granulosis* .These cysts appear as anechoic, rounded, unilocular structures with hypoechoic contents. The cystic material may be particulate or rounded. Cysts are generally of 2 to 5 cm diameter.

Scanning of Kidneys

- Kidneys in small ruminants are scanned in standing position.
- Lateral abdominal approach at paralumbar fossa keeping scan head cranio-dorsally is a good approach for scanning kidneys in small ruminants.
- The left kidney is located ventral to transverse process of L3, L5.
- The right kidney is located ventral to last rib and transverse process of L1-L3.
- Kidneys are easily located in transverse plane.

- Left kidney is well visualized. Three zones viz. hyperechoic central zone (representing fat), hypoechoic medulla and intermediate cortex can be recognized.
- Echo-texture of kidneys of small ruminants (Fig. 211) is comparable to that of canine.

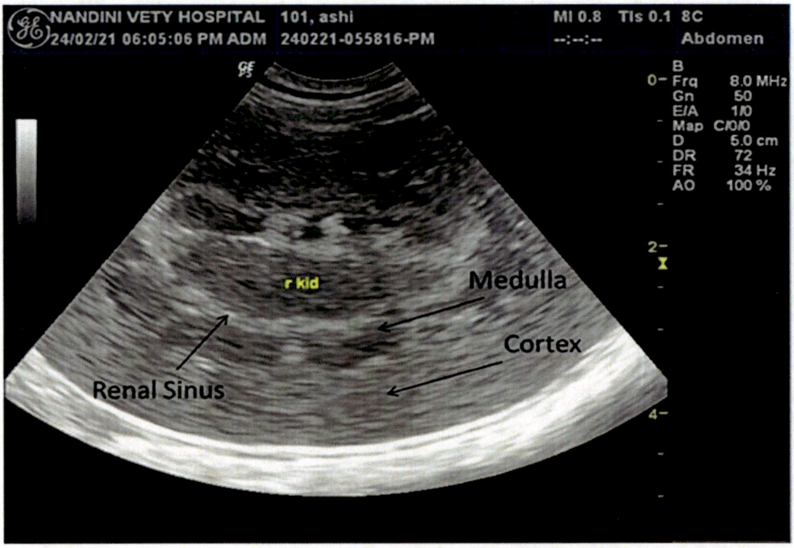

Fig. 211: Trans abdominal renal sonogram of a goat. Echo texture and echo pattern of goat kidney is similar to that of canines and large ruminants. The renal sinus is hyperechoic. Medulla is hypoechoic and cortex is relatively hyperechoic.

Scanning of Fore stomach

- Rumen wall appears as a thick echogenic line (Fig. 212) adjacent to left abdominal wall similar to large ruminants. Wall layering of rumen is not distinct. Internal reverberation artifacts suggests gaseous zone in dorsal rumen sac. Ingesta appears as anechoic to hypoechoic interspersed with gas and fluid (Fig. 212).

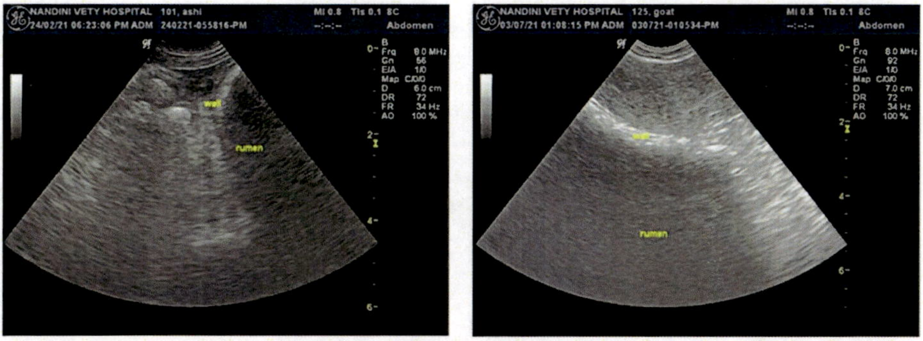

Fig. 212: Trans abdominal sonograms of a goat showing rumen, its wall and ingesta. In the right side sonogram spleen is also seen adjacent to rumen.

- Reticular wall (Fig.213 A) is slightly less thick than that of rumen.

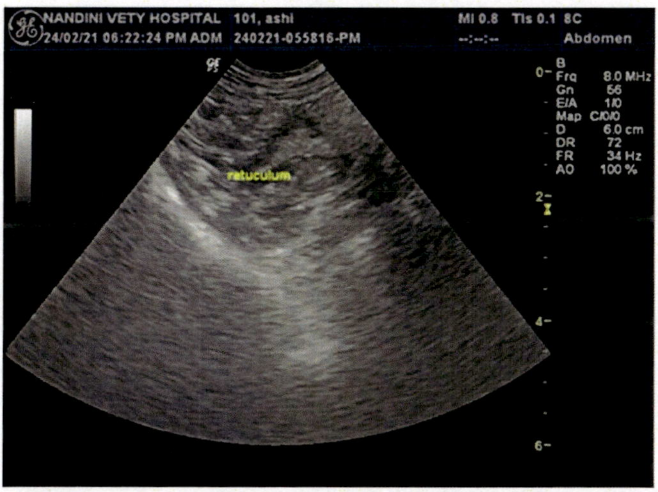

Fig. 213: A. Trans abdominal sonogram of a goat showing reticulum, its wall and ingesta.

- Omasal wall (Fig. 213 B) is slightly less thick than that of reticulum.

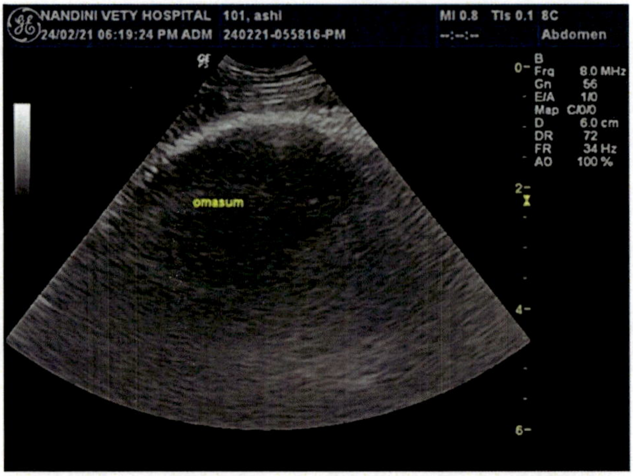

Fig. 213: B. Trans abdominal sonogram of a goat showing omasum, its wall and ingesta

Scanning of Spleen

- The spleen (Fig.214) is homogeneous in echo texture and contains small regular anechoic blood vessels.

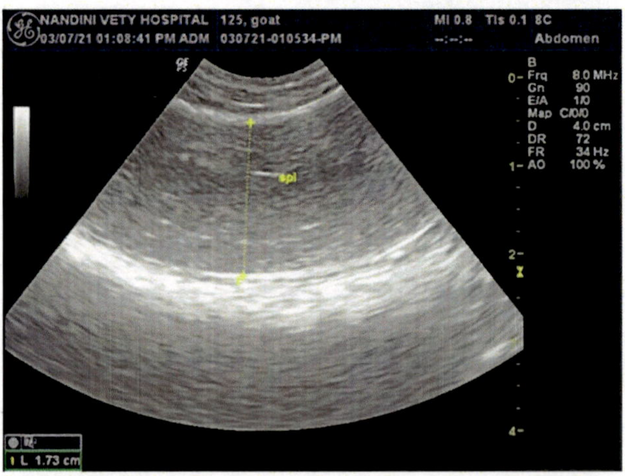

Fig. 214: Trans abdominal sonogram of the spleen of a goat. The spleen appears as homogeneously echogenic structure

Scanning of Udder

- The skin of goat udder is visualized as a hyper-echoic line. From this lamina several hypoechoic suspensory lamellae are detached dividing the mammary gland parenchyma into lobes. Lobes appear as a hyperechoic structure (Fig. 215).

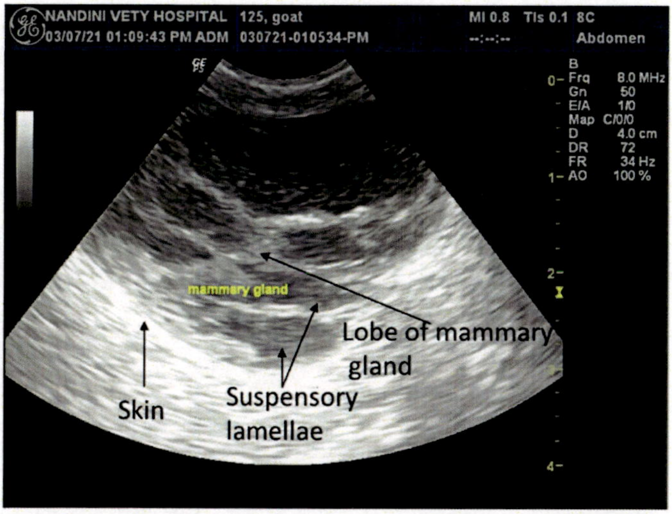

Fig. 215: Ultrasonographic image of mammary gland parenchyma of the goat showing skin as a hyperechoic line, suspensory lamellae as a hypoechoic structure and lobes as a slightly hyperechoic structure.

Other Indications of Sonography

- Ultrasonography can also be used to evaluate the testis, epididymis and scrotum in male goats and sheep.
- Normal testes are sonographically visualized as having thin, echogenic capsule and uniform hypoechoic parenchyma. Mediastinum testes are oriented along the longitudinal plane and are variably echogenic linear structure.
- Tails of epididymis are heterogeneous structure less echogenic than testicular parenchyma. The heads of epididymis appear similar to tails but are often obscured by anechoic loop shaped profile of the spermatic vessels.
- Testicular atrophy is visualized as smaller organ with over all reduced echogenicity in the parenchyma.
- Calcification is characterized by markedly hyperechoic areas with acoustic shadowing.
- Epididymitis in rams is characterized by enlarged hypoechoic space surrounded by thick hyperechoic capsule.
- Inguinal hernias appear as echogenic heterogeneous contents confined within bowel loop in spermatic cord (s). If visualization is continued for about a minute, variable peristalsis can also be seen.

- Anechoic fluid accumulation with in scrotal sac is seen in hernias, trauma and peritoneal effusion.

Thoracic Ultrasonography

- It has been used in small ruminants to detect thoracic diseases.
- For transthoracic ultrasonography a 5-6 cm wide strip on both side of the chest extending dorsally from point of elbow is prepared as usual detailed earlier. Generally 6-7th intercostals space is used to visualize lung surface and pleura.
- Normal visceral pleura appear as a moving echogenic line with reverberation artifacts.
- In normal sheep there is no pleural fluid.
- Latticework of fibrin and exudates between parietal and visceral pleural surface is suggestive of pleuritis.
- Abscesses on lung surface are visualized as encapsulated structure having echogenic fluid.

References

Bernier Gosselin, V., Babkine, M., Gains, M.J., Nichols, S., Arsenault, J. and Francoz,D.(2014). Validation of an ultrasound imagingtechnique of the tympanic bullae for the diagnosis of otitis media in calves. J. Vet. Internal Med. 28:1594-1601.

Cartee, R.A., Abrahim, A.K. and McLeary, D. (1986). B-mode ultrasonography of bovine udder and teat. In. J.A.Vet.Med.Ass. 188: 1284-1287.

Caruolo, E.V. and Mochrie, R.D.(1967). Ultrasonograms of lactating mammary glands. J. Dairy Sci.50:225-230.

Callesen, H., Greve, T., and Christensen, F. (1987). Ultrasonographically guided aspiration of bovine follicular oocytes. Theriogenol. 27:217-217.

Gleeson, D.E., O'Callaghan, E.J. and Rath, M.V. (2002).Effect of milking on bovine teat tissue as measured by ultrasonography. Irish Vet. J. 55: 628-632.

Klein, D., Flock, M., Khol, J.H., Franz, S., Stuger, H.P. and Baumgartner, W. (2005). Ultrasonographic measurements of bovine teat: breed differences and the significance of measurements of udder health. J.Dairy res. 72:296-302.

Kofler,J.1.,Geissbühler,U.and Steiner,A.(2014). Diagnostic imaging in bovine orthopedics. Vet. Clin. North. Am. Food. Anim.Pract.30: 11-53.

Munday, K. and Mudron, P. (2016).Abdominal ultrasonography in cattle. Folia Veterinaria 60: 34-60.

Ollivett, T.L., Caswell, J.L., Nydam, D.V., Duffield, T., Leslie, K.E., Hewson, J. and Kelton.D.(2015). Thoracic ultrasonography and bronchoalveolar lavage fluid analysis in Holstein calves with subclinical lung lesions. J. Vet. Intern. Med. 29:1728-34.

Pieterse, M.C., Vos, P.L.A.M., Kruip, T.A.M., Wurth,Y.A. and van Beneden, T.H. (1991). Transvaginal ultrasound guided follicular aspiration of bovine oocytes.Theriogenol. 35:857-862.

Pothmann, H., Erlen, A., Pichler, M., Huber, J. and Drillich, M. (2015). Relationship and repeatability of body condition scoring and Backfat thickness measurement in dairy cows by different Investigators. Berl. Munch. Tierarztl. Wochenschr. 128:319-25.

Seeh, C., Hospes, R. and Bostedt, H.1996).Use of visual methods (sonography/ endoscopy) in the diagnosis of a webbed teat in a cow, A case report. Tierarztliche Praxis. 24: 438-442

Wojtowski, J., Bielinska, S., Frackowiak, A., Ludwiczak, A., Krzysewski, J., Bagnicka, E. and Strzalkowska, N. (2010).Machine induced changes of caprine teats diagnosed by ultrasonography. Afric. J. Biotech. 9: 8698-8703.

Stadnik, L., Louda, F., Dezcek, J., Jezkova, A. and Rakos, M. (2010).Changes in teat parameters caused by milking and their recovery to their initial size. Arch. Tier. 53: 650-662.

Tharwat,M.I. and Buczinski,S. (2012). Diagnostic ultrasonography in cattle with abdominal fat necrosis. Can.Vet.J. 53:41-46.

Suggested Further Readings

Braun, U., Schefer, U. and Fohn, J. (1992). Urinary tract ultrasonography in normal rams and in rams with obstructive urolithiasis. Can. Vet.J. 33: 654-659.

Eilts, B.E., Pechman, R.D. and Taylor, H.W. (et al) (1989).Ultrasonographic evaluation of induced testicular lesions in male goats. Am.J.Vet.Res.50:1361-1364.

Gouletson, P.G., Amaridis, G.S., Cripps, P.J. (et al) (2003). Ultrasonographic appearance of clinically healthy testicles and epididymis of rams. Theriogenol.59: 1959-1972.

Scott, P. (2000). Ultrasonography of the urinary tract in male sheep with urethral obstruction. In Pract.22:239-334.

Scott, P.R. and Sargison, N.D. (2010). Ultrasonography as an adjunct to clinical Examination in sheep. Small Rim. Res. 92:108-119.

Sharkey, S., Callan. R.J. and Mortimer, R. (et al) (2001). Reproductive techniques in sheep. Vet. Clin.North Am. Food Anim.Pract. 17: 435-455.

Van Metre, D.C. and Smith, B.P. (1991). Clinical management of urolithiasis in small ruminants. Proc.9th Annual ACVIM Forum pp 555-558

22

Ultrasound in Equines

J.P. Varshney and P.S. Chaudhary

During last two decades significant advances have been made in diagnostic ultrasound .These advances have positively impacted on diagnostic imaging across all species of animals and have made ultrasound as an indispensable diagnostic modality in veterinary medicine. Since equines have been more a sport and pack animals, the ultrasound technique has long been utilized in the diagnosis of equine musculo-skeletal disorders. Recent years have witnessed its utility in the management of equine reproduction beside its use in the diagnosis of colic and other diseases.

Indications of Ultrasound in Equine Medicine

- Diagnosis of lameness, assessing wounds, joint surface, fractures, soft tissue injuries, and detection of back and pelvic injuries.
- Diagnosis of affections of tendons and ligaments of distal limb e.g. SDFT.
- Diagnosis of ilial wing fractures.
- Diagnosis of meniscal injury in stifle.
- Diagnosis of spine defects e.g. cervical facet joints.
- Pre breeding screening of uterus and ovaries.
- Diagnosis of pregnancy, foetal sexing, viability of foetus and ascertaining the number of foetus (s).
- Monitoring the health of the foetus.
- Visualizing liver, spleen and kidneys.
- Visualizing intestines in colic.
- Diagnosis of aortic-iliac thrombosis.
- Performing ultrasound guided biopsy.

- Evaluation of heart structure and its function to investigate cardiac murmurs, ataxia and sudden collapse.
- Evaluation of blood vessels.
- Evaluation of thoracic cavity including lungs.
- Diagnosis of lumps and bumps (haematomas or abscesses).
- Detection of foreign bodies.
- Examination of eye for periocular trauma, exophthalmos, corneal masses, corneal oedema, cataract, and anterior uveitis.

Ultrasound Equipment

- Portable ultrasound is most appropriate so that it can be taken at patient's site.
- Cart based or mobile ultrasounds can be used in hospital settings.

Suitable Transducers for Equines

- High frequency linear probe is appropriate for distal limbs and ophthalmic visualization.
- Low frequency convex (curvilinear) transducer is appropriate for pelvic and abdominal scanning.
- Rectal linear transducer is suitable for evaluation of reproductive tract, and diagnosis of pregnancy.
- Low frequency phased array (sector) transducer is suitable for cardiac evaluation.
- High frequency linear transducers are generally suitable for evaluating bumps and lumps.

Technique of Abdominal Ultrasound

- It is safe and non-invasive.
- It should not be performed in horses showing uncontrollable abdominal pain or fractious behaviour.
- Isopropyl alcohol is sprayed at the site to dampen the hairs.
- A coupling ultrasound gel is applied on the transducer to enhance image quality.
- A 3.5 MHz convex linear transducer can be used to visualize organs up to 25 cm depth.

- Sonographic examination of testis (Fig.216) can also be performed for the diagnosis of testicular diseases and scrotal hernias.

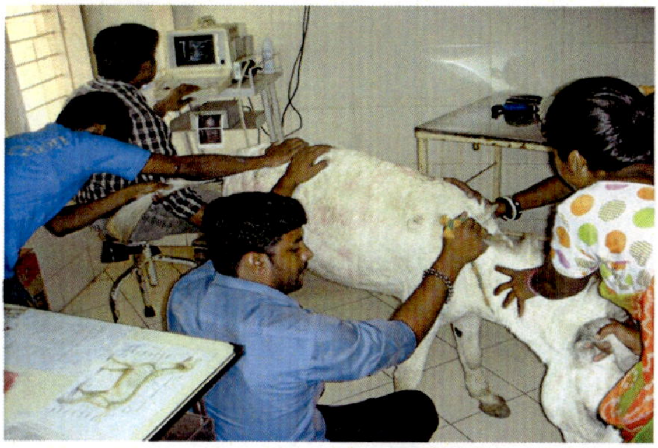

Fig. 216: Sonographic examination of testis of a donkey in standing position

Transrectal Ultrasound

- This window is commonly used to examine reproductive tract .
- For transrectal sonography in equines, linear transducers of 4.5 to 10 MHz frequency are more appropriate. Low frequency curvilinear rectal probes have greater penetration.
- A 5 MHz linear rectal transducer may be used to evaluate adult equine abdomen in cases of colic.
- Before using the transducer per rectum, acoustic gel is applied on the transducer and it is covered with plastic sleeve (Fig.217).

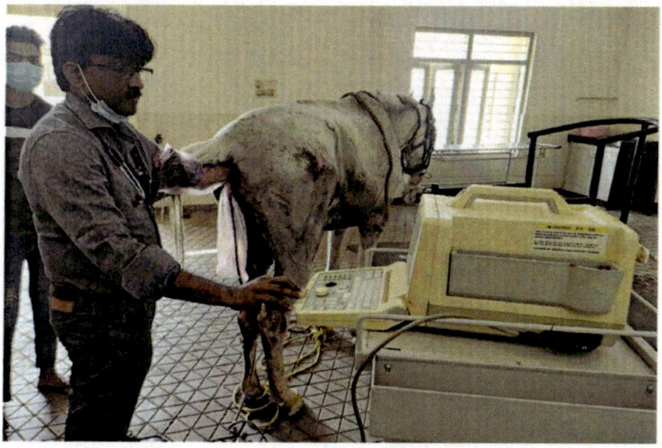

Fig. 217: Transrectal sonography in a horse

Visualization of Abdomen

- The abdomen is divided into three areas such as left paralumbar fossa, right paralumbar fossa, and ventral and inguinal regions (Fig.215). Each region may be further divided into 4 regions and all regions should be thoroughly examined.

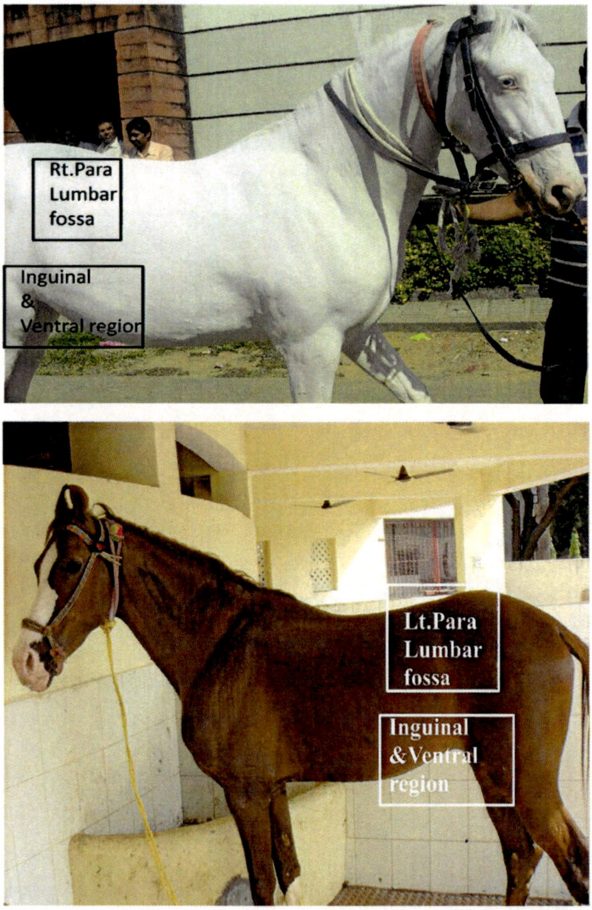

Fig. 218: Showing acoustic windows for transabdominal sonography

- Examination is started with visualizing through right paralumbar fossa, ventral and inguinal region, and then left paralumbar fossa.

Ultrasonographic Features in Diseases

- Horses with mild sand colic usually do not show distension of intestinal loops. In few cases ingesta with fluid is visible. Sand is better visualized in cases of sand colic with radiography.

- Abdominal ultrasound in sand colic cases may reveal brighter hyperechoic large colon wall in ventral abdomen. It may be due to reflection of sand in the colon.
- Ultrasonography is not ideal to detect enterolith in small and large colon .These can be better detected with radiography.
- Horses with peritonitis may show several slightly distended loops of small intestine with thickened wall in ventral and/or inguinal region. Grey or hazy abdominal fluid may be detected in ventral abdomen close to sternum.
- Intestinal ruptures in horses may have increased amount of abdominal fluid in ventral abdomen and varying stage of distended intestinal loops. Normal abdominal fluid is anechoic
- There is hardly any fluid detectable in normal stomach. Its outer wall is similar in appearance to the wall of large colon. Gastric distension in horses is characterized by fluid filled stomach between 10 and 13th rib on the left side of abdomen. Duodenum is also distended, amotile and oedematous in such cases.
- Strangulation of small intestine shows several distended loops adjacent to each other with slow or no peristalsis in the right lower paralumbar fossa region. Distended loops may be thickened and oedematous. Stomach may have more fluid due to reflux.
- Ultrasonographic examination in cases of large colon torsion or volvulus is difficult because of severe uncontrollable abdominal pain despite sedation. In case ultrasonographic examination is feasible, large colon may be visualized in right paralumbar fossa. The colonic vessels may be dilated and oedematous.
- Sonographic features of right dorsal colon displacement are not very conspicuous. Horses with left dorsal colon displacement may show fully or partially visualized left kidney, and colonic gas shadow is seen next to the dorsal edge of the spleen.
- Horses with nephro-splenic entrapment of large colon shows no visualization of left kidney and colonic gas shadow is seen next to the dorsal edge of the spleen. There may be varying amount of gastric fluid and slightly distended loops of small intestine with reduced peristalsis.

Ultrasonography in Equine Reproduction

In equines ultrasonography is being increasingly used for diagnosing pregnancy; monitoring foetal viability and its growth; detecting an early embryonic death; and detecting twins.

Pregnancy Diagnosis

- It is possible to detect an early conceptus of a single embryo between 9 to 16 days as an anechoic sphere with specular reflection sited ventrally and dorsally.
- The equine conceptus is mobile until implantation by 16 days post ovulation.
- Margin of conceptus become irregular from 19 to 24 days.
- Heart beat is visible around 22ndday after ovulation.
- Growth of allantois (starts from 24th day onwards post ovulation) lifts the embryo from the wall of conceptus.
- Allantoic membrane is visible as an echogenic line at each end of embryo.
- Allantois and embryo appear of almost similar size by day 30..
- By day 40, yolk sac is almost disappear and umbilicus can be detected attached to dorsal margin of the embryo.
- Limb buds are detectable from day 50 onwards.
- Foetal movements are also visible from day 50 onwards.
- Visceral organs (liver, lungs and heart valves) can be scanned.
- From mid late pregnancy onwards mineralization of osseous tissue is identifiable.
- Twins can be identified adjacent to each other or in separate position within uterine body or horn.
- Embryonic loss before 25 days post ovulation is sonographically characterized by small size of conceptus for the gestational age and failure of development.
- In practice single developing embryo can be confirmed by 35th day post ovulation.

Sex Determination

- Sex determination is done by adopting transrectal and transabdominal ultrasonographic approaches.
- A real time 5.0 MHZ and 3.5 MHz transducer are used.
- Sex determination during early gestation (59 to 68 days) can be done by transrectal sonography when foetus is in posterior presentation. Genital tubercle is identified. In male foals, it is in proximity to the umbilical cord. While in female foals, it is in the proximity to the tail. It needs expertise and experience.
- For sex determination after 68 days gestation, transabdominal approach is recommended as foetuses are deeply placed. Area from mammary gland to xiphoid on ventral abdomen is clipped and coupling gel is applied. Foetal heart beat is located. Then transducer is moved caudally and area caudal to umbilical cord is carefully scanned. Detection of prepuce or penis just behind umbilical cord suggests male foal. If there is presence of mammary glands and their two teats, female foal is suggested. In late stage of gestation transducer of 3.5 MHz is more appropriate.
- Sex determination can be accurately done from day 100 to 220 of gestation by employing both transrectal and transabdominal sonography.

Suggested Further Reading

Byars, T.D. and Halley, J. (1986). Use of ultrasound in equine internal medicine. Vet.Clin. NorthAm. Equine Pract. 2:253-258. doi: 10.1016/s0749-0739(17)30740-x.

Reef, V.B. (1998). Equine Diagnostic Ultrasound. W.B. Saunders Co, Philadelphia, London.

Wringley, R.H., Hendrickson, D. and Gibbons, D. (1998). Equine tendon and ligament ultrasonography. Equine teaching and research centre, Colorado State Uni., USA.

23

Ultrasound in Exotic Pets

J.P. Varshney and P.S. Chaudhary

Ultrasonography is being routinely practiced in canine and feline medicine for the diagnosis of diseases of the organs and also to confirm pregnancy. Its routine use in ruminant medicine is mainly restricted to pregnancy diagnosis. Recently the potential of ultrasonography is also being explored in zoo and wild animals as well as in exotic pets. Information available in companion and other domestic animals cannot be applied blindly to zoo and wild animals. There is a need to create basic sonographic data of different organs of healthy zoo and wild animals as a reference value so that any alteration in echo pattern from the normal can easily be detected. Ultrasonography in exotic pets can be used for sex determination of monomorphic species, assessing reproductive status, diagnosis of pregnancy and its monitoring , evaluation of organs in diseases, and to get ultrasound guided aspiration or biopsy.

Preparations Before Sonography

- In fur bearing animals either the fur is removed or sufficient amount of gel is applied to exclude the air.
- Small mammals are not to be excessively wet or chilled as hypothermia can be fatal.
- Alcohol based skin preparations are to be avoided.

Peculiar Problems Faced during Sonography

- Sonographic information available in humans, pet or domestic animals cannot be extrapolated as such.
- Restraints (physical and/ or chemical) for sonography in exotic pets and wild animals create an additional stress on animals. Therefore sonography is not a common practice in these animals.
- Anatomical peculiarities such as shell, plates, feathers, fur interfere with acoustic coupling of the transducer and skin.

- Air sacs in birds, thick skin, large subcutaneous fat etc. restrict penetration of ultrasound waves.
- Not much reference data is available on sonographic appearance of different organs in the exotic pets.

Reptiles

Lizards, snakes, and chelonian (turtle, tortoise, and terrapin) are the reptiles kept commonly as pets in urban dwellings. Ultrasonographic examination is very valuable and useful diagnostic modality in conjunction with radiography in reptiles also. It has not been widely utilized as diagnostic modality in reptile medicine. High resolution equipment is more desirable for ultrasonography in reptiles. As usual acoustic coupling gel is applied liberally on the skin and transducer. Animals less than 200 g weight require a standoff pad. Alternatively, the animals can partially be submerged in warm water and the transducer is placed underwater at an appropriate distance from the animal to achieve the optimum image

Indications for Ultrasonography

- Examination of swellings to differentiate tumour, abscess, trauma, parasitic cysts/worms, granuloma (bacterial/fungal).
- Parathyroid gland examination in metabolic bone disease or nutritional osteodystrophy.
- Examination of visceral organs for deposition of uric acid in gout. Affected organ reveals hyperechoic area of uric acid deposition.
- Diagnosis of respiratory disease is facilitated by detecting thick exudates or fluid in lungs.
- It can be used for the diagnosis of ocular and retrobulbar diseases.
- Sonography can also be used in the diagnosis of heart disease.
- Examination of kidneys to confirm renal disease.
- Diagnosis of egg retention or dystocia can be made. Calcified eggs are imaged.
- Diagnosis of intussusceptions or internal masses can be facilitated.

Imaging Procedure

- Aggressive or mobile snakes require sedation/ anesthesia.
- Snakes are scanned across the ventral body wall.

- In snakes heart is located by seeing heart beat ventrally in the caudal half of the first third of the length.
- Chelonians are placed in dorsal recumbenncy. Transducer is placed, after applying acoustic gel on it, in axillary, cervical, inguinal or prefemoral region.

Turtle/Tortoises

Imaging Procedure

- It is rather impossible to conduct sonographic examination in the small chelonians weighing few grams. Large chelonians (> 2.0 kg) are the better candidate for sonography.
- Fasting for 12 hours and chemical restrain (Ketamine @ 40 mg/kg and midazolam @ 2.0 mg/kg IM) is generally recommended for better results.
- Multifrequency transducer (2.5 to 5.0 MHz) can be used. Generally sector or convex transducers with small foot prints are advocated because they can fit well in cervical or prefemoral windows.
- The chelonians are kept in dorsal recumbency (Fig. 219) and acoustic gel is applied liberally on the skin and transducer.

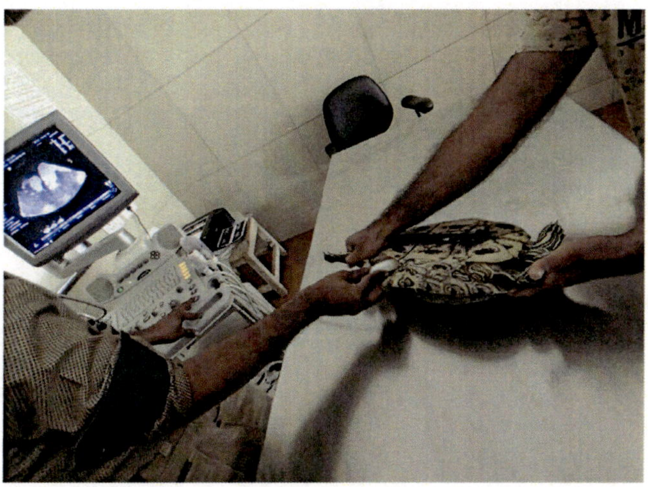

Fig. 219: Showing sonography is being done in a turtle. Turtle is placed upside down i.e. dorsal recumbency.

- Coelomic cavity is approached through ventral right and left cervical acoustic windows; and right and left prefemoral windows (Fig. 220).

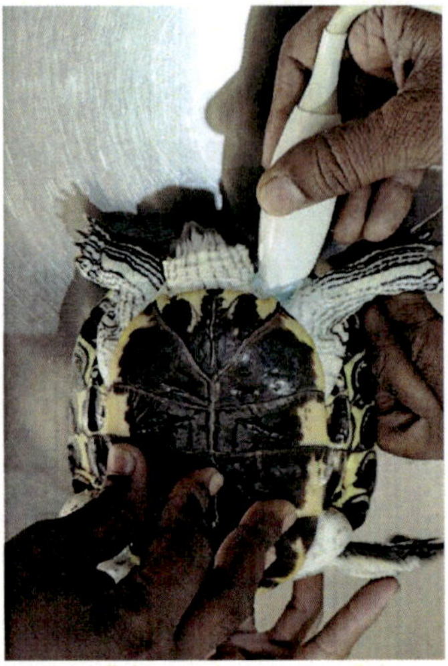

(A)

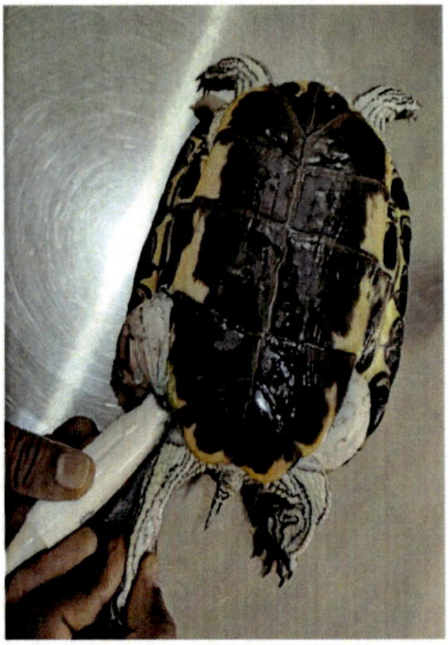

(B)

Fig. 220: Showing sonographic imaging of coelomic cavity of a turtle through cervical acoustic window **(A)** and prefemoral acoustic window **(B)**.

- Screening is done in longitudinal and transverse sections to the axis of chelonians.
- Diagramatic approximate position of the organs of chelonians is given in the Fig. 221 .
- Studies conducted by Meireles *et al.* (2016) in red footed tortoise showed that in cervical scans heart is seen in midline between liver lobes. Ventricle is 'V' shaped homogenously echogenic thick walled and two rounded atria. Thyroid is oval and hyperechoic, seen near heart in cardiac portion of the scan. In chelonians liver is bilobed. Right lobe is larger and anechoic gall bladder is attached to it. Liver (Fig. 222) is seen as a granular with homogenous hyperechoic parenchyma (relative to heart, intestines and kidneys) on the lateral edge to the mid line of cervical acoustic window.

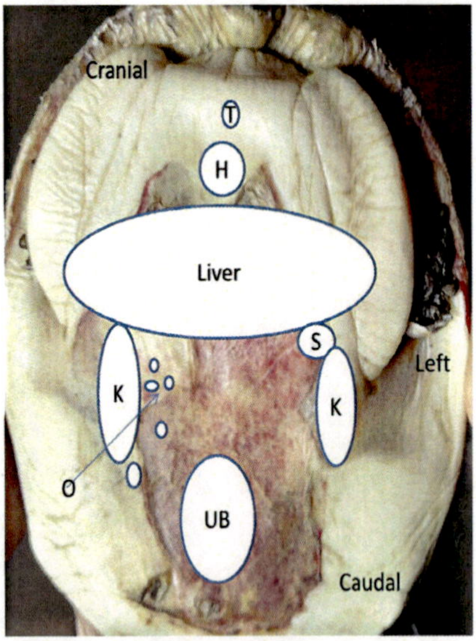

Fig. 221: A tortoise , placed in dorsal recumbency, is showing schematic representation of normal ultrasomographic location of different organs. The words T, H, S, O, K, UB denotes thyroid, heart, spleen, ovarian follicles, kidneys and urinary bladder respectively.

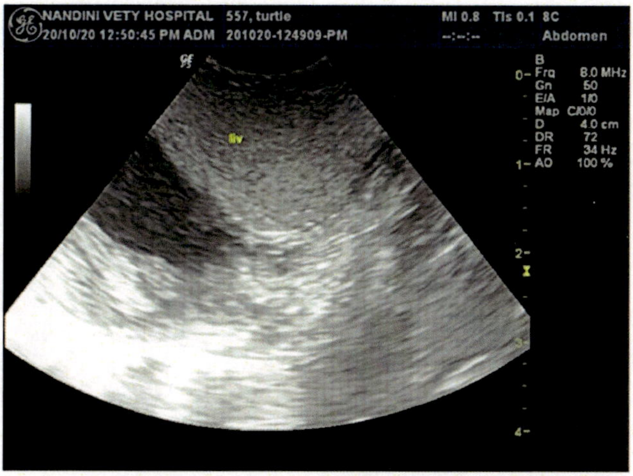

Fig. 222: Coelomic sonogram of a healthy normal turtle showing granular homogeneously hyperechoic hepatic parenchyma.

- Hepatic vessels (Fig. 223) are identified as tubular or sometimes tortuous structures with thin isoechoic or hyperechoic thin walls.

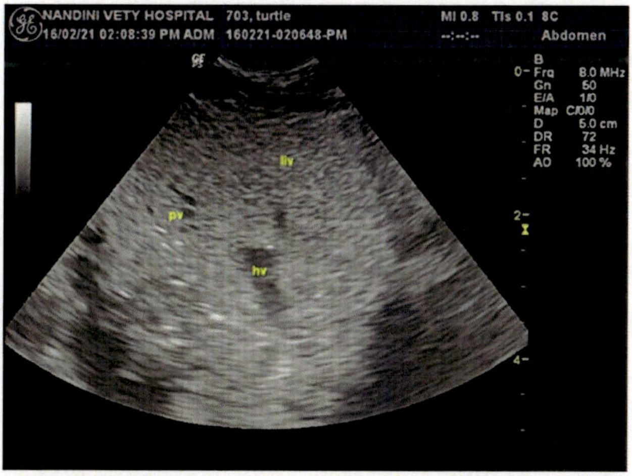

Fig. 223: Coelomic sonogram of a healthy normal turtle showing hepatic vessels.

- Gall bladder (Fig. 224) can be observed between liver lobes having hyperechoic to isoechoic thin wall with anechoic contents at the lateral edge of right cervical acoustic window scans. Gall bladder may be looked as rounded in cross section and slightly elliptical in longitudinal section.

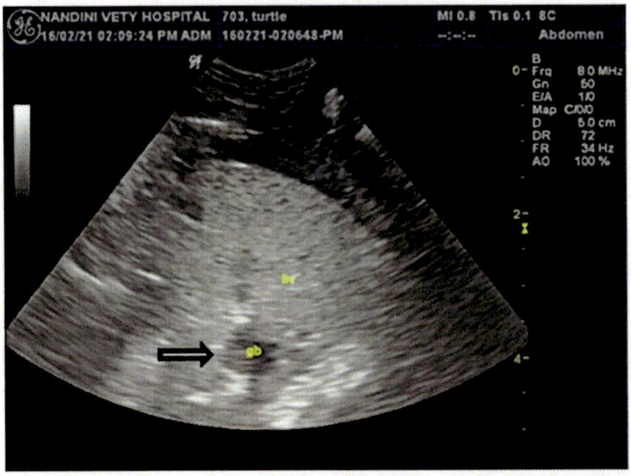

Fig. 224: Coelomic sonogram of a healthy turtle showing gall Bladder (arrow) as an elliptical thin hyperechoic walled structure with anechoic contents

- Stomach is seen in left cervical window scan as having hypoechoic thin wall with folds of varying sizes (Fig.225).

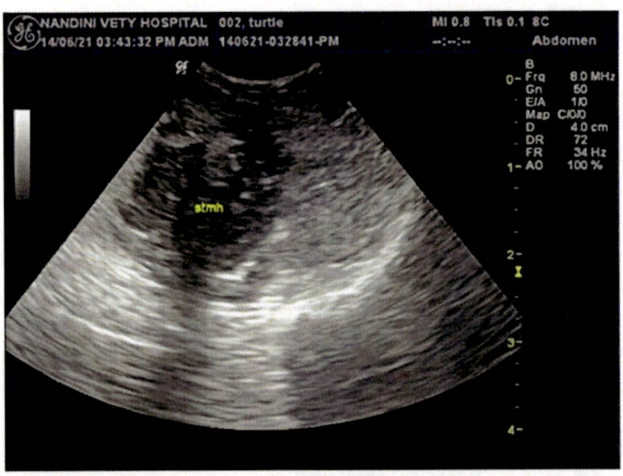

Fig. 225: Sonogram of a turtle taken from left cervical window. Stomach is a thin walled structure with folds as hypoechogenic lines. Anechoic fluid is also visible.

- Small intestine is visible in all four windows having parietal stratification in four layers. Intestines are better seen from right pre femoral window. Mucosal layer is thicker and hypoechoic. Muscular layer is thin and hypo to anechoic. Sub-mucosal and serosal layers are thin and hyperechoic. Stratification may not be visible in all cases. Large intestines are visible from the femoral acoustic windows as thin walled hypoechoic structures without parietal stratification.

- Spleen, pancreas and adrenals are difficlut to identify in normal condition. However, pancreas is an irregular strip extends along duodenum just past stomach. Spleen is an oval structure below the pancreas.
- Kidneys can be visualized through pre femoral acoustic window scans in dorsal caudal direction as compact hypoechoic structures with homogenous parenchyma, smooth margins. In longitudinal plane kidneys may appear somewhat triangular shape. Kidney may also appear as uniformly echogenic area, comma like without distinction of renal pelvis and capsule. The capsule and pelvis may not be visualized. Renal vasculature can be used as a land mark to identify kidneys.
- Visualization of urinary bladder (Fig. 226) may or may not be possible during the scanning through prefemoral windows as the format of urinary bladder varies according to its distention. It may be seen as thin hypoechoic line filled with anechoic contents. Echogenic dots floating in the anechoic fluid as seen in the Fig .226 may be due to urate crystals, parasites or faecal material.

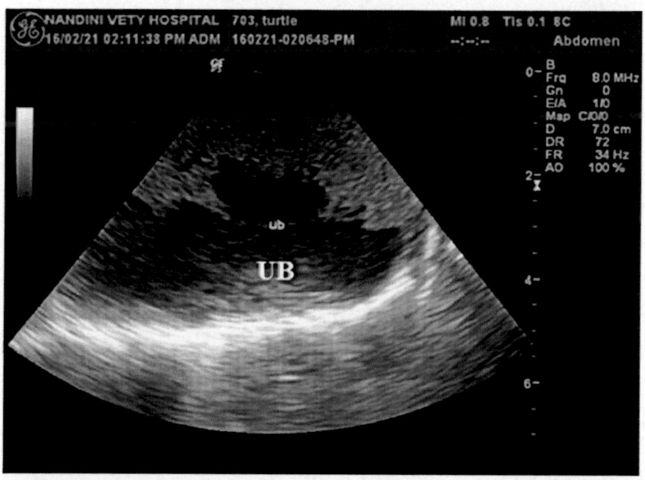

Fig. 226: Coelomic sonogram of a healthy turtle showing distended urinary bladder as a thin hypoechoic lined structure filled with anechoic contents. Hyperechoic floating particles visible in the anechoic fluid may be due to urate crystals, parasites or faecal material.

- Testes are seen as homogenous hyperechoic (in relation to parenchyma of the kidneys) and elongated well defined structures located slightly anterior and ventral to kidneys. Testes are more echogenic than kidneys. Sometimes it is difficult to see right testicle.
- Ovaries can be visualized through cervical and prefemoral windows. Ovarian follicles are observed as spherical hyperechoic structure (in

relation to oviduct) of different sizes (Fig. 227). Oviduct is generally seen as tubular structure with a sigmoid (Fig. 227) aspect between follicles and cranial to kidneys. The wall of oviduct is hypoechoic with poor boundaries.

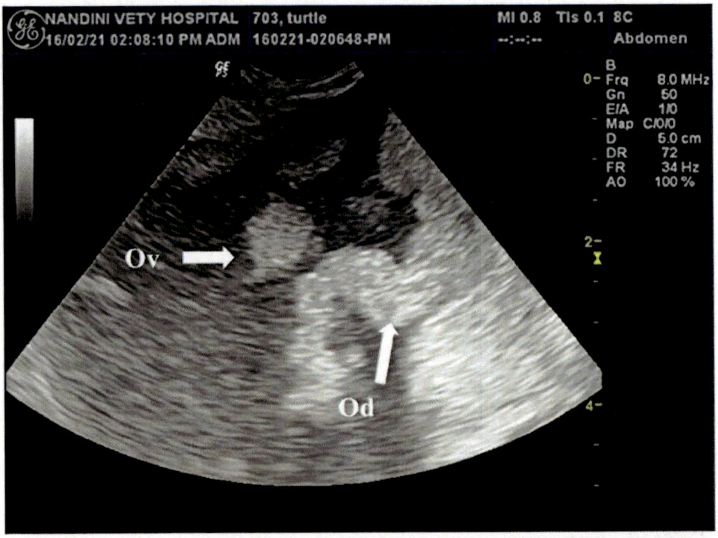

Fig. 227: Coelomic sonogram of a healthy normal turtle showing ovary (Ov) and ovi duct (Od). Ovary is spherical hyperechoic structure. Oviduct is sigmoid in appearance and is also echogenic.

- Eggs are visible as thin hyperechoic line with acoustic shadowing (Fig. 228 A) .In some chelonians a variable amount of free anechoic fluid may be seen in coelomic cavity. Ovulated eggs have hyperechoic yolk in the centre surrounded by the dark hypoechoic albumin (Fig. 225 B). With the deposition of shell, echogenicity of the egg shell is increased (Fig. 225 B).

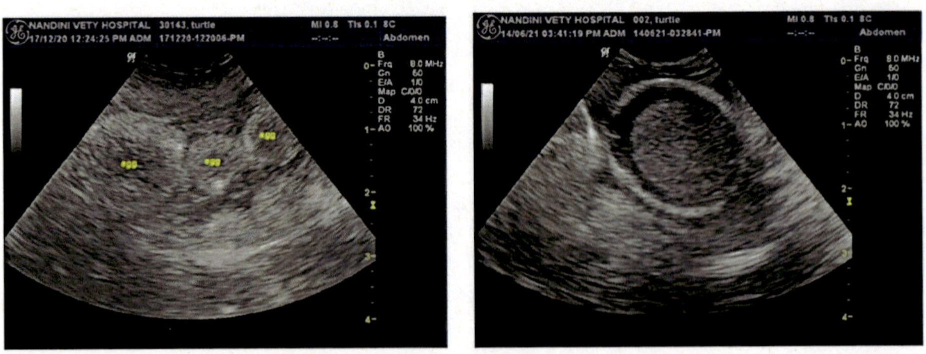

(A) **(B)**

Fig. 228: Coelomic sonogram of a female tortoise showing eggs. Eggs are visible as thin hyperechoic line with acoustic shadowing.

Abnormal Ultrasonographic Features in some Diseases in Chelonians

- Liver abscess appears as discrete disruption to the liver architecture.
- Differentiation between abscess and tumour requires hisopathology.
- Hepatic lipidosis appears as diffuse increase in echogenicity (Fig.229).

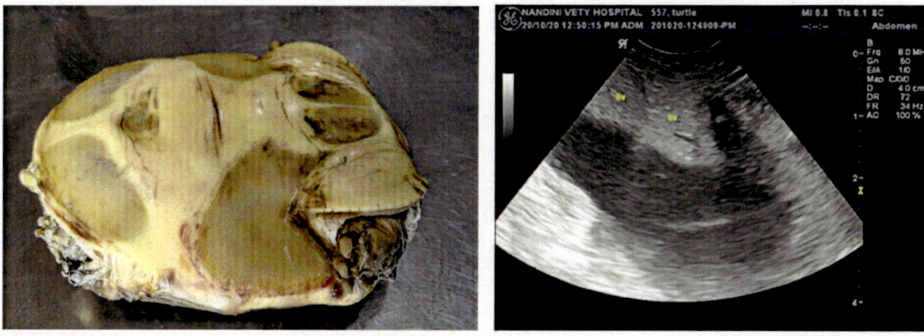

(A) **(B)**

Fig. 229: (A) Turtle showing yellowish discoloration **(B)** Its sonogram, viewed through cervical windows, is showing diffuse hyperechoic granular echo texture of the liver suggesting liver cirrhosis/fibrosis/ lipidosis.

- Uroliths appear as hyperechoic structure in bladder.
- Urinary bladder wall is seen when there is wall thickening.
- Hyperechoic deposits in kidneys and heart may indicate visceral gout.
- Gut stasis appears as distended loops filled with ingesta and liquid (Fig. 230).

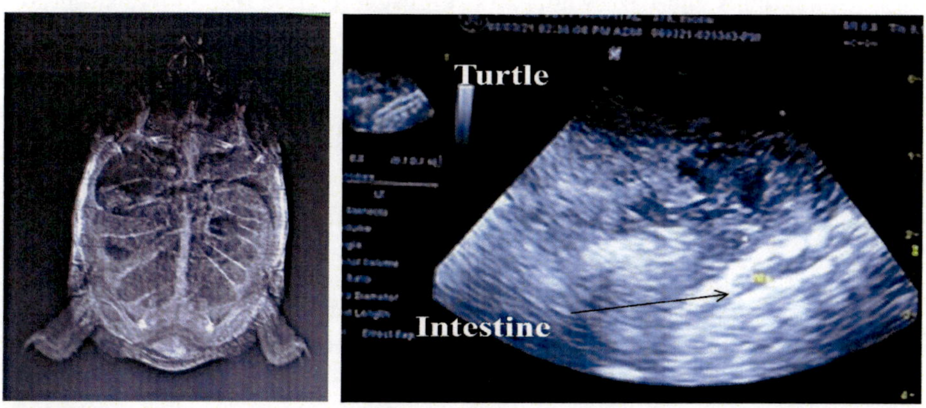

(A) **(B)**

Fig. 230: A turtle weighing 500 g with the history of vomiting and no passage of urine and faeces for a week was subjected to radiography and coelomic sonography. X-ray examination revealed gaseous distension of gastrointestinal tract **(A)**. Its sonogram **(B)** also showed distension of the gastrointestinal tract suggesting gut stasis.

Snakes

Ultrasonography is an important diagnostic tool for snakes and lizards also. Soft tissues can easily be evaluated.

- Snakes and lizards may be restrained manually but sometimes chemical restrain is necessary. They are placed with ventral side up for the sonographic examination (Fig. 231 A).
- For snakes and lizard linear transducers are generally advocated. For small reptiles transducers of 7.5 to 10 MHz and for large reptiles, transducers of 3.5 to 5.0 MHz are suitable.
- Ultrasonography may not be possible in snakes just prior to ecdysis due to the air trapped between the layers of cutis. Copious gel or a water bath is needed to reduce artefact caused by air trapped under the scales.
- Ultrasonography is suitable for the examination of heart, liver, gall bladder, urinary bladder, large intestines and gonads.
- In some animals examination of stomach, small intestine, spleen, pancreas and kidneys is also possible (Stetter, 2000).
- Because of longitudinal position of organs along the body axis in snakes (Fig.231 B), ultrasonographic examination should be started cranially beginning with the heart and ending with cloaca.
- The heart (Fig. 231 C) can serve as starting point. The heart is located and its chambers and valves are examined. Heart muscle is smaller than mammals and valves appear as highly reflective ribbon like structure.
- The liver is caudal to heart in cranial part of the abdomen and can be seen as a moderately hyperechoic organ (Fig. 231D).
- The stomach, spleen, pancreas and gall bladder can be seen caudal to the liver.
- The gall bladder in snakes is not very well developed. It may be located at relatively long distance from the caudal tip of the liver.
- The spleen is only visualized in large snakes as circular organ more hyperechoic than liver. The spleen is located caudal to liver and cranial to gonads (Sainsbury and Gill, 1991).
- The pancreas is generally not visible. When visualized it is less hyperechoic.

- Gonads can be detected as hyperechoic structures. Gonads can be visualized easily in gravid female. The size of ovary may vary from the size of spleen to filling the entire coelomic cavity depending on the stage of reproduction. Ovaries are anechoic.
- The kidneys are located caudal to gonads. As compared to left kidney, right kidney is more cranial. Echotexture of the kidneys (Fig. 231 E) is somewhat similar to the liver .
- Major blood vessel appears as hypoechoic tubular structure with thin echogenic wall (Fig. 231 F).
- Visualization of testicles in males is difficult.
- Eggs contain two layers (upper one consists of anechoic albumin and lower consists of highly echoic yolk).The kidneys in snakes are situated caudally to gonads. Right kidney is cranial to left kidney. Both kidneys are cylindrical in shape with homogenous granulated echo-texture that is more echogenic than body fat. Distinction between sinus, medulla and cortex is difficult (Tenhu *et al.*,1995). Snakes do not possess urinary bladder (Redrobe, 2006). The shape of anal sac is round or oval depending upon its contents and may be seen as anechoic or hyperechoic. Uric acid particles may be seen as snowflakes or conglomerated structures. The image of intestine varies depending upon dietary nature of the snake (herbivore or carnivore). Carnivore snakes have large stomach with longitudinal folds and short intestine. While herbivore snakes have small thin walled stomach and elongated intestines showing mucosal folds. In some snakes it may not be possible to examine organs in coelomic cavity because of lungs reaching almost caudal to pelvis.

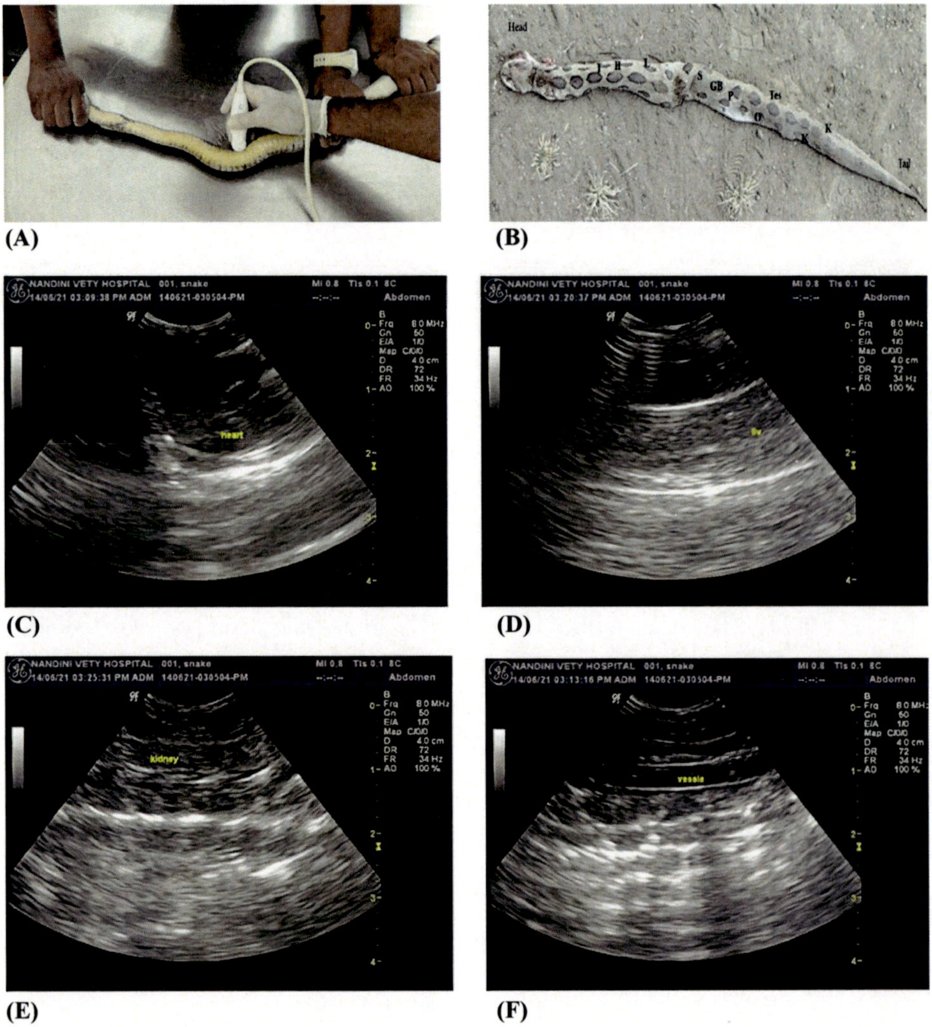

Fig. 231: Showing positioning of snakes for sonographic examination **(A)**, schematic representation of normal ultrasomographic location of different organs of the snake (B) and sonograms of different organs **(C,D,E and F)**. The words T, H, L,S, GB,P,O,Tes.,K in Fig. B denotes thyroid, heart, liver, spleen, gall bladder, pancreas, ovarian follicles, testes and kidneys respectively. Sonograms of heart **(C)**, liver **(D)**, kidney **(E)** and major blood vessel **(F)** of a normal rat snake can also be seen.

Abnormal Ultrasonographic Features in Some Disease of Snakes

- Gall bladder is easily visualized in anorectic snake as a greatly enlarged organ filling approximately one third diameter of snake.

- Anal sac abscess can be visualized as hyperechoic structure. Though gastrointestinal tract is not readily identified, masses in the tract can be identified.

Birds

Ultrasonography plays an important role in pet birds also. Small size and air sac system in birds poses some restriction on the use of ultrasonography. It is generally used to provide additional information on soft tissue structures and space occupying lesions.

Indications for Sonography

- It is usually indicated for the examination of liver, subcutaneous swelling, visceral gout, dystocia, urogenital and cardiovascular system.
- The diagnosis of cardiomegaly, hydropericardium, neoplasia, cysts, egg binding, laminated eggs is facilitated by the use of ultrasonography in birds.
- Fine needle ultrasound guided biopsy is another common use of ultrasound in birds.

Transducer

- A micro-convex transducer (with small foot print) of 7.0 to 12.0 MHz is an ideal choice for the use in birds.

Sonographic examination

- Examination time should be kept as short as possible.
- For cardio-vascular evaluation, device should have a frame time of at least 100 frames per second so as to distinguish the diastolic and systolic phases.
- For psittacine birds, fasting of 1 to 2 hours before ultrasonography is sufficient. While in pigeons or raptors a longer fasting (> 24 hours) yields good results.
- Anesthesia is required to avoid the risk of stress and also in case of Spectral Doppler ultrasonography where handling can influence the heart action and blood velocity.
- Ventro-median approach is most common coupling site where transducer is placed on the skin behind the sternum. If there are feathers in this area, plucking is needed (Fig. 232A) Gel is applied liberally on the skin in

usual manner. The birds should be kept in upright position. In pigeons and raptor flank area (parasternal approach or lateral approach) is another site for ultasonographic examination. In this approach birds are held in lateral position with legs stretched caudally and gentle pressure is applied to compress the caudal thoracic air sac.

- Diagrammatic representation of normal sonographic anatomy of the bird is shown in the Fig. 232 B.
- Liver is examined first followed by heart, gastrointestinal and urogenital system. Scanning of liver is facilitated by hepatomegaly. In pigeons gall bladder is absent. Liver may not be seen if surrounding organs are enlarged. Liver has a medium degree of echogenicity and is finely homogenously granulated with sharp margin (Fig.232 C). Hepatic vessels are seen as tubular structure. For visualization of gall bladder a fasting of 1 to 2 days is recommended.
- Spleen is less echogenic than the liver. Spleen can be visualized better through lateral coupling site. If there is splenomegaly, spleen may look round or oval.
- Lungs look echogenic due to air (Fig. 232 D and E).
- Crop and esophagus is generally not visible in majority of cases.
- Ventriculus or gizzard can be recognized by its contents. Grit in the gizzard is seen as hyperechoic particles with distal acoustic shadowing. Grit may be surrounded by hypoechoic material (Fig.232 F). Muscle layer in ventriculus may be seen as round to oval hypoechoic zone and an acoustic shadow can be seen behind ventriculus due to reflection of sound wave. Koilin layer of ventriculus can only be seen and assessed if transducer is of more than 12 MHz. Proventriculus is cranial to ventriculus and have medium degree of echogenicity and hyperechoic contents.
- Intestines (Fig. 232 G) are generally identified by peristalsis. Layering of intestinal wall is discernable only to certain degree.
- Aspacer is useful for imaging pancreas as it is located immediately under skin. Generally normal pancreas is not visualized sonographically. It is hyperechoic structure lying between duodenal loops. There is blood vessel in the centre of the pancreas that helps in its recognition.
- Kidneys of normal shape and size are generally not visible with transcutaneous coupling site. However, enlarged kidneys can be identified.

- Transcutaneous ultrasonography has been proved to be a useful, noninvasive, and fast diagnostic tool, especially in imaging laminated eggs and changes of the oviduct (Hofbaur and Krautwald-Junghanns, 1999).
- To overcome the problems associated with transcoelomic ultrasonography in birds, transcloacal and transintestinal ultrasonography employing high resolution miniaturized probes are being increasingly considered superior.
- Visualization of the gonads and genital tract is far better in trans-intestinal ultrasonography. Use of transcloacal ultrasonography is restricted to the visualization of caudal genital tract.
- Ovaries can only be scanned when there is a follicle, abscess or granuloma. Inactive ovaries and testicles are not identifiable in transcutaneous sonography. The bursa fabricus is seen only in juvenile birds.
- There is no urinary bladder and diaphragm in birds.
- Echocardiography is the best for examining cardiovascular system. B-mode echocardiography can be performed in partially upright position without sedation or anesthesia. Heart is generally examined from ventro-median position. In pigeons parasternal approach (between last rib and pelvis) may also be used in addition to ventro-median approach as this approach provides several long and short axis views. Echocardiography is helpful in the diagnosis of pericarditis and pericardial effusions.
- Ultrasound guided aspirate from pericardial sac may also be obtained for cytological or microbial examinations.
- Ultrasonographic examination is also appropriate for the diagnosis of arteriosclerosis in large vessels near heart.

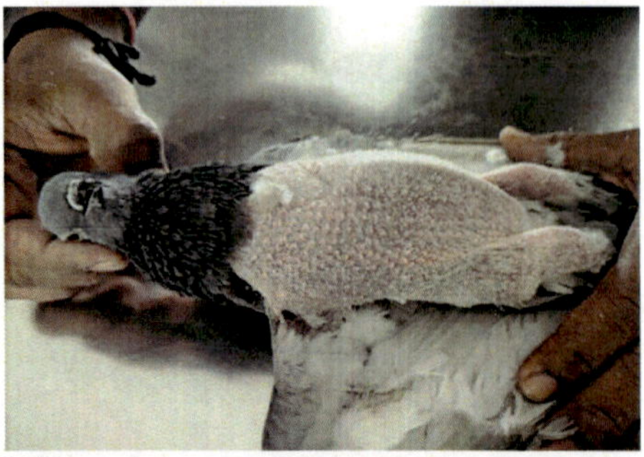

(A)

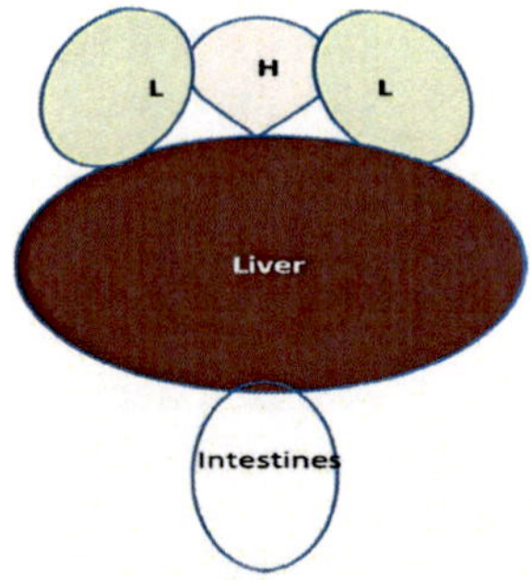

(B)

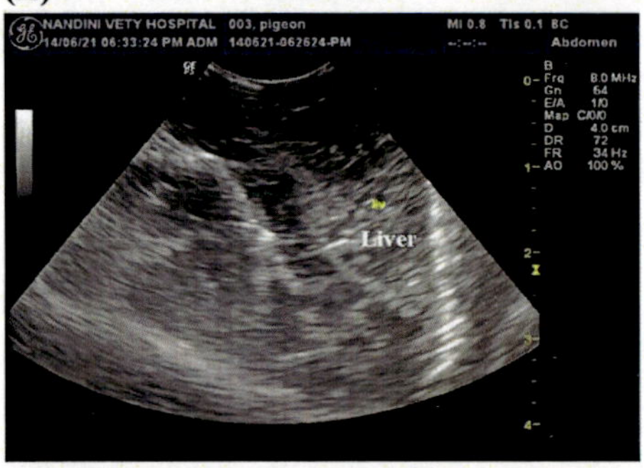

(C)

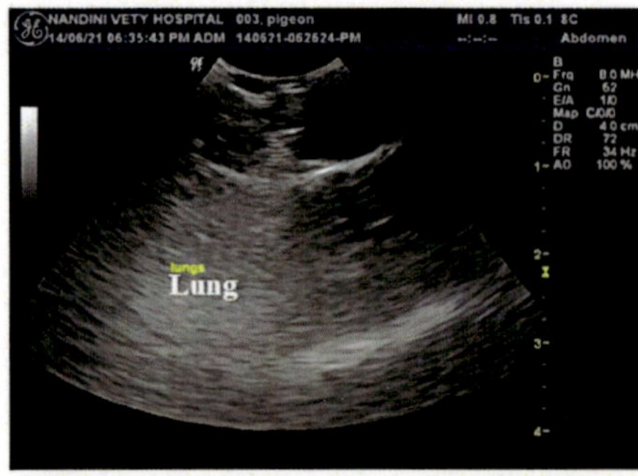

(D)

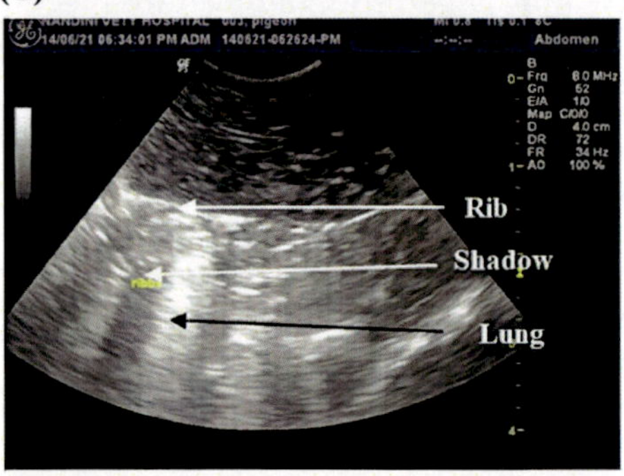

(E)

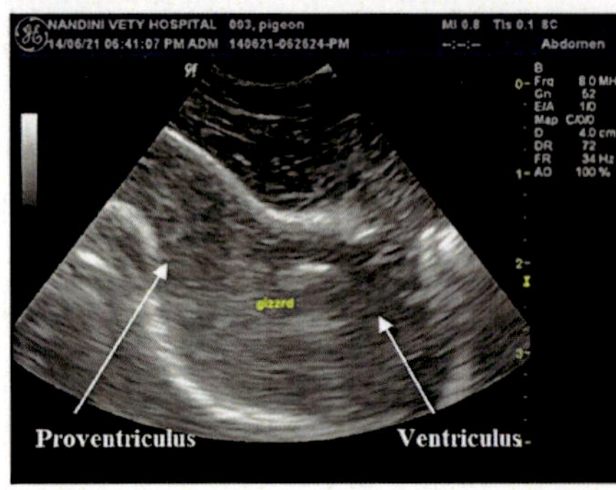

(F)

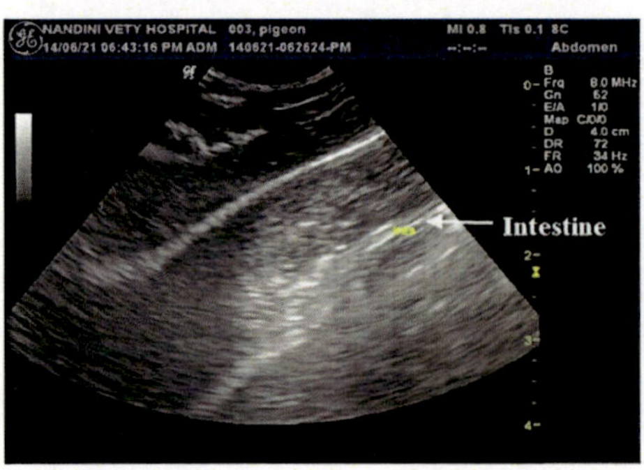

(G)

Fig. 232: Showing preparation of the pigeon for sonography **(A),** schematic diagram **(B)** and sonograms of Liver **(C)**, Lung **(D)** , ribs and lung **(E)**, proventriculus and ventriculus **(F)** , and intestines **(G)**.

Abnormal Ultrasonographic Features in Birds

- Multiple discrete abscesses are associated with yersiniosis or biliary tree neoplasm.
- Air filled sacs restrict visualization of normal ovaries, however, enlarged ovaries (due to normal folliculogenesis, tumor or granuloma) can be visualized .
- Tumours may appear as masses of mixed echogenicity/hyperechogenicity with irregular margins (Fig. 233).

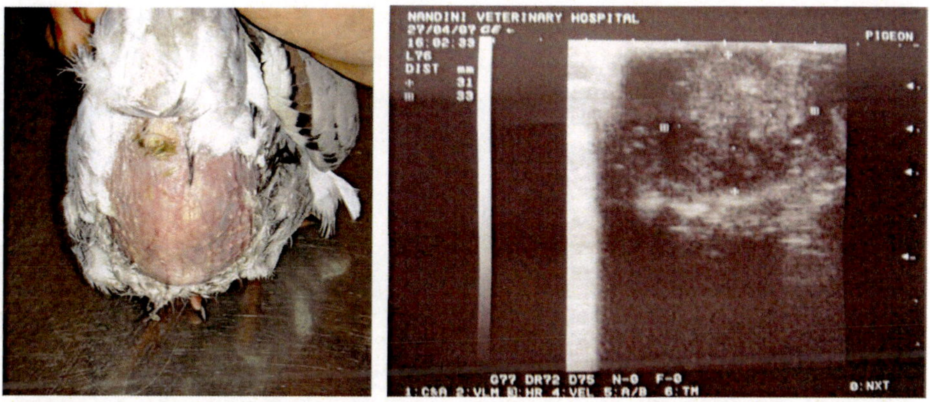

(A) **(B)**

Fig. 233: A pigeon having hard swelling in perianal region **(A)**. The transabdominal sonogram of the pigeon revealed a mass of mixed echogenicity with irregular margines suggesting tumour **(B)**.

Small Exotic Mammals

Ultrasound in exotic species can be used for sex determination of monomorphic species, assessment of reproductive status, pregnancy diagnosis and monitoring of foetus, detecting abnormalities in organs and structures, and for getting biopsy of lesions in the organs.

Points of Consideration

- In general, the anatomy of small exotic mammals is similar to that of familiar domestic species.
- Positioning of small exotic mammals and placement of transducer is similar.
- Stress of restrain for ultrasonography and risk of trauma to animal and handler should be taken into consideration.

- Sedation or general anesthesia in small exotic mammals can avoid the stress of restrain and risk of trauma.
- Large hind gut in herbivore may hinder ultrasonographic examination of abdomen in small exotic mammals.
- Ultrasonography of bladder, uterus, liver, spleen, kidneys and ovaries can also be done percutaneously via ventral abdomen.

Abnormalities Needing Ultrasonographic Examination

- Hepatic lipidosis is relatively common sequel to anorexia in rabbits, guinea pigs.
- Urolithiasis with bladder wall thickening is also common abnormality in small exotic mammals.
- Urethral obstruction due to prostatic hyperplasia is common in male ferrets.
- Ovarian cysts have been reported in guinea pigs.
- Uterine adenocarcinoma and pyometra needs to be differentiated in rabbits.
- Diagnosis of subcutaneous (cervical adenitis) and abdominal masses (abdominal lymph node abscessization) in guinea pigs.
- Intraocular abscess and neoplasia in small exotic mammals.
- Cardiomyopathy and septal defects in rabbits, and cardiomyopathy in ferrets needs cardiac ultrasound examination.

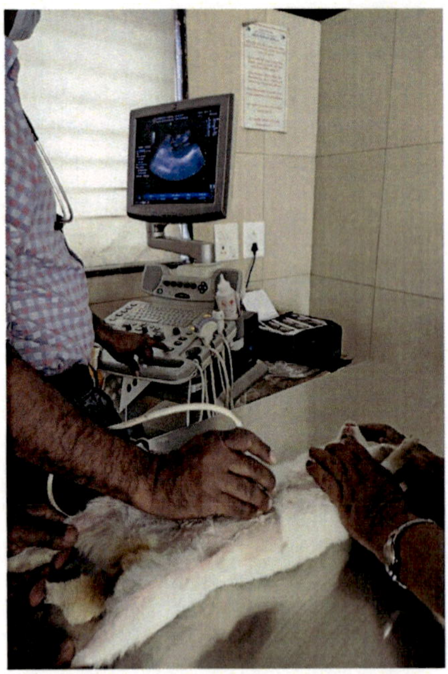

Fig. 234: Transabdominal sonography in a rabbit. The rabbit is placed in a leg up position.

Rabbits

- In rabbits ultrasonography is being increasingly used for the diagnosis of pregnancy and determining the live and dead status of the foetus.

- The diagnosis of pregnancy in rabbits can be made after the 7th day of pregnancy.
- Rabbits are positioned in a leg up position; abdominal area is applied with alcohol (Fig. 234).
- The transducer is placed on the area moving gently from skull to tail or side to side up to get clear images on screen.
- Ultrasonography is also undertaken to assess the movement of the small intestine of rabbits. High definition transducers (7.5-20 MHz) with small foot print (< 2 cm) are more suitable for rabbits.
- Sonograms of liver, intestine, spleen, colon and urinary bladder of a healthy rabbit are shown in the Fig. 235.

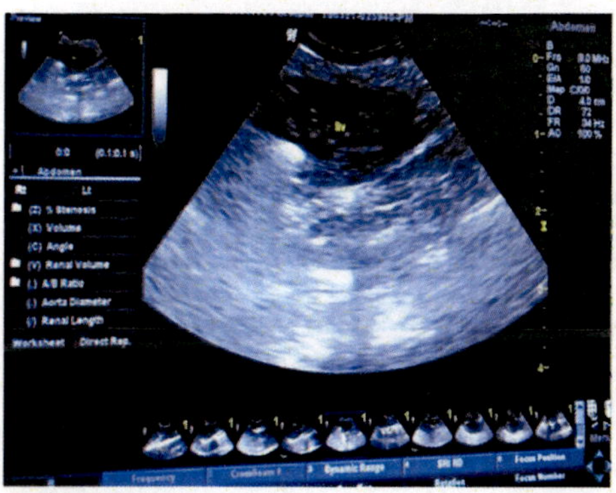

(A)

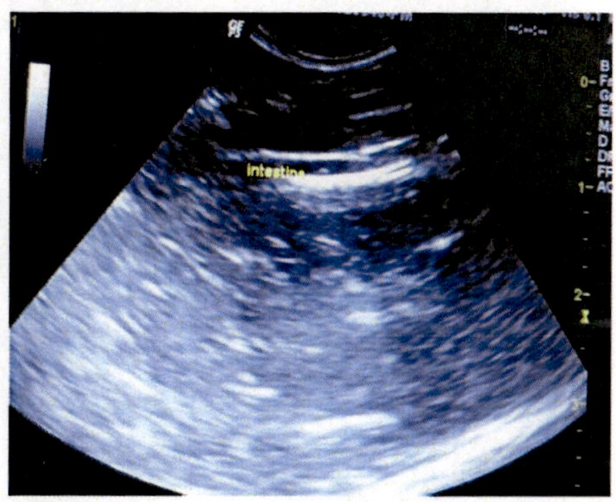

(B)

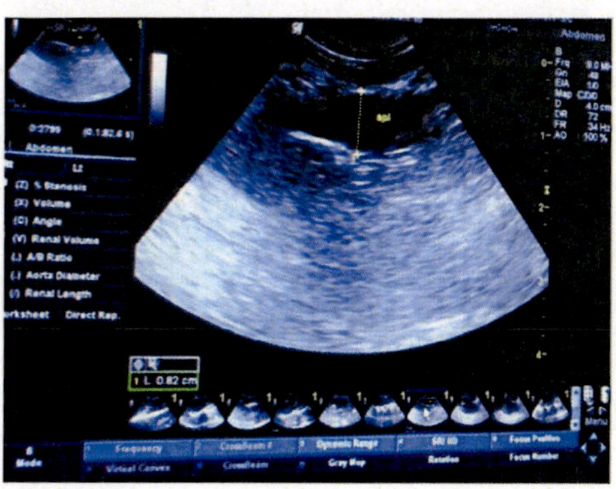

(C)

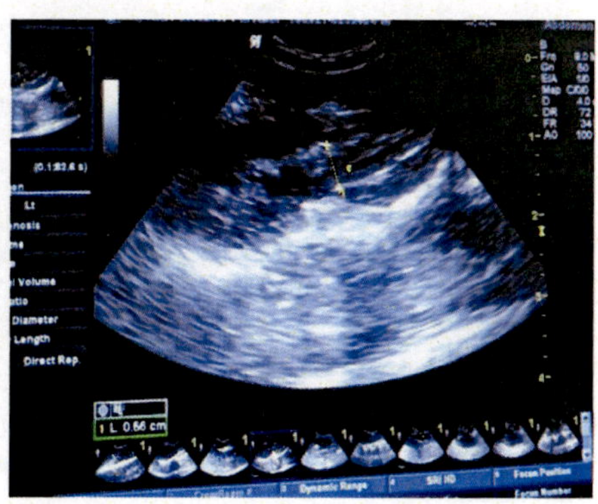

(D)

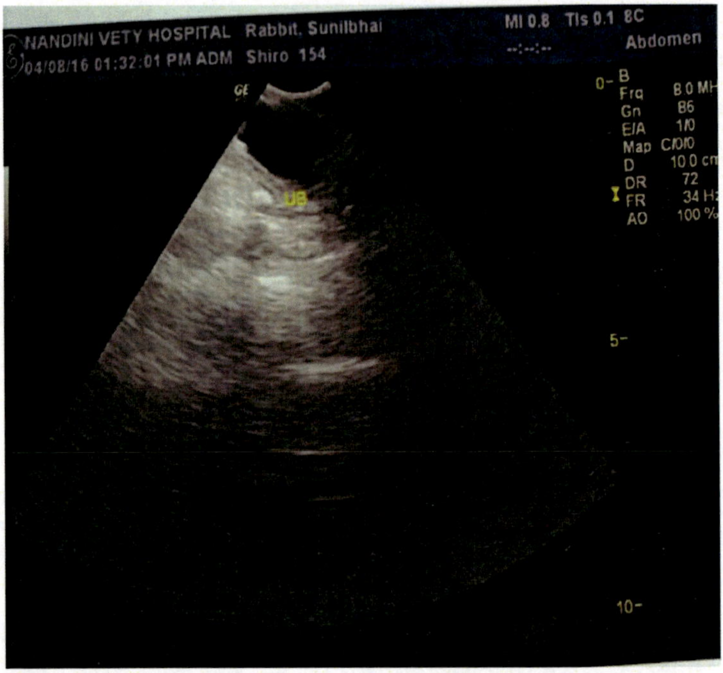

(E)

Fig. 235: Transabdominal sonogram of an adult healthy rabbit showing liver **(A)**, intestine **(B)**, spleen **(C)**, colon **(D)** and urinary bladder **(E)**.

- Abdominal ultrasonography is also very useful in rabbits for the diagnosis of liver lobe torsion, hepatic coccidiosis, haematuria, pyometra / endometritis, uterine tumour, proptosis and gut stasis.
- In hepatic coccidiosis, dilation of hepatobilliary tree is markedly seen.
- Homogenously increased echogenicity of liver is seen in hepatic lipidosis.
- Ultrasonography can help in differentiating various causes of haematuria (urolithiasis, cystitis, urinary bladder tumour, uterine tumour, renal infection or normal pigment porphyrin).
- Uterine tumour appears as echogenic mass attached to uterine wall and projecting into uterine lumen (Fig. 236)

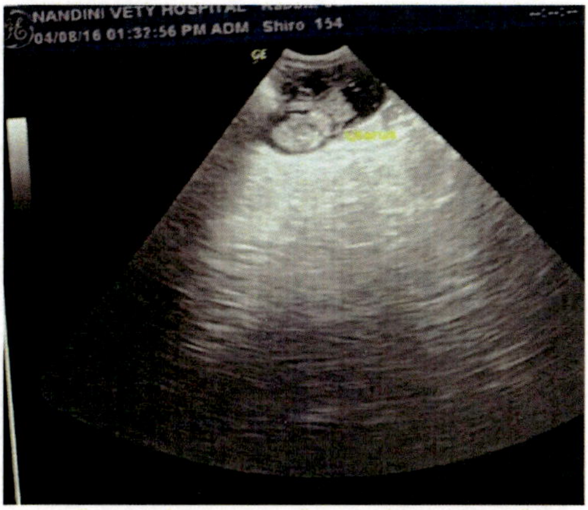

Fig. 236. Sonogram of a female rabbit with haematuria showing hyperechoic mass attached to uterine wall and projecting into uterine lumen suggesting uterine tumour.

- Gut stasis is common in rabbits. It is clinically characterized by anorexia, distended abdomen, scanty or no faeces, marked weakness and abdominal pain. Radiographic imaging is most useful in cases of gut stasis. Abdominal sonography is also being performed in the diagnosis of abdominal diseases. But the presence of large amount of gas in gastro-intestinal tract restricts its utility without reducing the gas. Sonographically gut stasis may appear as generalized distension of intestines with anechoic fluid and hyperechoic gas in the lumen (Fig. 237).

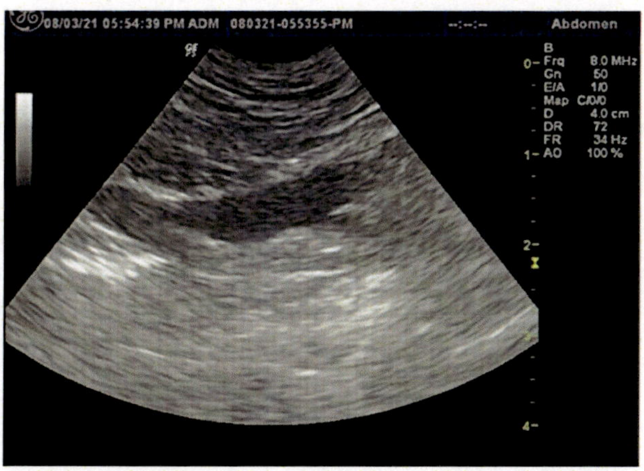

Fig. 237: Abdominal sonogram of an adult rabbit with anorexia, marked weakness, scanty faeces and abdominal pain showing distension of intestines with anechoic fluid and hyperechoic gas in the lumen with loss of intestinal layering suggesting gut stasis.

Pregnancy Diagnosis

- In rabbits gestation period is typically between 31 to 33 days.
- Ultrasonography (Real time) has been used effectively to diagnose pregnancy in rabbit doe(s) as early as day 7 of gestation.
- A 5 MHZ transducer is suitable for pregnancy diagnosis in rabbit does.
- Ultrasonographic examination of uterus of rabbits is performed transcutaneously. The site is prepared by clipping hairs and acoustic gel is applied liberally on skin and transducer. The doe is restrained in dorsal recumbency. Transducer is positioned externally against the abdominal wall in front of pubic bone. The transducer is held in sagittal plane. Scanning is done from caudal to cranial area.
- On day 7, a low echogenicity area located in the uterine lumen has been regarded as indication of pregnancy (Ypsilantis and Saratsis, 1999).
- On day 8, embryonic vesicles with a diameter of about 8 mm have been identified .It size reaches to 12 mm on day 9 and 17 mm on day 10; and embryonic pole becomes identifiable (Ypsilantis and Saratsis, 1999).

Rodents

- Transducers of 20 and 55 MHz are generally used for rodents.
- Transducers of 15–20 MHz (image depth 3–4 cm), 30–40 MHz (image depth 10–20 mm) and up to 50 MHz (image depth 9 mm) are used for adult rats, adult mice and neonatal mouse respectively.
- B- mode imaging is most commonly used in rodents.
- For heart and its valve evaluation M-mode imaging is done.
- Ultrasound technique is also used for dynamic study of ovarian structures.
- Transabdominal and transrectal ultrasounds have been used to measure aortic diameters in rodent model of aneurysm disease (Knipp *et al*., 2003).
- In guinea pigs ultrasonography can be a valuable aid in the diagnosis of pregnancy and determining the status of fetus; various causes of haematuria; lymphadenopathy (main cause is *Streptococcus zooepidemicus*): cystic ovaries and uterine abnormalities.

References

Hofbauer, H. and Krautwald-Junghanns, M.E. (1999). Transcutaneous ultrasonography of the avian urogenital tract. Vet. Radiol.Ultrasound 40:58-64.

Knipp, B.S., Ailawadi, G., Sullivan, V.V., Roelofs, K.J., Henke, P.K., Stanley, J.C. and Upchurch, G.R.(2003).Ultrasound measurement of aortic diameters in rodent.Models of aneurysm disease. J.Surg. Res.112:97-101.

Meireles, Y.S., Shiniki, F.S.,Matte, D.R., Morgado, T.O., Kempe, G.V., Correa, S.H.R., de Souza, R.L. and Nespoli,P.B. (2016). Ultrasound characterization of the coelomic cavity organs of the red footed tortoise (Chelonoidis carbonaria). Cienc. Rural 46 :1. Online version ISSN 1678-4596. (https://doi.org/10.1590/0103- 8478cr20150876).

Redrobe, S. (2006). Ultrasonography of Exotic Animals. In : Diagnostic Ultrasound in Animal Practice. Mannion, P. (ed.), Blackwell Science Ltd, A Blackwell Publishing Company, Oxford, U.K. ,p 314.

Sainsbury, A.W. and Gill, C.I.S. (1991). Ultrasonographic anatomy and scanning technique of Coelomic organs of the Bose Monitor .J. Zoo Wild Med. 22:421-433.

Stetter, M. (2000). Diagnostic imaging of reptiles. In :Current Veterinary Therapy XIII: Small Animal Practice, Kirk, R. (Ed.) .W.B. Saunders, Orlando, Florida, pp.1163—1168.

Tenhu, H., Schildger, B.J. and Gever, B. (1995). Ultraschalluntersuchungen des Grunen Leguans,Iguans iguana, (Ultrasound Investigations In green Iguanas, Iguana Iguana). Verhber Zootiere, 37:319-323.

Ypsilantis, P. and Saratsis, Ph. (1999). Early pregnancy diagnosis in the rabbits by real time ultrasonography. World Rabbit Sci. 7: 95-99.

Further Readings

Mannion, P. (2006). Diagnostic Ultrasound in Animal Practice. Blackwell Science Ltd, A Blackwell Publishing, Company, Oxford, U.K.

Section 4: Therapeutic Ultrasound

24

Therapeutic Ultrasound

J.P. Varshney and P.S. Chaudhary

- Utility of ultrasound has extended from diagnostic realm to alternate therapies. Therapeutic ultrasound is also known as ultrasound physiotherapy. It is a commonly used modality for the rehabilitation of the soft tissues of the musculoskeletal system.
- Therapeutic ultrasound is a non-invasive therapeutic modality being employed to enhance and facilitate healing owing to its thermal, mechanical and chemical effects in both dogs and cats. It decreases pain and muscle spasms as well as speed up healing process. Therapeutic ultrasound can be used along with pain killers and other pain management measures.
- Ultrasound is being used in human medicine for therapeutic purpose since 1940s.
- Its therapeutic use in veterinary medicine dates back to 1970s.
- Therapeutic ultrasound relies on variety of power setting in therapeutic ultrasound machine manufactured by different manufacturers.
- The ultrasound unit consists of a generator unit, a programmer to control parameters and a transducer head (Fig. 238). Ultrasound therapy device should regularly be calibrated at least once a month to ensure that ultrasonic power is indicated with an accuracy of ± 20% (Rivest *et al.*, 1986).

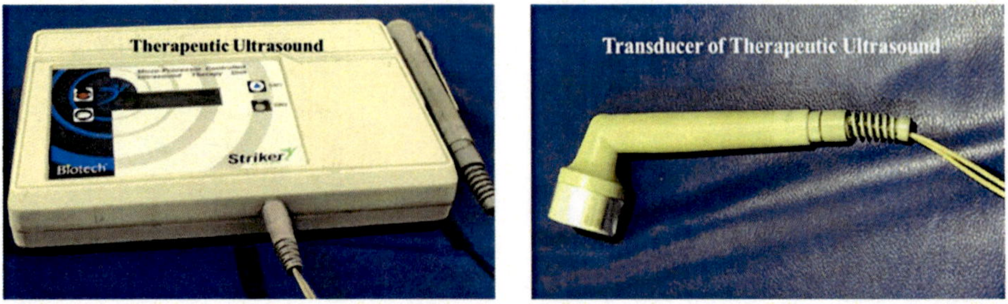

(A) **(B)**

Fig. 238: Therapeutic Ultrasound Unit **(A)** and Transducer **(B)**

- Crystal in the probe begins to vibrate at a specific frequency when an electric current is applied. The vibrations of the crystal generate pulsed or continuous pressure waves (energy) that pass through the skin and vibrate the tissues.
- The physical effects resulting from compression and rarefaction of energy are acoustic streaming and acoustic cavitation. These non-thermal phenomena accelerate the inflammatory phase of wound healing (Tsai *et al.*, 2011), promote ion transport, increase cellular permeability (Dinno *et al.*,1989), increase fibroblast protein synthesis (Ramirez *et al.*, 1997, and Doan *et al.,* 1999), and promote shifts in extracellular ion concentration gradients (terHaar, 1999).
- Thermal effects vary and are correlated to the magnitude of tissue warming. Thermal effect is due to absorption of energy from the waves when ultrasound beam penetrates into the tissues. Tissue warming has been shown to increase collagen extensibility and improve flexibility.
- For therapeutic purpose 1 MHz probe is used for the treatment of tissues deep up to 8 cm and 3 MHz probe is used for the treatment of superficial tissues
- Recently a low frequency therapeutic ultrasound (38 kHz) is being used to produce much deeper and much more intense effect than traditional high frequency therapeutic ultrasound (1 to 3 MHz) for an effective treatment of muscles, tendons, ligaments, joints and bone conditions in horses and dogs both in acute and chronic stages.
- The power ranges from 0.2 to 3.0 watts/square cm
- The ultrasound probe is applied directly against the pet's skin using water-soluble ultrasound gel.

- Therapeutic ultrasound is used to soften and break down scars, to reduce pain and inflammation through its thermal effect that in turn increases blood supply.
- Usually no sedation is needed for dogs and cats. Nevertheless, proper restrain is mandatory. Area to be subjected to therapeutic ultrasound is prepared by shaving and applying ultrasound gel. Therapeutic ultrasound probe is applied directly on the area and is moved steadily over the area in overlapping manner.
- Generally a session lasts for 10 to 20 minutes. Treatment is given 2 to 3 sessions per week till condition improves.
- Therapeutic ultrasound provides relief in injuries as it has potential to reduce inflammation, reduce pain, increase blood supply, and to increase motion in old injuries of tendons and ligaments.

Therapeutic ultrasound is indicated in the management of tendon injuries, ligament injuries, bursa injuries, scar tissue management, preventing post operational scars, acute swellings, muscle injuries, and slow healing wounds. Continuous ultrasound followed by pulsating ultrasound is used for the management of fibrosis of muscles, tendons or ligaments for good antifibrotic effect. Muscle spasms can be reduced by the application therapeutic ultrasound.

- Therapeutic ultrasound can also be used in the management of chronic problems such as hip dysplasia, elbow dysplasia, osteoarthritis and chronic pain.
- Therapeutic ultrasound can also be employed for controlling inflammation and post-surgical problems such as a torn cranial cruciate ligament or patellar dislocation.
- In the 1980s, high pressure-amplitude shockwaves came into use in humans for mechanically resolving kidney stones, and "lithotripsy" rapidly replaced surgery as the most frequent treatment choice.
- The use of ultrasonic energy for therapy is continuing to expand, and other applications include uterine fibroid ablation, tumour ablation, cataract removal (phacoemulsification), surgical tissue cutting and haemostasis, transdermal drug delivery, and bone fracture healing in humans. For tumour ablation, high intensity focused ultrasound (HIFU) is used.
- Prospective new areas of the application of therapeutic ultrasound are being explored continuously in human medicine. One such area is direct

sonothrombolysis using external typically low frequency ultrasound for the treatment of thrombotic diseases such as stroke (Siegal and Luo, 2008). Micro bubble based therapeutic ultrasound is another new area being researched for targeted therapy. Another area is the cavitation mechanism that is also being exploited to create a new tissue-ablation method known as histotripsy (Kieran *et al.*, 2007).

- Application of therapeutic ultrasound is contraindicated over orthopaedic implants, bone plates, tumours (malignancies), infected areas, gravid uterus, open spinal cord, growth plates of young one's bones, eyes, skull, testicles, heart, brain, open wounds, skin rashes, eczema, over areas of decreased sensation, around eyes and sex organs, and over an area of acute infection. Ultrasound should also be not used on unconscious patients.
- Undesirable bio effects (burns) can occur for thermal-based therapies and significant haemorrhage for mechanical-based therapies (e.g. lithotripsy).
- Though therapeutic ultrasound is an alternate therapy due to their low risk of complication, superficial burns may be associated with prolonged exposure time of low intensity ultrasound. Therefore it is necessary that ultrasound band remains in motion when in contact with the skin.

References

Dinno, M.A., Crum, L.A. and Wu, J. (1989). The effect of therapeutic ultrasound on electrophysiological parameters of frog skin. Ultrasound Med. Biol. 15:461–470.

Doan, N., Reher Meghji, P.S. and Harris, M. (1999). *In Vitro*e ffects of Therapeutic ultrasound on cell proliferation, protein synthesis, and cytokine poduction by human fibroblasts, osteoblasts, and monocytes. J. Oral Maxillofacial Surg. 57:409–19.

Kieran, K., Hall, T.L., Parsons, J.E., Wolf, J.S., Jr. Fowlkes, J.B., Cain, C.A and Roberts, W.W. (2007). Refining histotripsy: defining the parameter space for the creation of nonthermal lesions with high intensity, pulsed focused ultrasound of the in vitro kidney. J Urol. 178:672–676.

Ramirez, A., Schwane, J.A., McFarland, C. and Starcher, B.(1997). The effect of ultrasound on collagen synthesis and fibroblast proliferation *in vitro*. Med. Sci. Sports. Exerc. 29:326–32.

Rivest, M., Girardi, C.Q.D., Seaborne, D. and Lambert, J. (1886). Evaluation of therapeutic ultrasound devices: performance stability over 44 weeks of clinical use. Physiotherapy Can.39:77-86.

Siegel, R.J. and Luo, H. (2008). Ultrasound thrombolysis. Ultrasonics 48:312–320. terHaar, G. (1999). Therapeutic ultrasound. Eur. J. Ultrasound. 9:3–9.

Tsai, W.C., Tang, S.T. and Liang, F.C. (2011). Effect of therapeutic ultrasound on tendons. Am. J. Phys. Med. Rehabil. 90:1068–1073.

Suggested Further Reading

Saini, N.S., Roy, K.S., Bansal, P.S., Singh, B. and Simran, P.S. (2002). A preliminary study on the effect of ultrasound therapy on the healing of surgically severed Achilles tendons in five dogs. Vet.Med. A. Physiol. Pathol.Clin.Med. 49:321-328.

Section 5: Case Studies

25

Sonograms in Different Diseases of Animals: Case Studies

J.P. Varshney, P.S. Chaudhary and Neetu Saini

Sonograms of animals suffering from different diseases are presented along with other investigations as case studies to provide a comprehensive picture of the disease.

Canines

Ascites

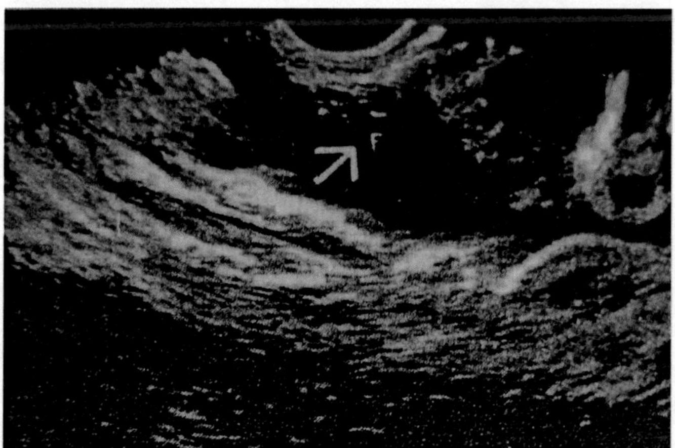

Fig. 239: Trans abdominal sonogram of a dog with canine monocytic ehrlichiosis showing an increased amount of anechoic fluid in the peritoneum suggesting ascites (Kumar and Varshney, 2006).

Cardiac Diseases

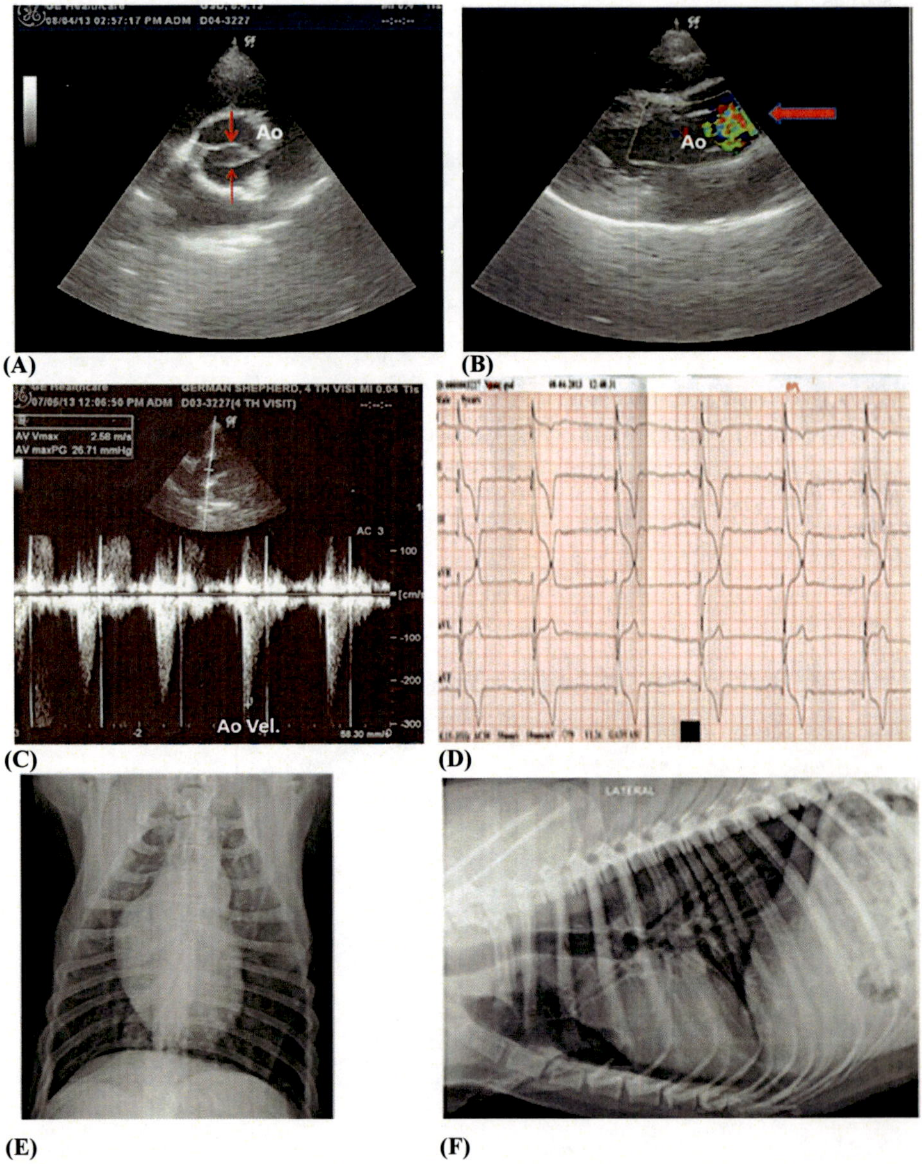

Fig. 240: Echocardiogram, electrocardiogram and radiographs of a nine year old male German Shepherd with exercise intolerance, malaise, lethargy, weakness and fever for one month. 2-D echocardiogram right parasternal short axis view **(A)** is showing two cusps of unequal size in the aortic valve giving "fish mouth like" appearance more pronounced in systole. Normally aortic valve has three cusps. Colour flow Doppler right parasternal long axis view **(B)** at aortic valve revealed large eccentric jet of aortic regurgitation. The aortic flow velocity, measured

Contd.

from left apical five-chamber view with continuous-wave Doppler **(C)** was high (2.58 m/sec) as compared to the normal reference value (1.02±0.143m/s). Electrocardiogram **(D)** is showing wide QRS suggestive of left bundle branch block(LBBB). Radiograph in ventro-dorsal view is showing a bulge between 1 and 2 O' clock position **(E)** and radiograph in right lateral recumbency is showing prominence at the level of the cranial waist of the heart **(F)** . Based on these investigations the dog was diagnosed with aortic insufficiency due to bicuspid aortic valve (Saini *et al.*, 2018).

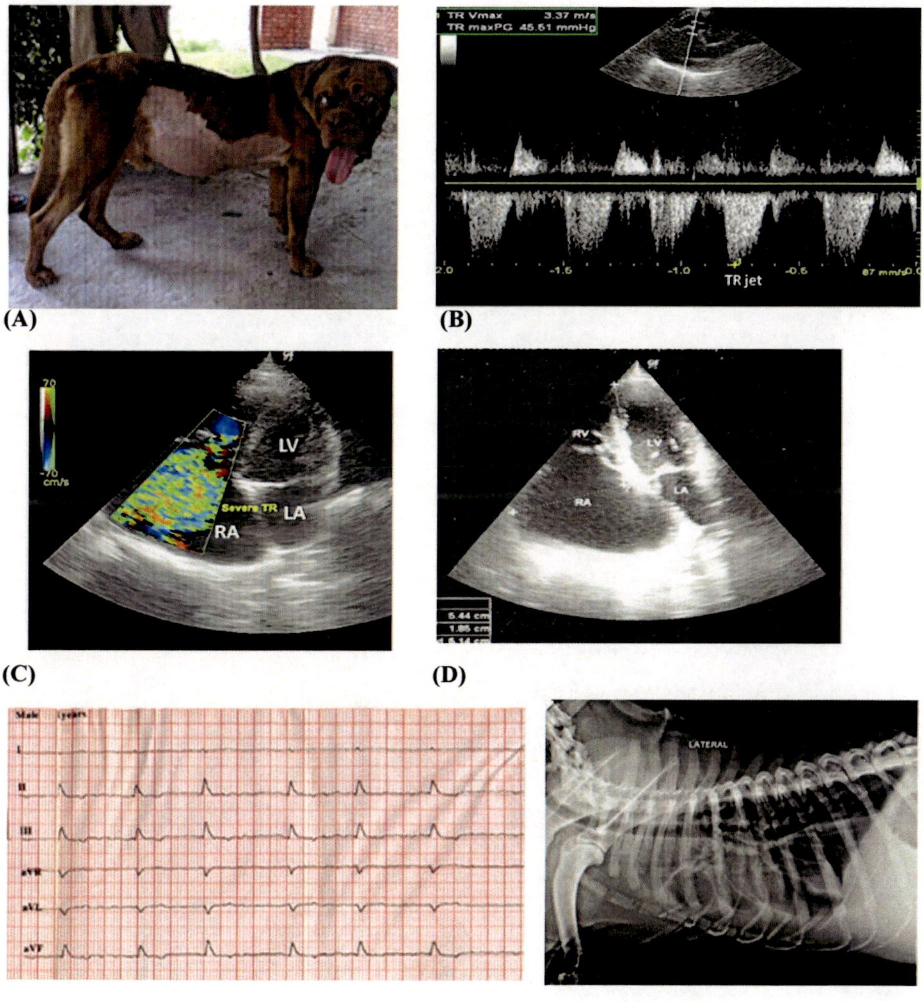

(A) **(B)** **(C)** **(D)** **(E)** **(F)**

Fig. 241: Showing echocardiogram, electrocardiogram and radiographs of one year old male French Mastiff **(A)** with exercise intolerance, anorexia, ascites, lethargy and weakness. Continuous wave Doppler **(B)** examination revealed high tricuspid regurgitant velocity (3.37 m/s) indicating an increased pressure gradient between right atrium and right ventricle (45.51 mm Hg). Colour Doppler examination **(C)** is showing severe tricuspid regurgitation into right atrium

Contd.

and severely enlarged right atrium (left apical four chamber view). TR= Tricuspid regurgitation, RA= Right atrium, LA= Left atrium and LV= left ventricle. The ventrally displaced tricuspid septal leaflet is seen in the left apical 4 chamber view **(D)** indicating Ebstein's anomaly. The total length of right ventricle is 5.44 cm with 1.86 cm atrialised right ventricle. Interventricular septum is pushed towards the left side due to elevated pressure in right cardiac chambers RV= Right ventricle, RA = right atrium, LV = left ventricle, LA =left atrium. Electrocardiogram of the dog **(E)** is consistent with low voltage complex and atrial fibrillation .Tracheal elevation, increased tracheal bifurcation angle, mild pleural effusions and pulmonary edema are evident in the radiograph **(F)**.The diagnosis of Ebstein's anomaly is based on detection of tricuspid valve regurgitation with severe right atrial enlargement and downward displacement of tricuspid valve leaflets into right ventricle on Doppler echocardiography (Saini et al., 2017).

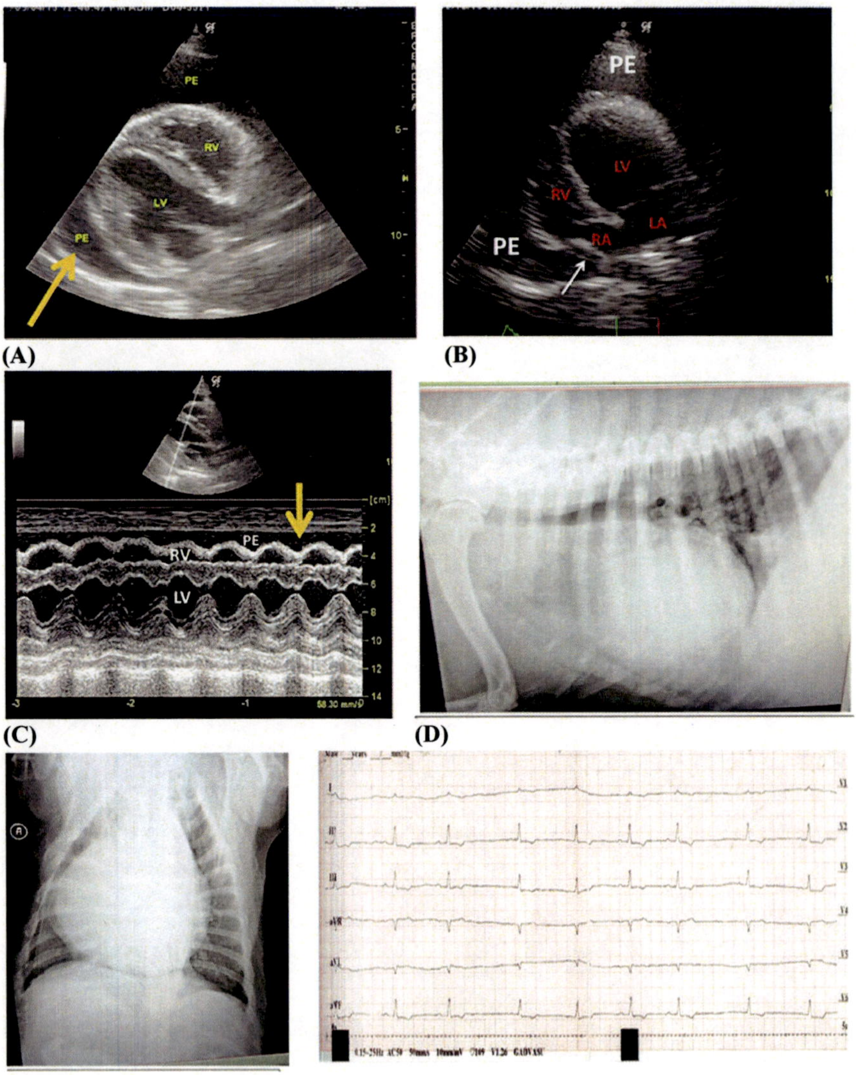

Fig. 242: Showing echocardiogram, electrocardiogram and radiographs of a seven year old male Labrador with exercise intolerance, dyspnoea, ascites and lethargy. The large echo-free space of pericardial effusions surrounds the heart of this dog in right parasternal long axis view **(A)**. PE = pericardial effusions, RV = right ventricle, LV = left ventricle. Left apical four chamber view **(B)** is showing right atrial diastolic collapse indicating cardiac tamponade (white arrow). M-mode image at right parasternal long axis view **(C)** is showing right ventricular diastolic collapse (arrow) indicating cardiac tamponade. PE = pericardial effusions, RV = right ventricle, RA = right atrium, LV =left ventricle, LA = left atrium . Globoid heart occupying five intercostal spaces with alveolar pattern in cranial lung lobe in right lateral **(D)** ; and enlarged heart occupying more than 75% space in ventro-dorsal thoracic **(E)** radiographs is evident. Low voltage complexes in electrocardiogram **(F)** is also suggested pericardial effusions. Based on echocardiographic, electrocardiographic and radiographic investigations the Labrador was diagnosed with pericardial effusion due to cardiac temponade.

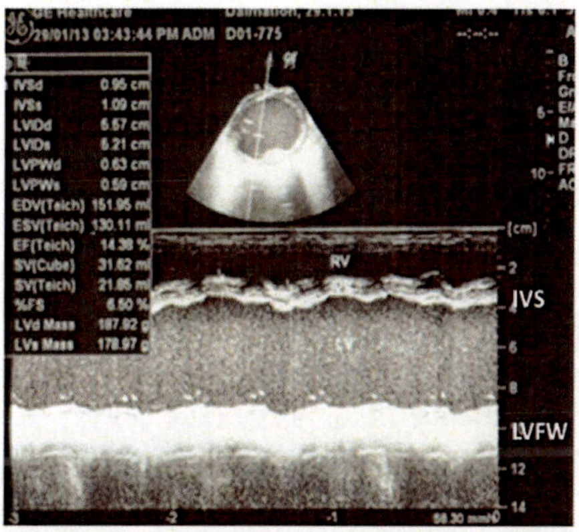

(A)

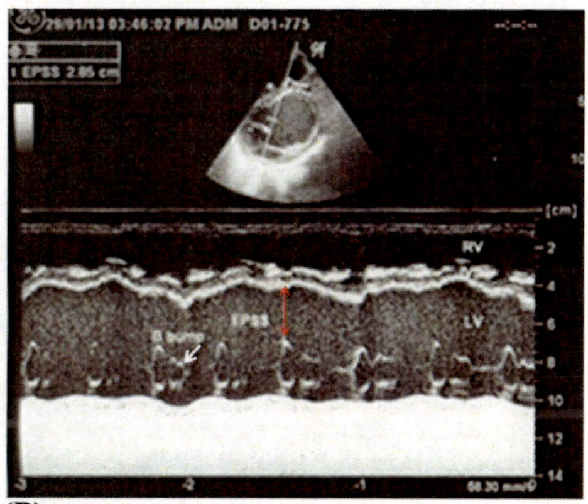

(B)

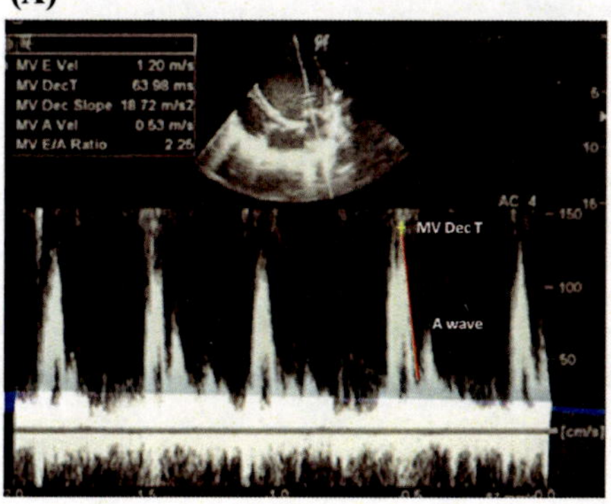

(C)

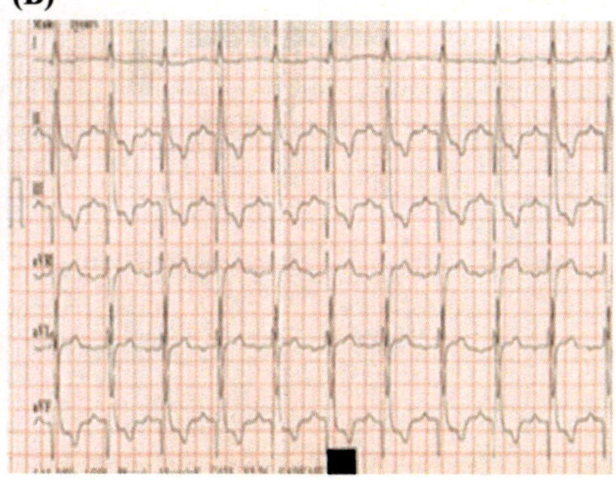
(D)

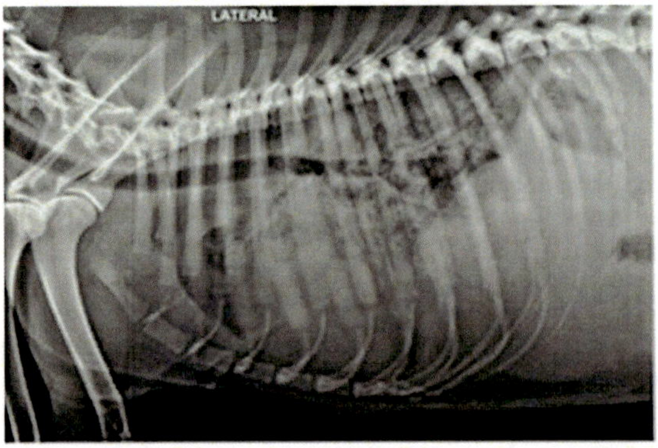

(E)

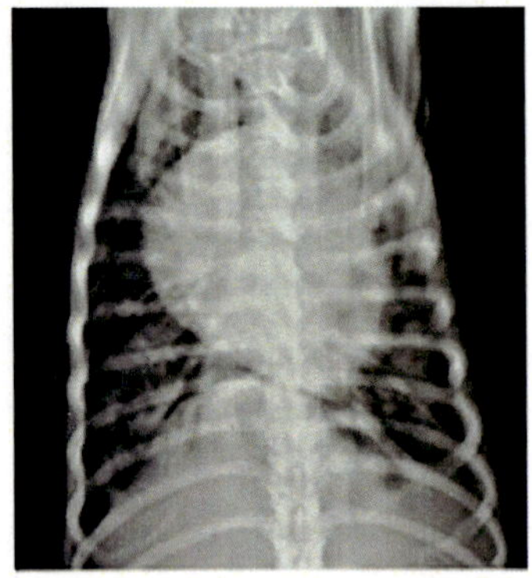

(F)

Fig. 243: Showing echocardiogram, electrocardiogram and radiographs of one year old male Dalmatian with episodic coughing, severe progressive dyspnoea, panting, pyrexia, exercise intolerance, lethargy and nasal discharge for 10-15 days. M mode echocardiography at the level of chordae tendinae **(A)** revealed dilation of left ventricle while at the level of mitral valve **(B)** indicated increased EPSS (2.85 cm) and a 'B' bump at the end of mitral valve diastolic motion indicating a delayed closure and an increased end diastolic left ventricular pressure. The EF % (Ejection Fraction) and FS % are 14.38 % and6.5 % respectively indicating systolic failure. RV = right ventricle, LV =left ventricle, IVS = Interventricular septum, LVFW = left ventricular Free wall. FS%- Fractional shortening and EF%-Ejection Fraction. Pulse Doppler echocardiography at mitral valve **(C)** is showing restrictive filling pattern.Rapid early mitral valve deceleration time (63.98msec) and a lower A wave velocity are associated with poor survival in dogs with dilated cardiomyopathy. MV DecT = Mitral valve deceleration time. Tall (2.8 mV) and wide (0.08 s) 'QRS' with deep Q (0.8 mV) was consistent with bi-ventricular enlargement **(D)**. Radiographs of chest confirmed severe perihilar edema masking the cardiac shadow and alveolar pattern indicating pulmonary edema in caudal lung lobe **(E)**, shifting of the apex of heart to left side, dilation of pulmonary vein at the level of 9th rib and increased tracheal bifurcation angle **(F)** further confirming cardiomyopathy. Based on echocardiographic, electrocardiographic and radiographic investigations the dog was diagnosed with dilated cardiomyopathy.

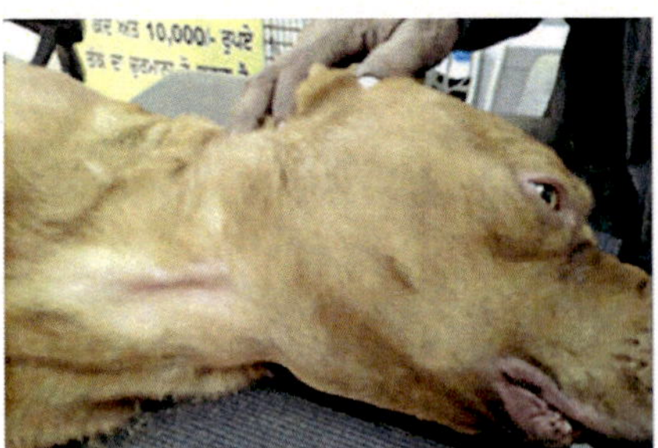

(A)

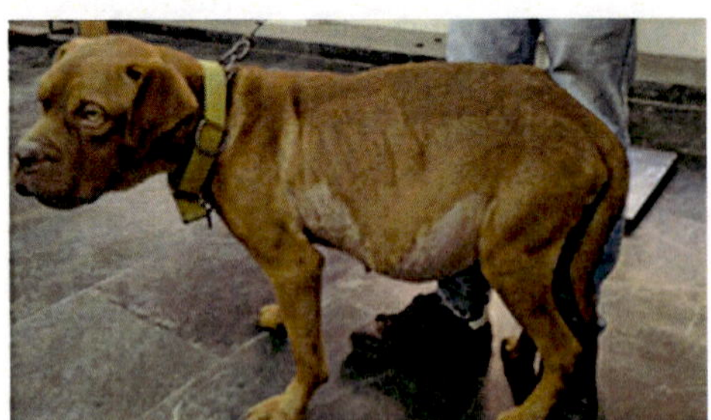

(B)

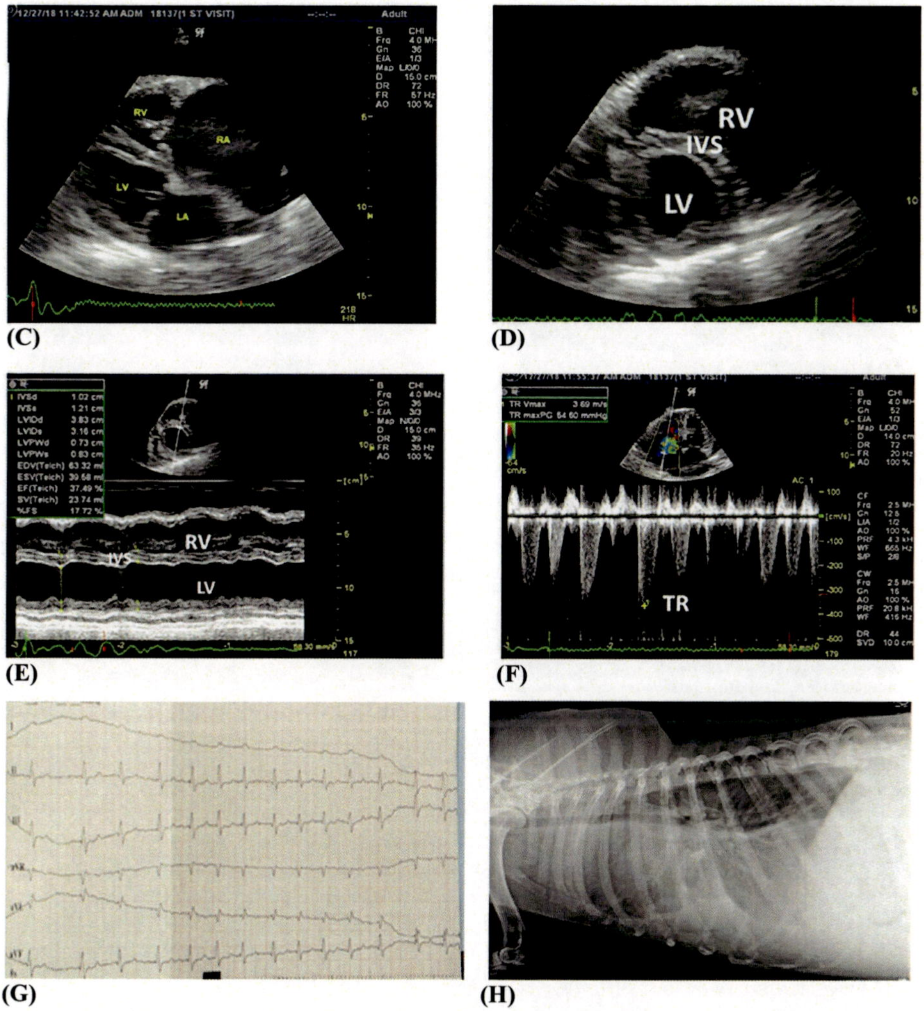

Fig. 244: Showing echocardiogram, electrocardiogram and radiographs of a two year old male French Mastiff with jugular distension **(A)**, abdominal distension **(B)**, exercise intolerance, and respiratory distress. 2- D echocardiogram at right parasternal long axis view is showing severe enlargement of right cardiac chambers **(C)**. There is flattening (bowing) of the ventricular septum towards the left ventricle due to elevated pressure in right cardiac chambers. RV = right ventricle, RA = right atrium, LV = left ventricle, LA =left atrium. Right parasternal transverse image **(D)** is showing enlarged right ventricle (RV) and flattening of interventricular septum. Right ventricular enlargement with poor ventricular function is also evident in M-mode electrocardiography **(E)**. Continuous wave Doppler at tricuspid valve **(F)** is showing high tricuspid regurgitant velocity of 3.69 m/s indicating an increased pressure gradient (54.60 mm Hg) between right atrium and right ventricle .Electrocardiogram **(G)** is showing low voltage complexes. Severe pleural effusion is seen in right lateral chest radiograph **(H)**. Based on investigations the dog was diagnosed with right ventricular cardiomyopathy.

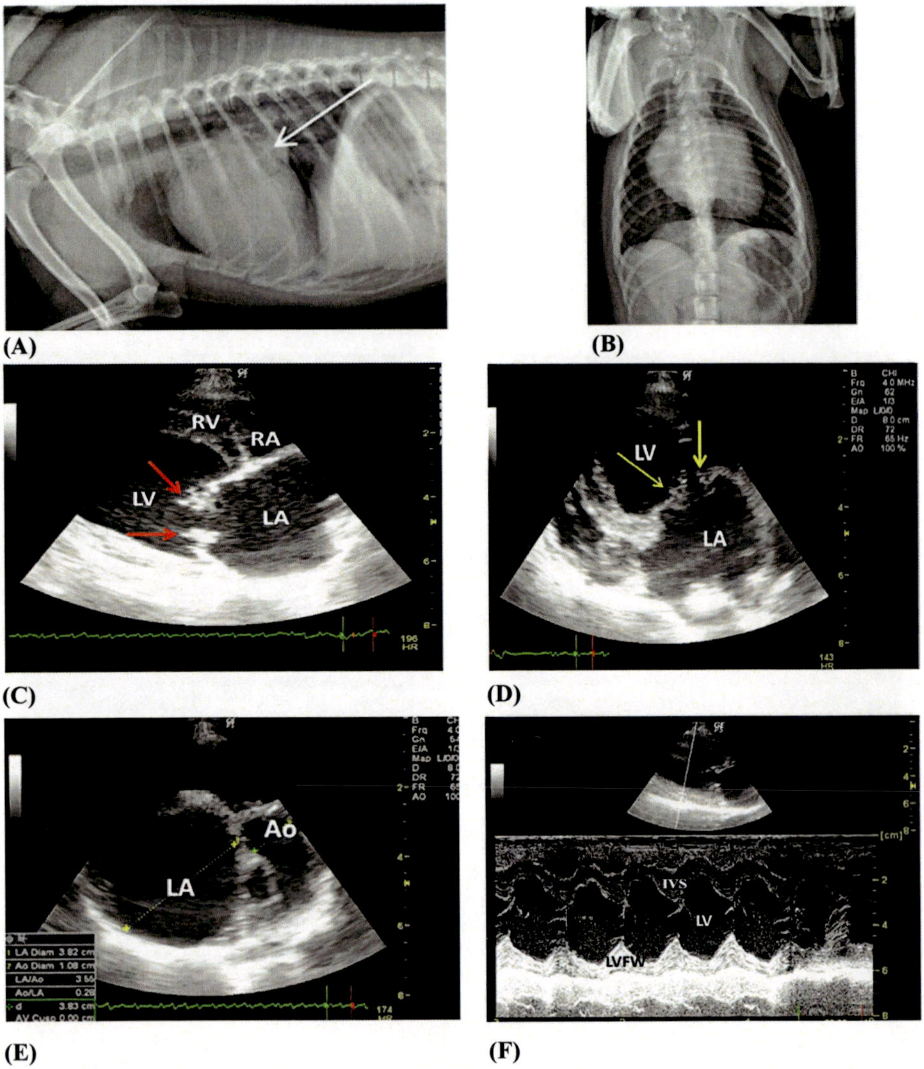

Fig. 245: Showing echocardiogram and radiographs of a six year old male Pomeranian with exercise intolerance, dyspnoea, lethargy and chronic coughing for one month. Radiographs taken in right lateral recumbency**(A)** and ventrodorsal **(B)** views showed left atrial enlargement. 2-D echocardiogram in right parasternal long axis view **(C)** and left apical four chamber view **(D)** are showing thickened mitral valve leaflets (arrows) suggesting chronic mitral valve disease(CMVD). Another 2-D echocardiogram **(E),** taken in right parasternal short axis view at the level of aorta, is showing severe left atrial enlargement. LA: Ao ratio is 3.56. M -mode echocardiography **(F)** is showing hyperkinetic interventricular septum (IVS) and left ventricular free wall (LVFW). Based on echocardiographic and radiographic findings the dog was diagnosed with chronic mitral valve degenerative disease.

The characteristic M mode echocardiographic changes in right parasternal short axis view at the level of mitral valve in this case are exaggerated movement of inter-ventricular septum and hyper- dynamic left ventricular systolic functions with an increased EF% and FS% .

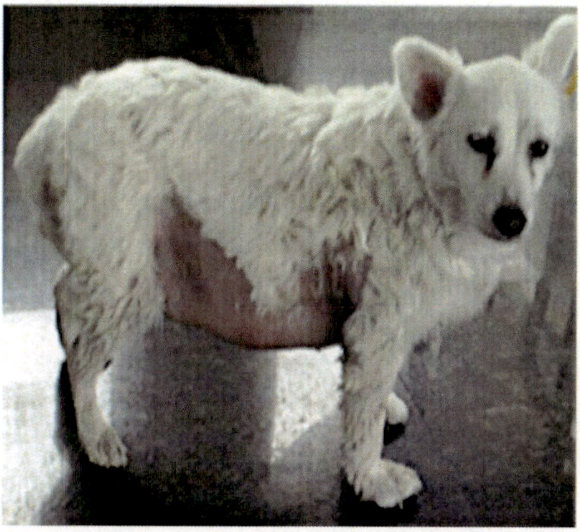

(A)

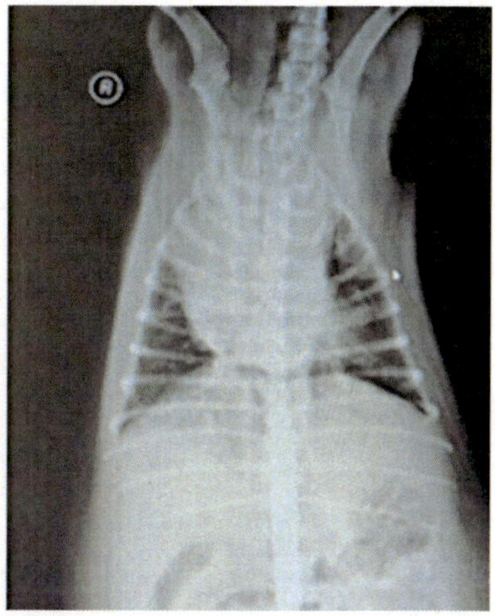

(B)

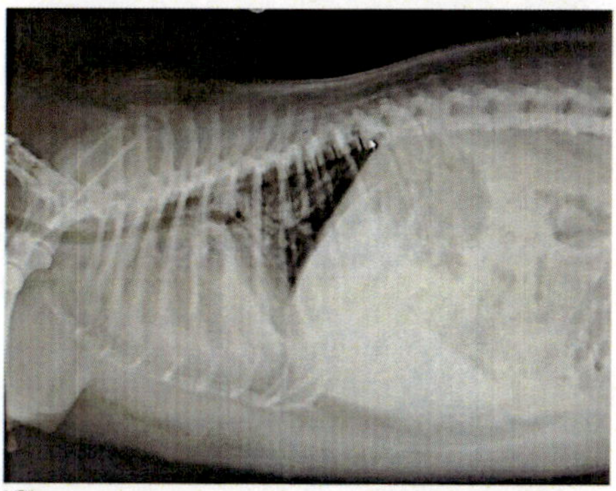

(C)

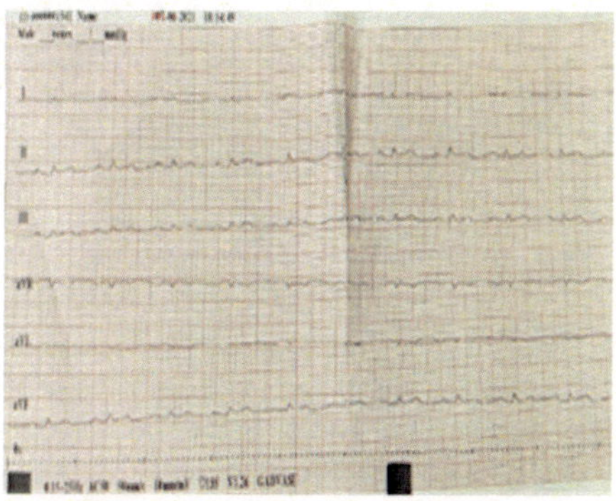

(D)

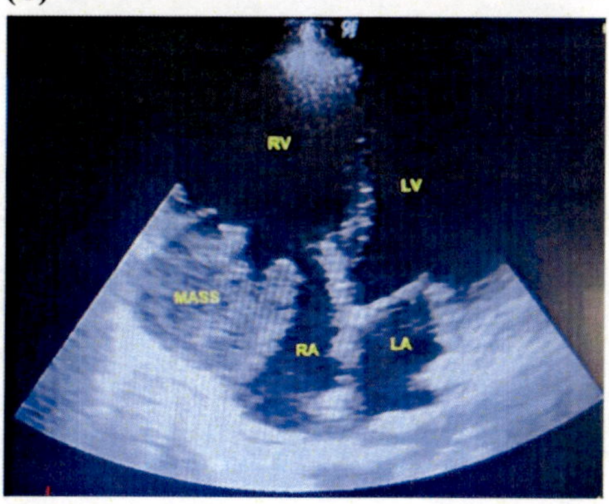

(E)

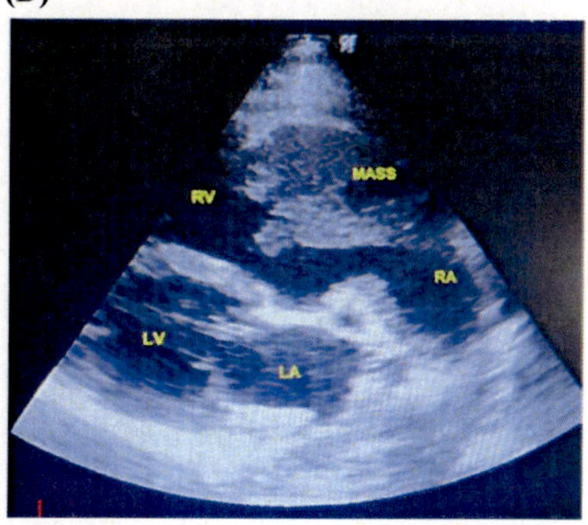

(F)

Fig. 246: Radiographs, electrocardiogram and sonograms of a nine year old Pomeranian dog **(A)** with the history of abdominal distension, hind limb oedema and ventral body line edema, exercise

Contd.

intolerance and lethargy. Radiographs are showing soft tissue density in cranial mediastinum and pleural fissure line in ventro-dorsal view (B); and hazy cardiac silhouette, dorsally pushed up trachea, severe interstitial lung pattern in caudal lung lobe and pleural effusions in right lateral view (C). Low voltage complex with sinus rhythm and heart rate of 130 bpm is evident in the electrocardiogram (D). Left apical 4 chamber view (E) and right parasternal long axis view (F) are showing hyperechoic irregular margined mass in the right atrium with the enlargement of both right atrium and right ventricle. Based on these investigations the dog with hind limb and ventral body line oedema was diagnosed with cardiac mass in the right atrium.

Diaphragmatic Hernia

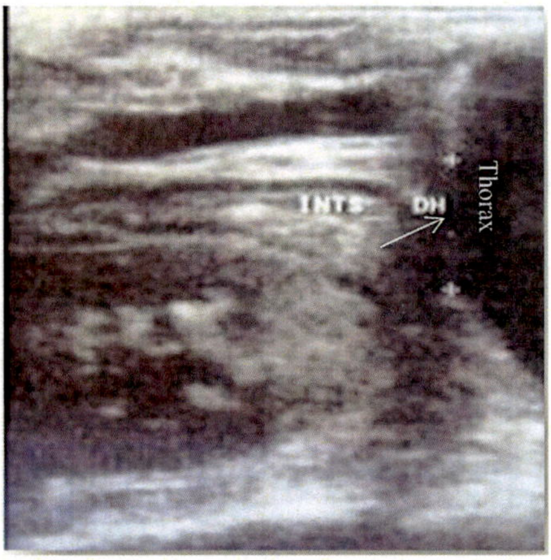

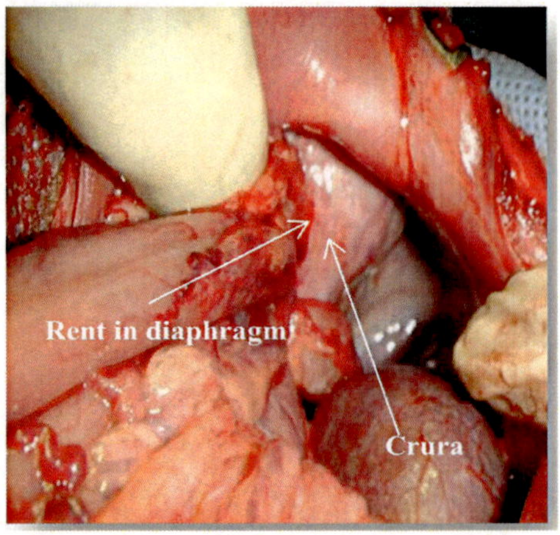

(A) **(B)**

Fig. 247: Trans abdominal sonogram of a dyspneic stray dog revealed breach in the diaphragm and invading intestines in the thorax suggesting diaphragmatic hernia **(A)**. Surgical intervention confirmed rent in the crura **(B)**.

Gastro-intestinal System

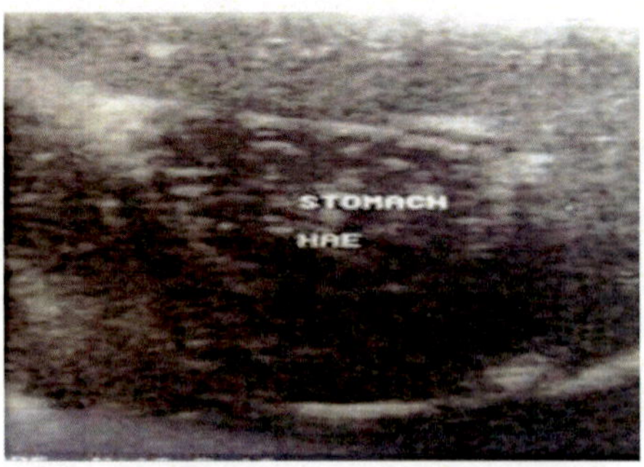

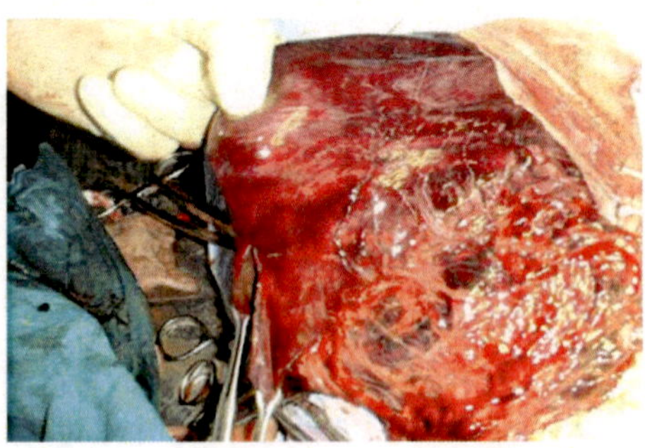

(A) **(B)**

Fig. 248: Trans abdominal sonogram of a Labrador with blood mixed vomiting showing focal hyperechoic zones of increased gas accumulation or blood clots at gastric mucosal surface **(A)** suggesting gastric ulceration and hemorrhages. Surgery confirmed gastric ulceration with hemorrhages **(B)**.

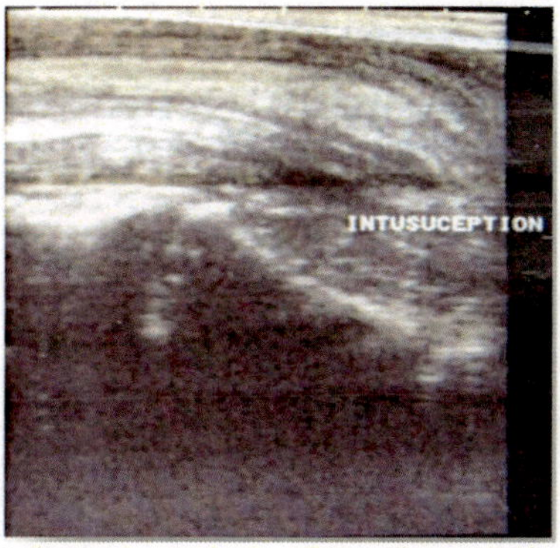

(A)

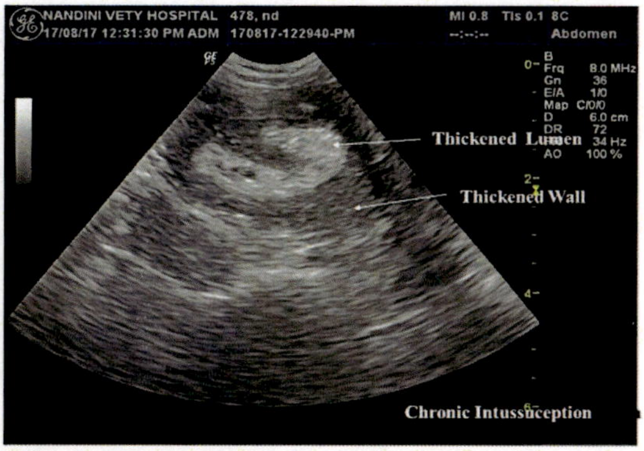

(B)

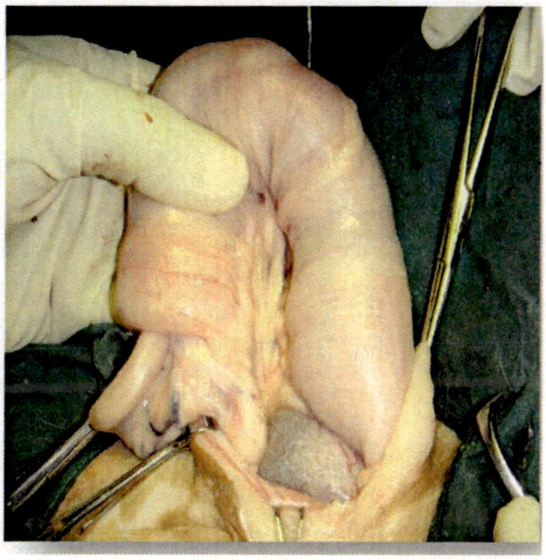

(C)

Fig. 249: Trans abdominal sonogram of a dog with abdominal pain showing multilayered concentric ring appearance of intestines **(A)**, thickening of intestinal wall and lumen **(B)** suggesting chronic intussusception. Laparotomy confirmed intussusception **(C)**.

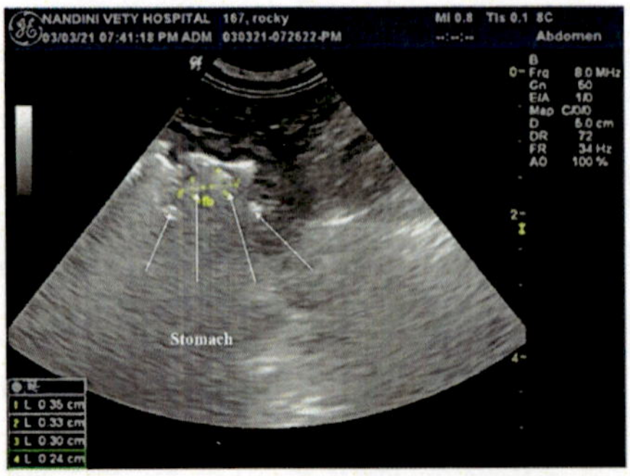

(A)

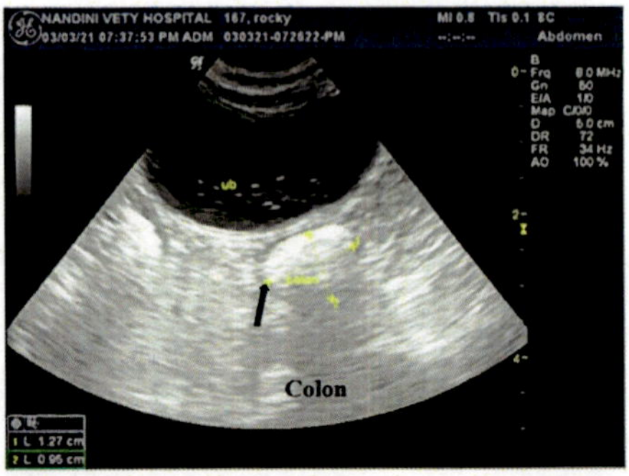

(B)

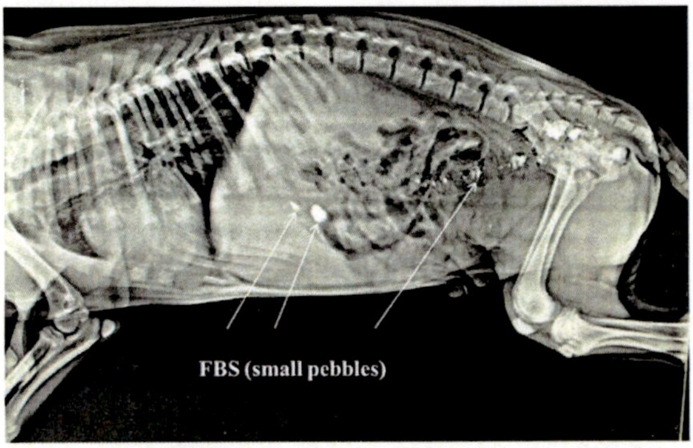

(C)

Fig. 250: Trans abdominal sonogram **(A and B)** and radiograph **(C)** of a male Siberian Huskie with vomiting and abdominal pain. Sonogram revealed small hyperechoic irregular shaped material with shadowing in the stomach **(A)** and colon **(B)** suggesting small pebbles (foreign bodies). Radiograph also confirmed multiple small variable size and shaped foreign bodies resembling with small pebbles in the stomach and intestines.

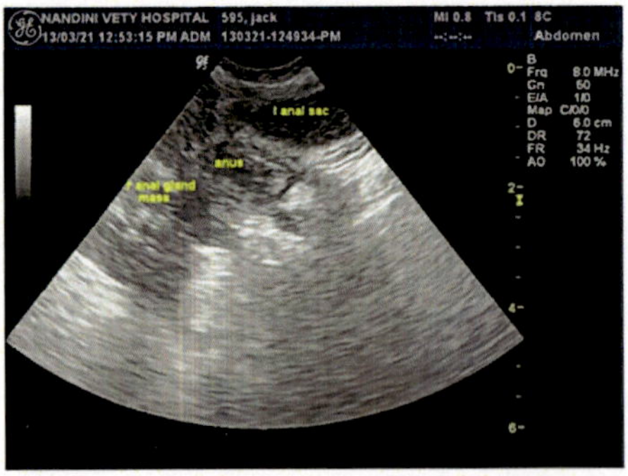

(A)

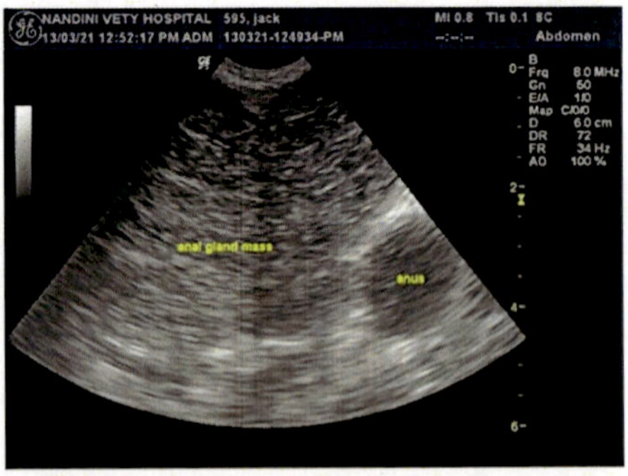

(B)

Fig. 251: Sonogram of anal sacs, in dorsal recumbency, of a seven year old male Labrador with anal bleeding, difficult passage of faeces and painful palpable anal mass showing echogenic circumscribed structure in the right anal sac **(A, B)** suggesting an anal sac tumour. Biochemical

Contd.

investigations revealed the values of serum creatinine, blood urea nitrogen, total serum proteins, serum albumin, serum alkaline phosphatase, ALT, AST, total serum bilirubin, direct bilirubin and serum calcium as 1.2 mg/dl, 20.0 mg/dl, 8.0g/dl, 3.0g/dl, 94U/L 35 IU/L, 27.0 IU/L, 0.9 mg/dl, 0.2 mg/dl, and 7.2 mg/dl respectively.

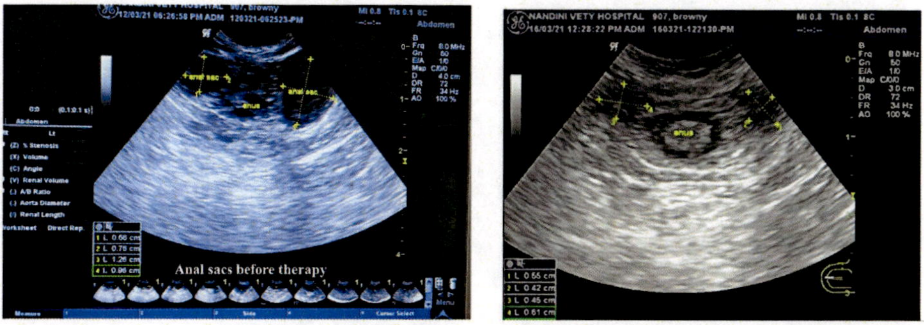

(A) (B)

Fig. 252: Sonogram of a male non-descript dog with anal scooting and, pyogenic discharge from anus showing distended anal sacs (Left 0.76 x 0.66 cm; Right 1.26 x 0.96 cm **(A)** having hypoechoic fluid with diffuse point like hyperechoic debris suggesting anal sac infection. The dog was treated with parenteral enrofloxacin and meloxicam with povidone iodine solution anal flushing after anal sac squeezing daily for 7 days. Post therapy sonogram **(B)** showed regression in the size of anal sacs (Left 0.66 x 0.42 cm; Right 0.61 x 0.45 cm) and sac contents became anechoic.

Hepatobiliary system

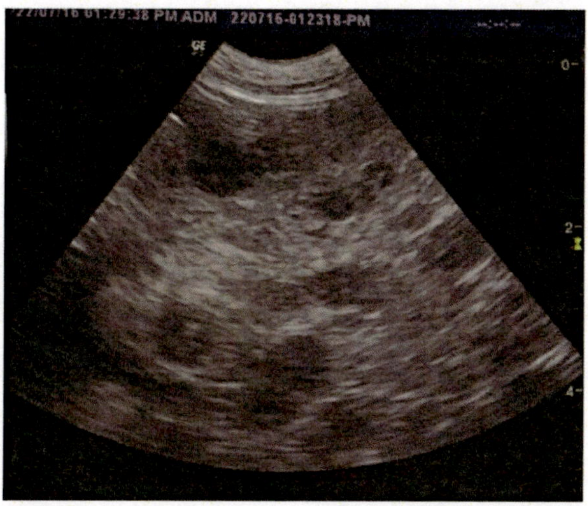

Fig. 253: Sonogram of a 3.5 year old male Great Dane with vomiting, anorexia, polydipsia, polyuria, progressive increase in total bilirubin (1.8, 2.6, 3.7, 3.9, 6.8, 8.7 mg/dl), blood urea (39.6,46.0, 56.0, 60.7, 68.2, 78,6 mg/dl), serum creatinine (0.95, 0.98, 1.3 ,2.0, 2.8, 3.4 mg/dl); progressive decrease in Hb (16.6, 15.0, 13.0 , 12.7, 10.7,10.0 g/dl), PCV (50,45,38,36,33, 31%), RBC (7.18, 6.2, 5.59, 5.5 ,5.1, 4.0 x10^6/mm^3) and blood platelet count (128000, 117000,110000, 89000, 80000, 58000 /mm^3) showing multiple hypoechoic patches of variable size in liver lobe suggesting hepatic nodular hyperplasia.

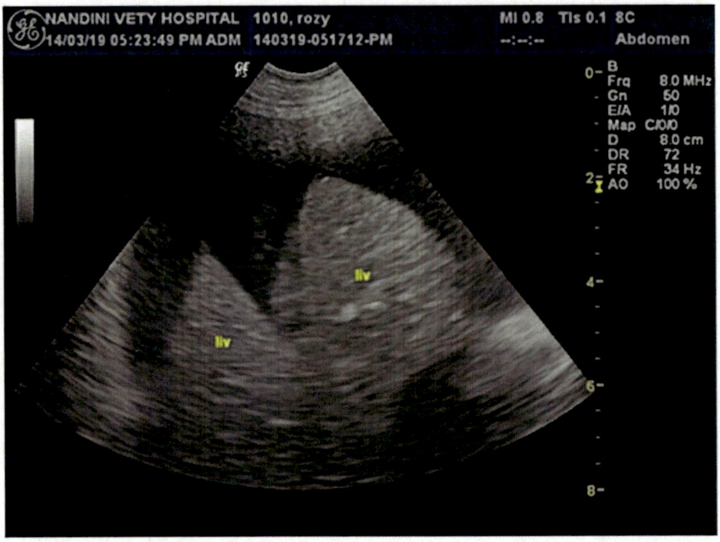

Fig. 254: Trans abdominal sonogram of a six year old Golden Retriever bitch with ascites showing hyperechoic liver suggestive of liver cirrhosis / liver fibrosis. Values of serum creatinine (1.8mg/dl), blood urea nitrogen (25.0 mg/dl), ALT (26 U/L), AST (18 U/L), SAP (100 U/l), total bilirubin (.0.8 mg/dl), direct bilirubin (0.3 mg/dl), total serum proteins (6.3 g/dl), serum albumin (2.9 g/dl) were within normal range. The liver enzymes were towards lower margin of normal value.

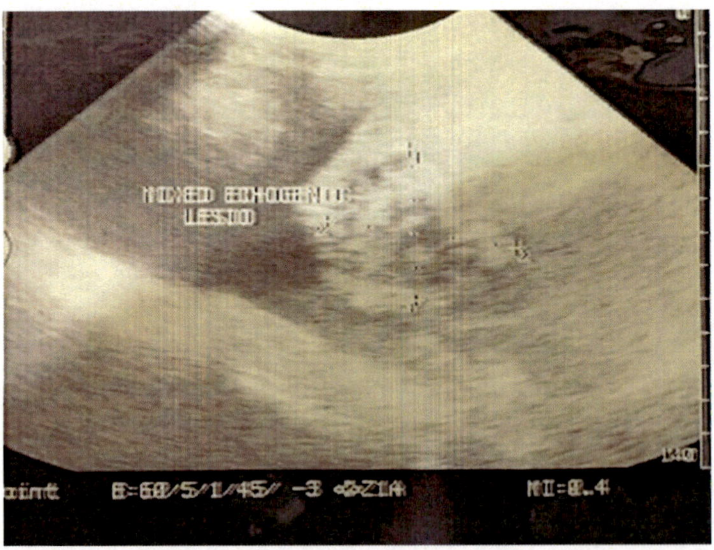

Fig. 255: Trans abdominal sonogram of a 14 month old male Pomeranian with muscular twitching, melena, jaundice, vomiting, anorexia and increased values of ALT (2062 IU /l) and AST(1870 IU/l.), anaemia (Hb 6.8 g/dl ,total erythrocytes 2.88 x 10^6 / mm^3, packed cell volume

Contd.

19.7%), leukocytosis (total leukocytes 36480 / mm^3), thrombocytopenia (platelets 56000/ mm^3) showing sludge in gall bladder, mass of echogenicity measuring 50.5 x 50.1 mm involving under surface of the left lobe of the liver abutting pancreas and medial aspect of spleen suggestive of possible malignant lesion.

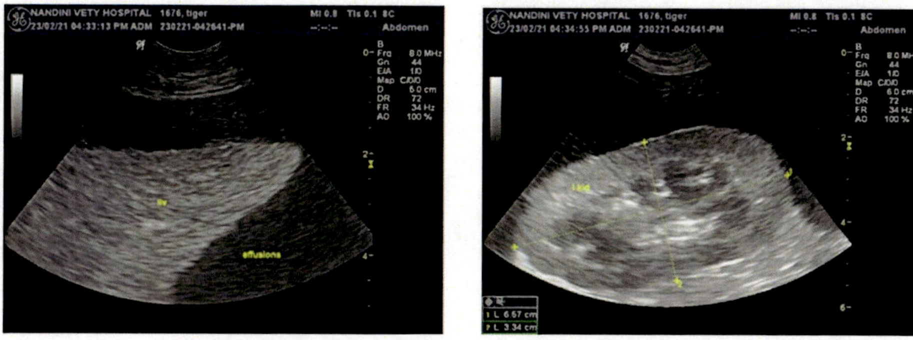

(A) **(B)**

Fig. 256: Trans abdominal sonogram of a ten year old male German shepherd dog with ascites, hind limb odema, scrotal odema showing hyperechoic liver with anechoic fluid in the abdomen **(A)** and normal left kidney **(B)**. Right kidney could not be visualized due to an excess peritoneal effusion. Serum biochemistry revealed normal values for serum creatinine (1.4 mg/dl), blood urea nitrogen (23 mg/dl), ALT (41.0 IU/L), SAP (89 U/L), AST (35 IU/L), sodium (142 mEq/L), potassium (4.1 mEq/L), chloride (107 mEq/L); lower values for serum protein (5.4 g/dl), albumin (2.2 d/dl); and increased protein level in ascetic fluid (0.38 g/dl). Hyperechoic liver with within range ALT, SAP and high protein ascetic fluid suggested hepatic cirrhosis/fibrosis with post hepatic or post sinusoidal portal hypertension.

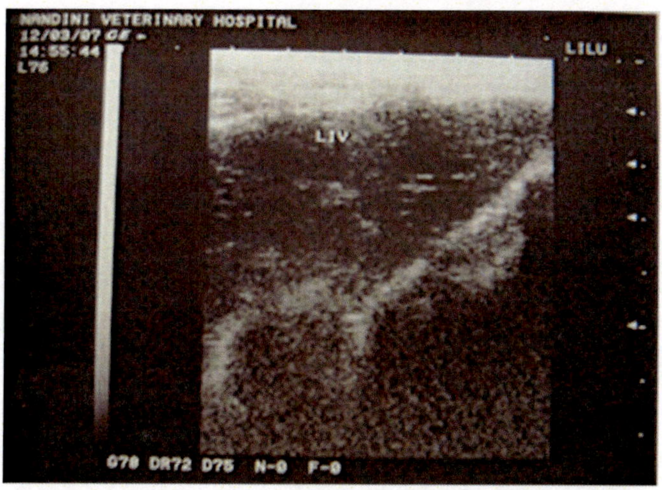

Fig. 257: Trans abdominal sonogram of an epileptic Pomeranian male dog on anti-epileptic drug treatment with phenobarbitone having elevated liver enzymes (ALT 240 IU/L, SAP 200 U/L) showing diffuse hypoechoic liver.

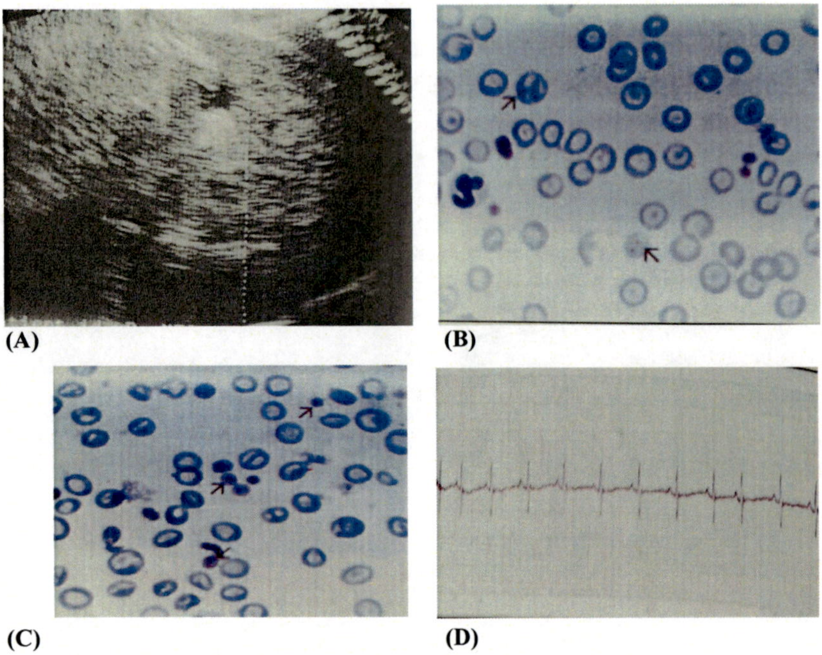

Fig. 258: Trans abdominal hepatic sonogram **(A)** of a one month old non-descript pup with a concurrent infection of Babesia canis **(B)** and Ehrlichia platys **(C)** showing enlarged liver (size 10.7 cm, weight 1010 g) and fluid in liver lobes. Plasma ALT (204 IU/L) and SAP (412.6 IU/L) values were elevated. Electrocardiogram **(D)** revealed sinus rhythm (HR 150 bpm), and almost equal amplitude of 'R' (0.5 mV) and 'S' waves (0. 5 mV) with flattened 'T' wave (Varshney et al., 2004).

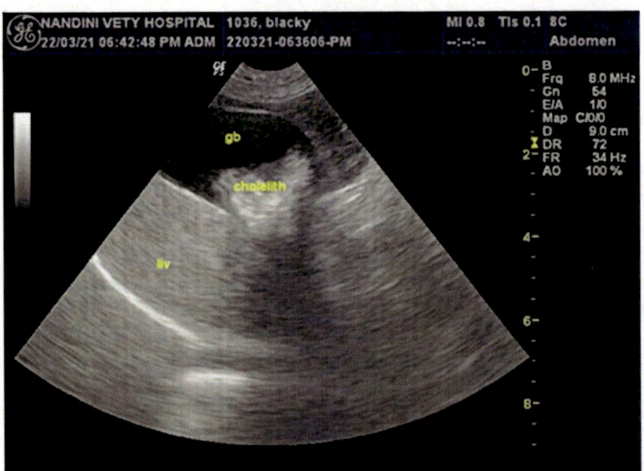

Fig.259: Hepato-biliary sonogram of a two year old male Labrador showing hyperechoic liver and a hyperechoic image with acoustic shadowing in the gall bladder suggesting cholelith with hepatic cirrhosis/fibrosis. ALT (168 IU/L), AST (168 IU/L) and serum amylase (978 U/L) levels were elevated but serum lipase (27.77U/L) was low.

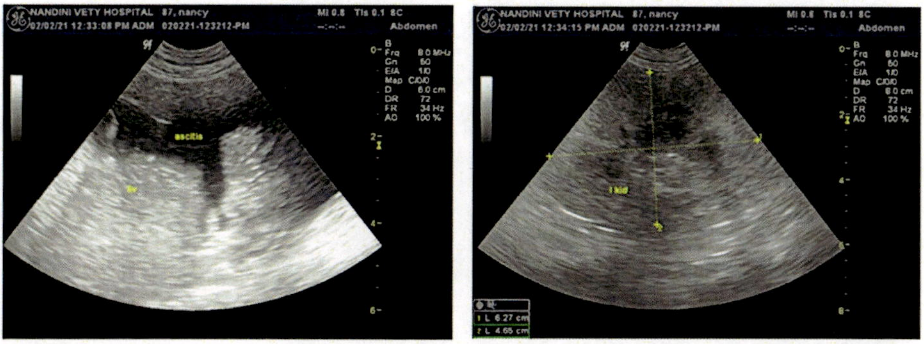

(A) **(B)**

Fig. 260: Trans abdominal sonogram of a three year old male Labrador with jaundice and ascites showing hyperechoic liver with fliud in abdomen **(A);** and hyperechoic atrophied left kidney with loss of demarcation between cortex and medulla **(B)** suggestive of hepatic cirrhosis/fibrosis with atrophied kidney. Haemato-biochemical investigations revealed anaemia (haemoglobin 10.2 g/dl, total erythrocytes 4.45 x10^6/mm^3, haematocrit 28.9%); leukocytosis (43400/mm^3), normal platelet count (217,000/mm^3); lower side values of ALT (30.2U/L), total proteins (4.6 g/dl), albumin 1.3 g/dl) and A/G ration (0.39); with increased total bilirubin (3.34 mg/dl), serum creatinine (13.41 mg/dl) and blood urea nitrogen (89.2 mg/dl) confirming decrease in normal hepatic cells due to fibrosis/cirrhosis; and renal failure.

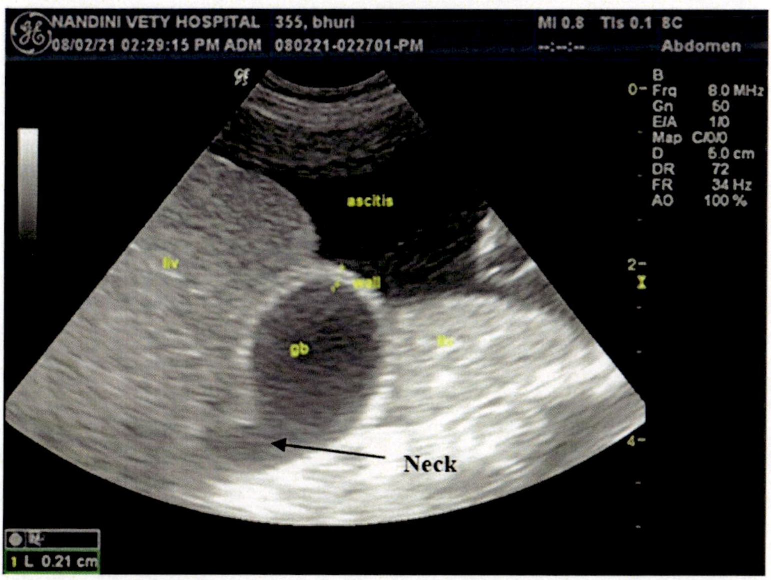

Fig. 261: Trans abdominal sonogram of an adult dog (Bhuri) with ascites showing hyperechoic liver, anechoic fluid in the abdomen and thickened hyperechoic gall bladder wall (> 3 mm) suggesting cirrhosis/fibrosis with cholecystitis. Tapering neck of the gall bladder can also be seen (black arrow). Biochemical investigation revealed lower values of ALT (16.0 U/l), total serum proteins (3.8 mg/dl) and albumin (1.6 g/dl).

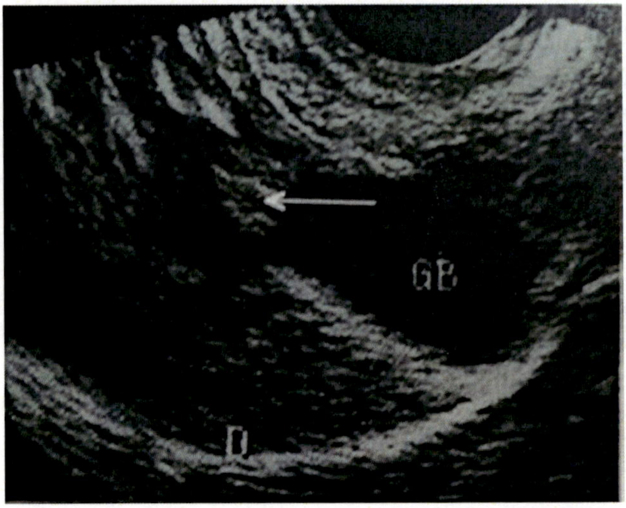

Fig. 262: Trans abdominal sonogram of a dog with jaundice showing a hyperechoic structure with acoustic shadow in the duct of gall bladder suggesting calculi in theduct (Tiwari et al., 2001).

Pancreas

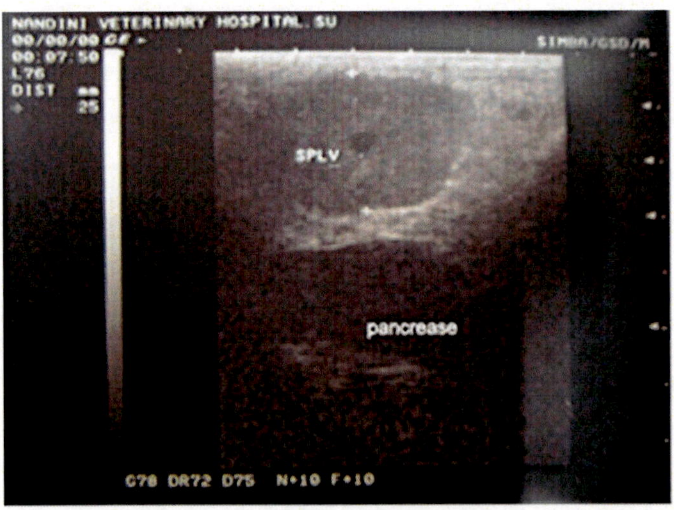

Fig. 263: Sonogram of a two year old male German Shepherd with babesiosis, caused by B. gibsoni,showing inflamed hypoechoic pancreas.Biochemical investigations revealed increased values of blood urea nitrogen (118.61 mg/dl), , serum creatinine (8.92 mg/dl), blood glucose (197.0 mg/dl), serum ALT (190.0 U/L) serum lipase (627 IU/L) and serum amylase (2159 IU/L); low values of total serum protein (3.55 g/dl), serum albumin (1.86 g/dl), and serum globulin (1.69 g/dl); within range values of serum alkaline phosphatase (144.0 U/L), total bilirubin (0.45 mg/dl), direct bilirubin (0.15 mg/dl) and indirect bilirubin (0.30 mg/dl) .Sonographic and biochemical findings suggested acute pancreatitis.

Prostate Glands

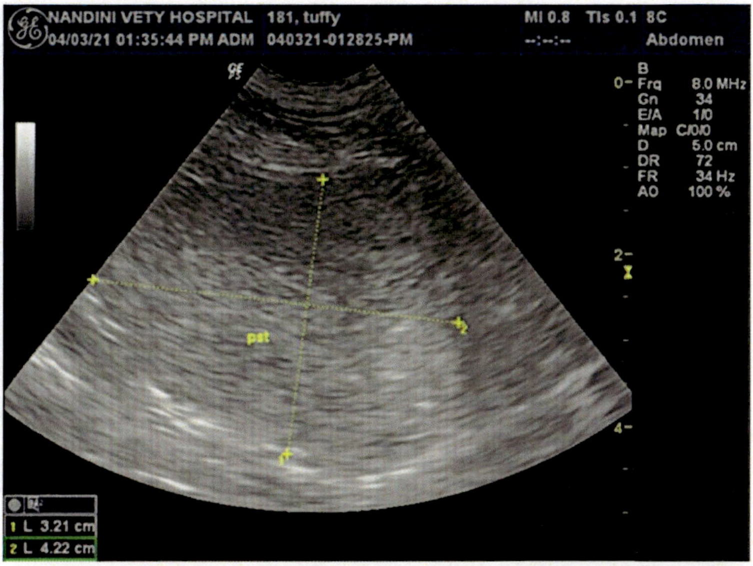

Fig. 264: Sonogram of an eight year old Shitzu with constipation and urinary incontinence, showing prostatomegaly (32.1 x 42.2 mm) with smooth contours and multiple hyperechoic areas suggesting benign prostatic hyperplasia. Lower level of prostate specific antigen (<0.1ng/ml) ruled out prostatic tumour.

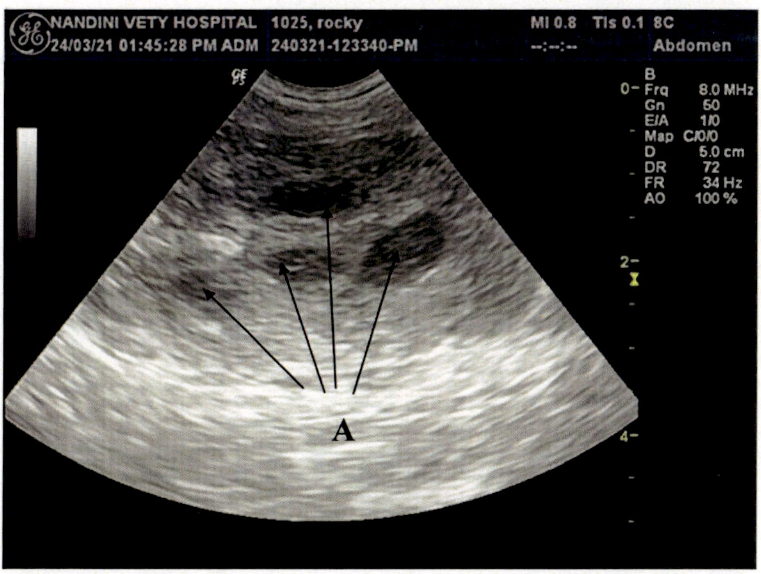

(A)

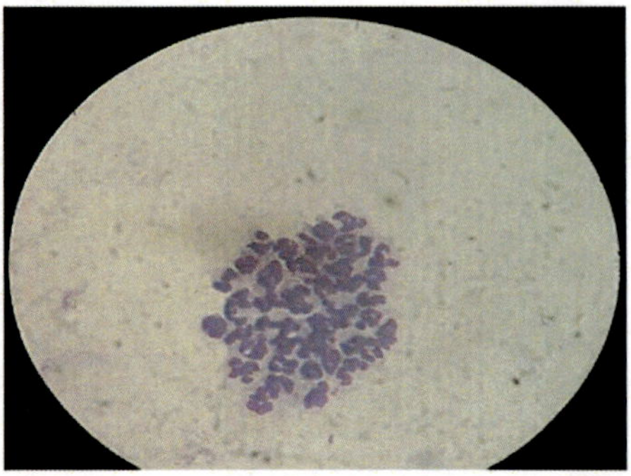

(B)

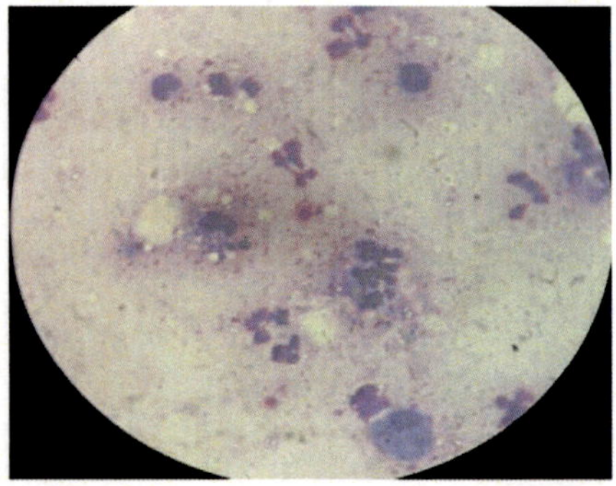

(C)

Fig.265: Trans abdominal sonogram of prostate of a 12 year old crossbred dog with constipation, haematuria showing multiple thick walled anechoic cavity structures **(A)** with posterior acoustic enhancement deep to the cavity lesion suggesting prostatic abscesses. Prostatic fluid cytology **(B and C)** revealed preponderance of leukocytes and cocci.

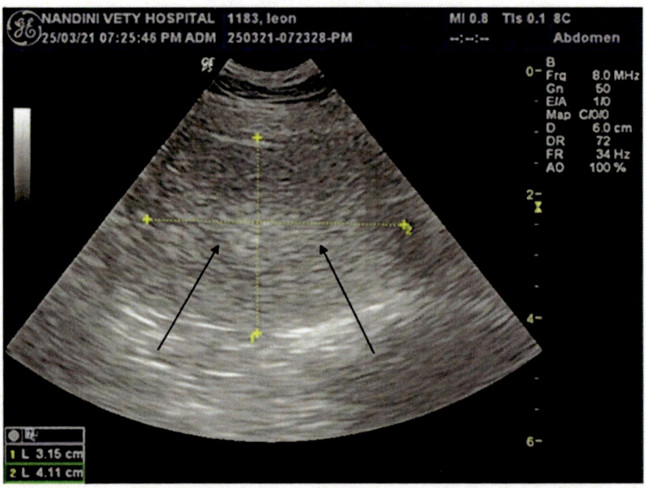

Fig. 266: Trans abdominal sonogram of prostate of a 10 year old Labrador with retention of urine showing diffuse hyperechogenicity as well as mixed echogenic pattern and enlarged prostate (41.1 x 31.5 mm) suggesting chronic prostatitis. Catheterized urine revealed the abundance of erythrocytes.

Spleen

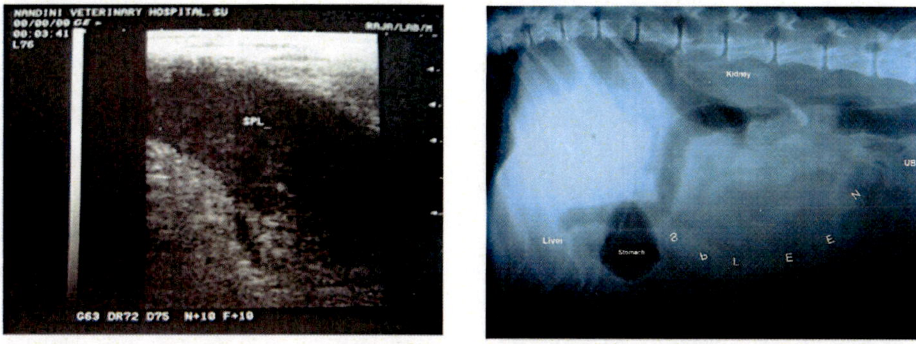

Fig. 267: Splenomegaly in an adult male 5 year old Labrador with concurrent infection of *B. gibsoni* and *E. canis*. Serum creatinine (1.0 mg/dl), BUN (24 mg/dl), BUN:Creatinine ratio (24), total bilirubin (0.2 mg/dl), direct bilirubin (0.1 mg/dl), ALT (62 IU/ l), AST (24 IU/l), and SAP (70 U/l), were within normal range. Transabdominal sonogram is showing (A) hypoechoic enlarged spleen covering > 40 % area of left abdomen suggesting splenic inflammation/ congestion . X-ray of the same dog also confirmed very much enlarged spleen **(B)**.

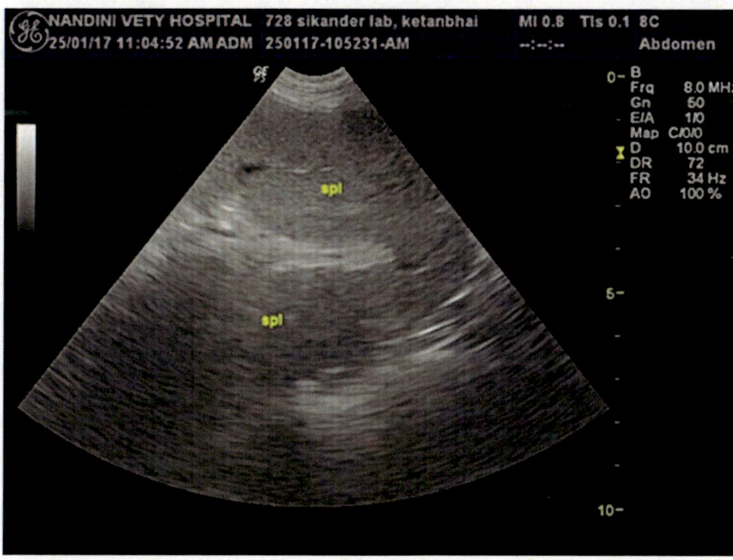

Fig. 268: Trans abdominal splenic sonogram of an adult male Labrador showing hypoechoicity with hyperechoic spackles suggesting splenic torsion.

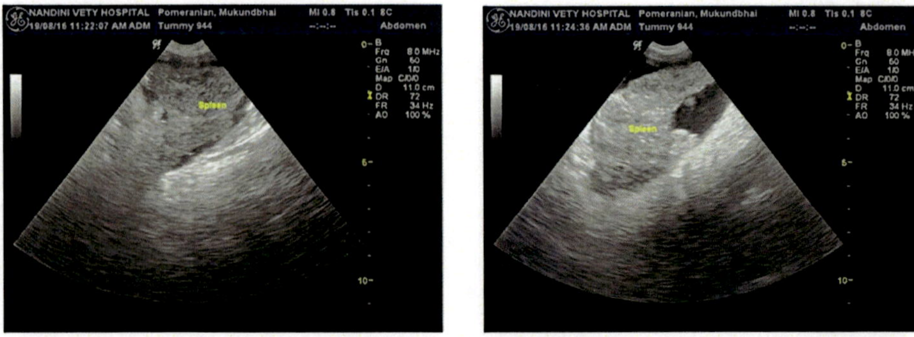

Fig. 269: Trans abdominal sonogram of a 5 month old Pomeranian dog with ascites showing hyperechoic and enlarged spleen with two nodular hyperechoic foci and very irregular margin suggestive of splenic nodular hyperplasia.

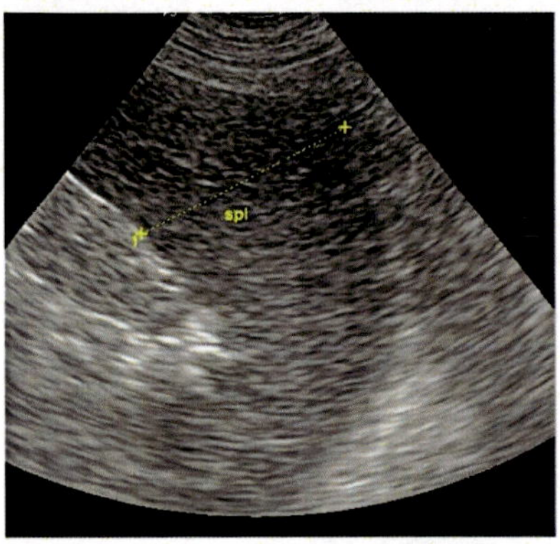

(A)

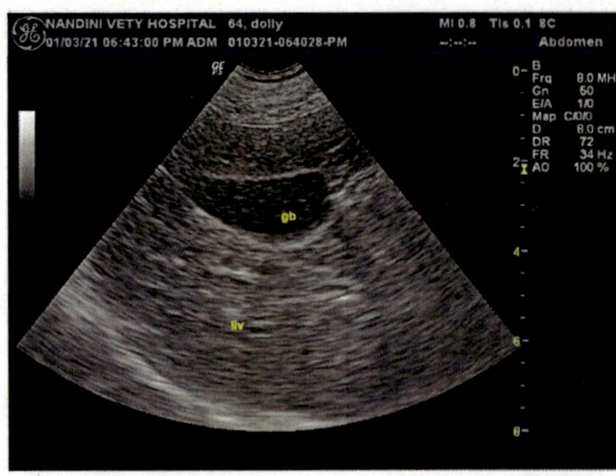

(B)

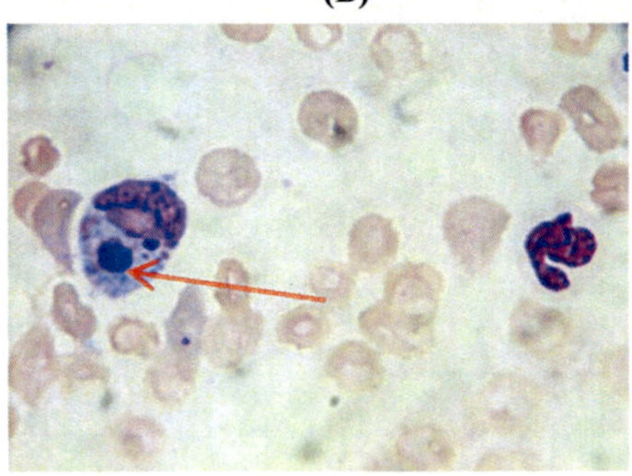

(C)

Fig. 270: Trans abdominal sonograms of an eight year old bitch with pyrexia (103.2 ^{0}F) and palpable spleen in left abdomen showing enlarged and hypoechoic spleen **(A)**; and slightly hypoechoic liver and an elliptical anechoic fluid filled gall bladder **(B)** suggesting infectious splenitis. Haemato-biochemical investigations revealed the presence of *E. canis* morula in the monocytes **(C)**, normal values for serum creatinine (1.4 mg/dl) , blood urea nitrogen (20 mg/dl), serum alkaline phosphatase (95 U/L), AST (17 IU/L), ALT (25 IU/L);slightly increased serum bilirubin (total 0.9mg/dl, indirect 0.7 mg/dl), total leukocytes (12.2 x 10^3/mm^3); and lowered values of haemoglobin (9.6 g/dl), total erythrocytes (4.0x10^6/mm^3), and total serum proteins (5.2 g/dl) suggesting ehrlichiosis with leukocytosis. Based on investigations, hypoechoic enlarged spleen (infectious splenitis) in the bitch was due to ehrlichiosis caused by *E.canis*.

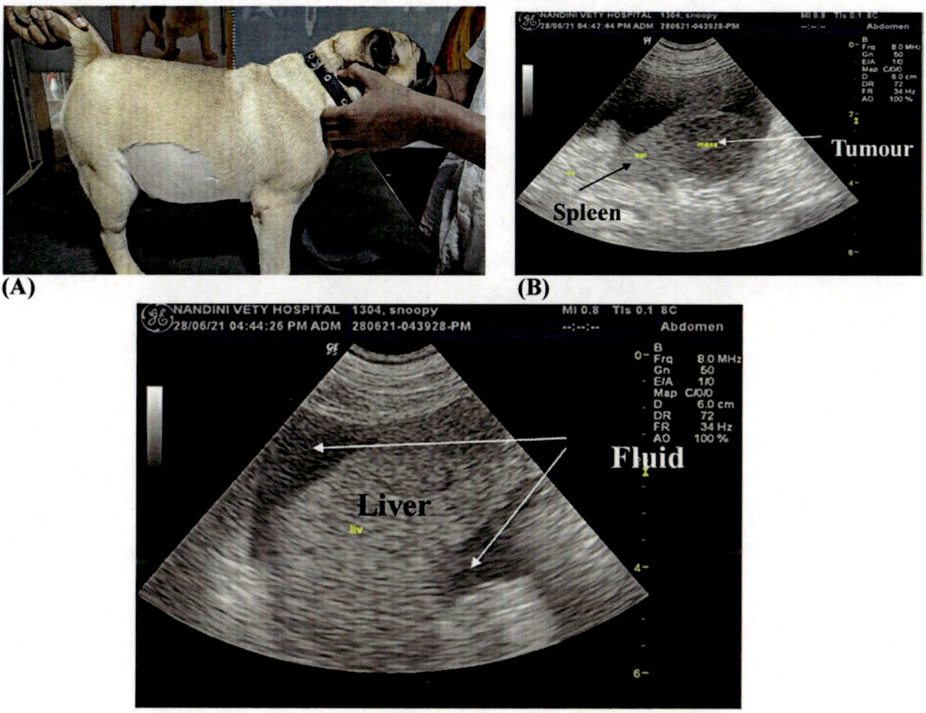

(A) **(B)** **(C)**

Fig. 271: Sonograms of a six year old male Pug with abdominal distension **(A)** showing poorly margined hypoechoic mass (white arrow) in hyperechoic spleen **(B)** and hyperechoic liver **(C)**. Haemogram revealed normal values of haemoglobin (11.10 g%), total erythrocytes (5.49 x 10^6/mm^3), packed cell volume (35%), MCHC (31.45%), RDW (16.20%), platelet count (187,000/mm^3); lower values of MCV (64.30 fl), MCH (20.22 pg), neutrophils (20%), monocytes (2%), eosinophil (2 %); and increased values of total leukocyte count (24100/ mm^3) and lymphocytes (76%). Biochemical investigation revealed normal value of serum creatinine (0.9 mg/dl); lowered value of total serum protein (5.9 g/dl) and albumin (2.4 g/dl); and increased values of ALT (215 IU/L), ascetic fluid total protein (0.4 g/dl), ascetic fluid albumin (0.18 g/dl) and serum ascites albumin gradient (SAAG)(2.22). Values of SAAG >1.1 are suggestive of portal hypertension. The diagnosis was arrived at splenic tumour, hepatic cirrhosis and ascites with portal hypertension.

Stomach

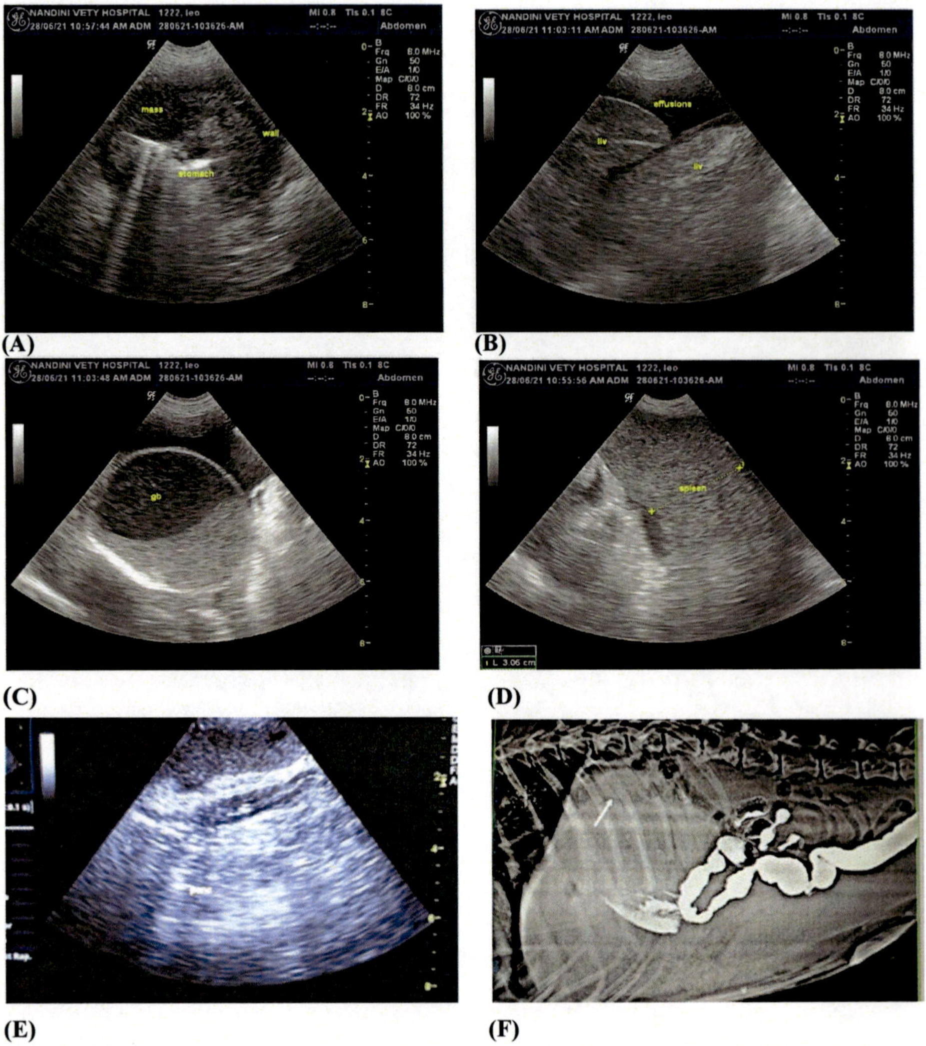

Fig. 272: Trans abdominal sonograms and abdominal radiograph of a nine year old male Labrador with the history of weight loss (7.0 kg in one year), recurrent vomiting, and erratic appetite for one year. The dog was teated symptomaticaly with no tangible results. Sonogram **(A)** is showing loss of wall layering of the stomach and a hypoechoic mass in the lumen of the stomach in fundus area. Gas and fluid is also visible. Hyerechoic liver with fluid is seen in sonogram at B.Markedly distended gall bladder with sludge **(C)**, hyperechoic and enlarged spleen **(D)** and pancreas **(E)** are also visible in sonograms. An elliptical radiopaque structure of 28.6 x 24.5 mm size is visible in the radiograph **(F)**.Conspicuous haemato- biochemical changes consisted of neutrophilia (93% neutrophils), lowered value of ALT (26 IU/L); increased values of serum amylase (549 U/L) and lipase (749 U/L); and within range value of blood glucose (86 mg/dl). Investigations were suggestive of a mass in the stomach with cirrhotic liver, distended gall bladder with sludge, enlargd spleen and sonographically visible pancreas.

Testis and Scrotum

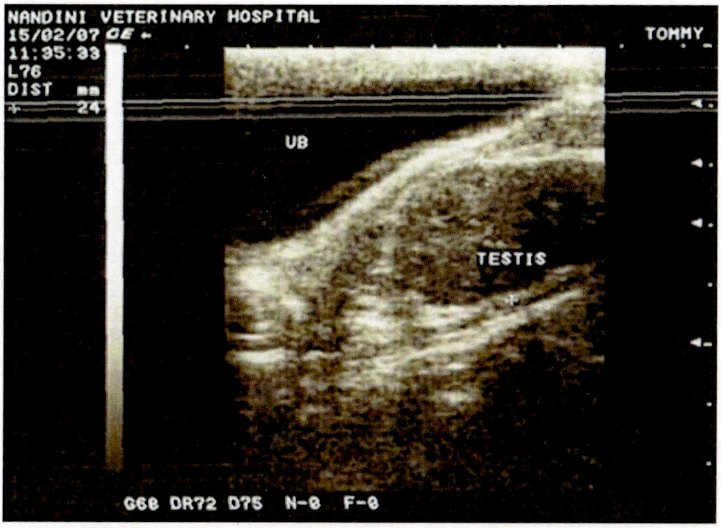

Fig. 273: Trans abdominal sonogram of a cryptorchid young dog showing retained testis just lateral to the urinary bladder trigone area. The retained testis is small, oval, echo poor structure uniform in echogenicity.

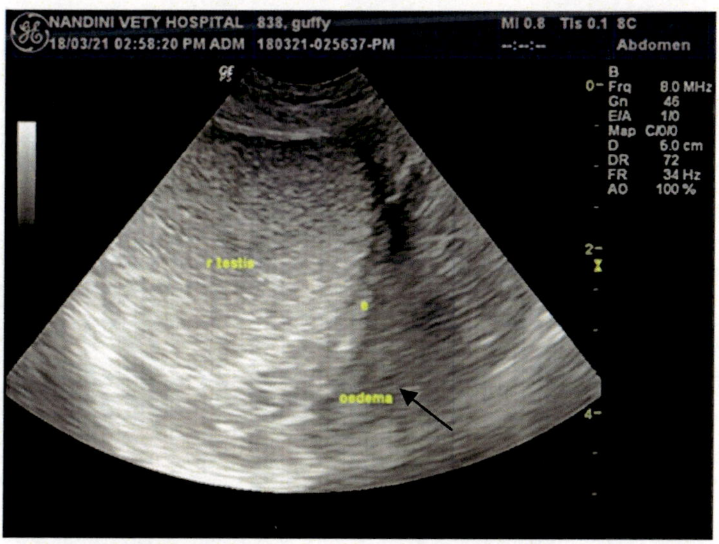

Fig. 274: Scrotal sonogram of a two year old male Golden Retriever with swelling of right side scrotum showing anechoic/hypoechoic (arrow) echotexture of subcutaneous tissues with normal echotexture of right testis suggesting subcutaneous odema.

Urinary System

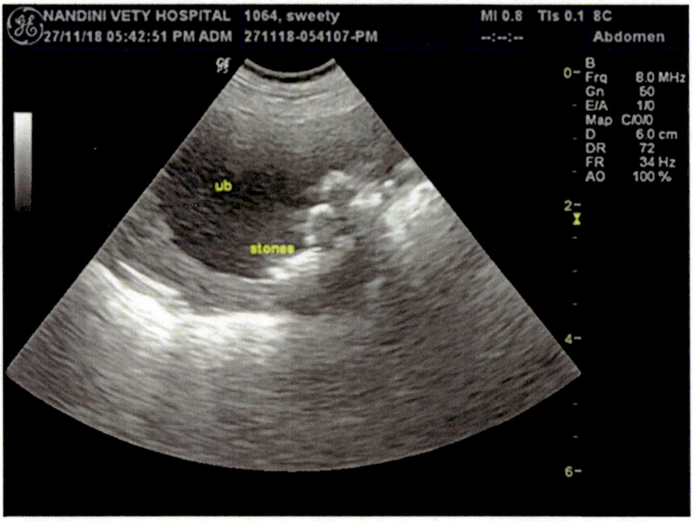

Fig. 275: Trans abdominal sonogram of a five year old male Pomeranian with urinary incontinence and hematuria showing hyperechoic curvilinear structures with acoustic shadowing in the urinary bladder suggesting cystoliths.

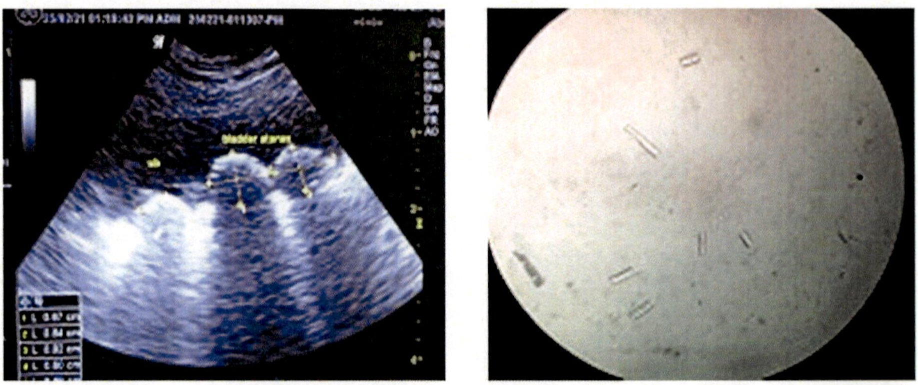

(A) **(B)**

Fig. 276: Trans abdominal sonogram of urinary bladder **(A)** of a 10 year old male Labrador with haematuria and dysuria showing cystoliths (hyperechoic) submerged in urine with shadowing **(A)**. Urine microscopy revealed proponderance of Picket Fence calcium oxalate monohydrate crystals and erythrocytes **(B)**.

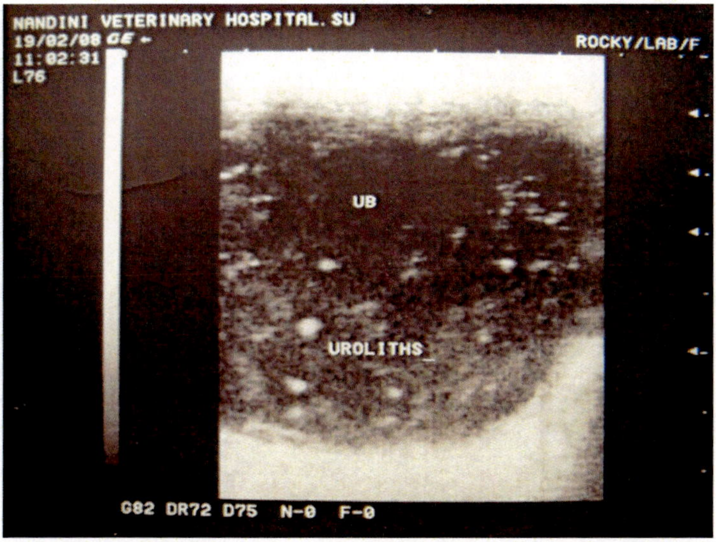

Fig. 277: Trans abdominal sonogram of an adult male Labrador with urinary dribbling showing multiple hyperechoic small liths in the urinary bladder suggesting multiple cystoliths.

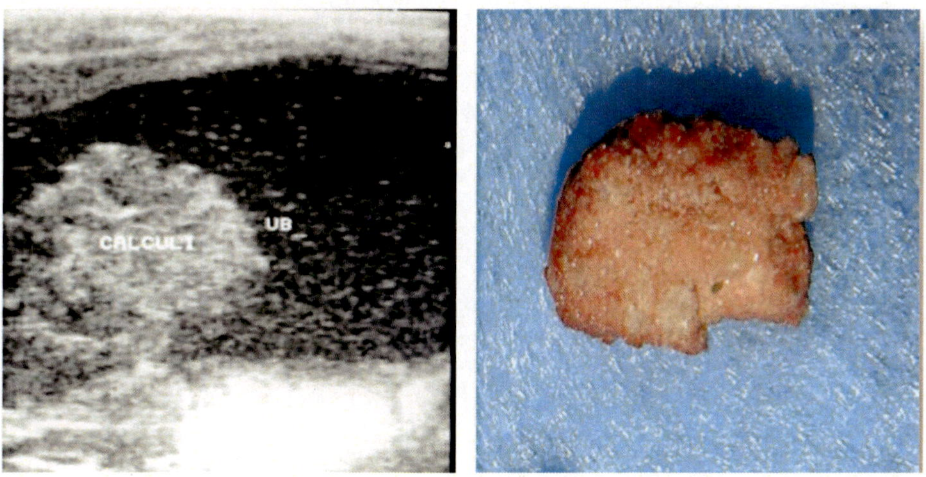

(A) **(B)**

Fig. 278: Trans abdominal sonogram of a male Great Dane showing hyperechoic small crystals and a large hyperechpoic calculi with rough margins suggesting cystolith **(A)**. A large stone **(B)** was removed from the bladder after surgery.

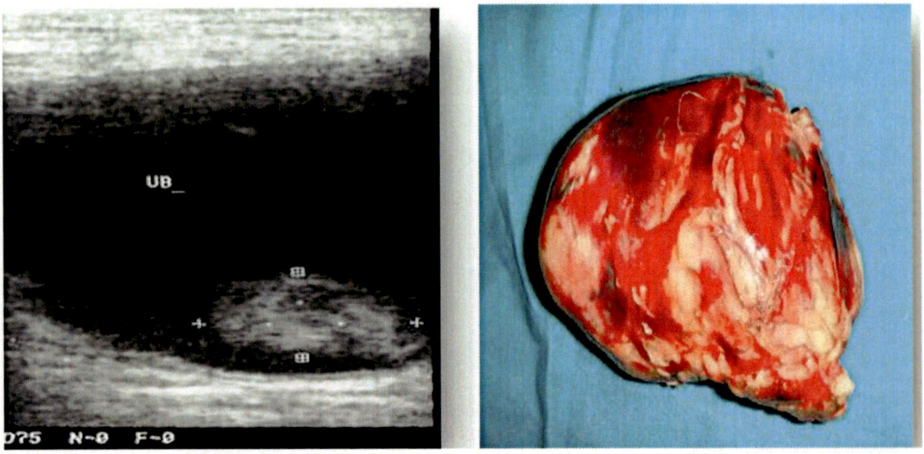

(A) **(B)**

Fig. 279: Trans abdominal sonogram of a male Great Dane with haematuria, dysuria showing broad based irregular echogenic mass attached to bladder wall without acoustic shadowing suggesting tumour in the urinary bladder **(A)**. Surgery confirmed a mass in the bladder **(B)**.

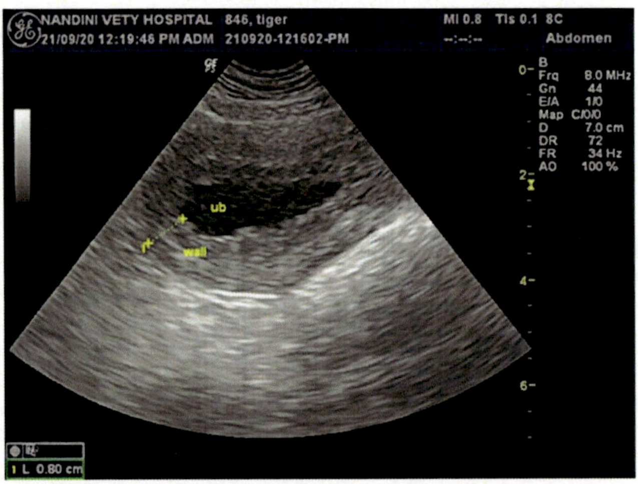

Fig. 280: Trans abdominal sonogram of a male Labrador with micturition and haematuria showing thickened (> 3 mm) hyperechoic urinary bladder wall. *E.coli* was isolated on cultural examination of urine. Based on cultural and sonographic examination the diagnosis of bacterial cystitis was arrived at.

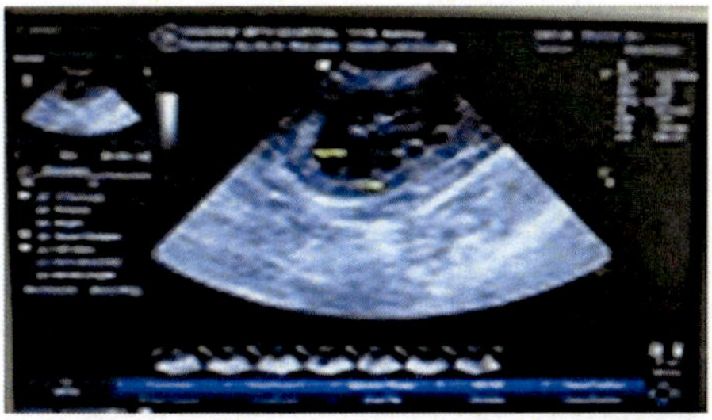
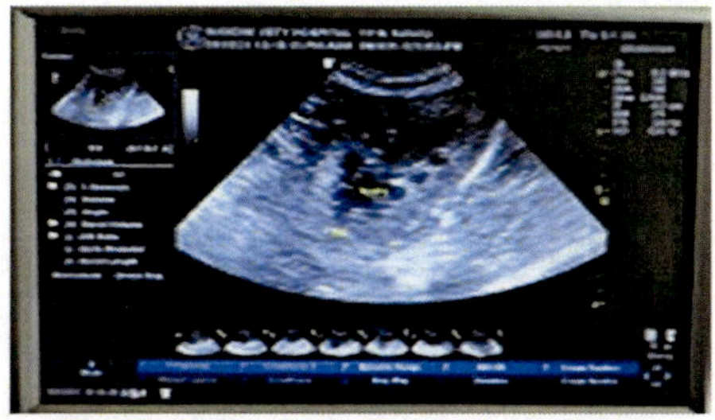

(A) **(B)**

Fig. 281: Trans abdominal sonogram of a ten year old female Pomeranian dog with persisting vomiting, anorexia, lethargy showing marked dilation of renal pelvis with anechoic fluid in left **(A)** and right **(B)** kidneys suggesting hydronephrosis. Biochemical investigations revealed grade 4 renal failure (serum creatinine 7.9 mg/dl, and BUN 61 mg/dl, sodium 142 mEq/L, potassium 4.6 mEq/L , chloride 105 mEq/L).

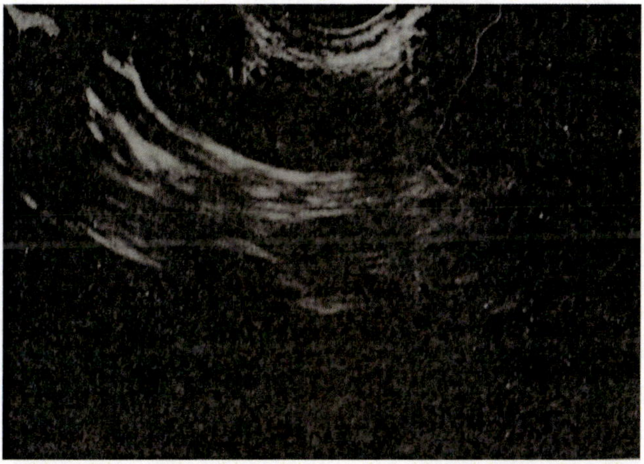

Fig. 282: Trans abdominal renal sonogram of a 10 month old male Doberman with increased thirst, frequent urination and weight loss for 40-45 days showing hypoechoic echo texture of left kidney with loss of demarcation between cortex and medulla (Varshney *et al*., 2003). Biochemical estimations revealed glucosuria (1%) with low level of blood glucose (67 mg/ml). Repeat examination on next day revealed increased glucosuria (2%), low specific gravity of urine (1.004), proteinuria (+ ve), crystals of cysteine, uric acid and phosphate; and normal glucose metabolism (fasting glucose 90 mg/dl, postprandial glucose 123 mg/ml). Ultrasonographic picture of the kidney, presence of glucosuria but normal blood glucose level, led to the diagnosis of Fanconi's syndrome. It is a multiple renal tubular defect.

Uterus

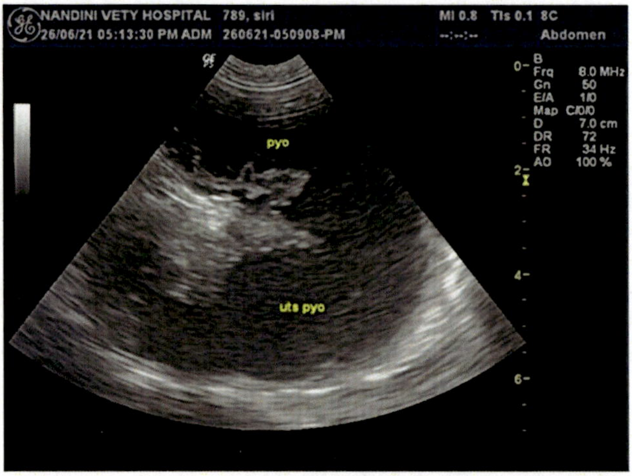

Fig. 283: Trans abdominal sonogram of an adult Labrador bitch with vaginal discharge showing anechoic fluid accumulation in uterine horns suggesting hydrometra/mucometra/ pyometra.

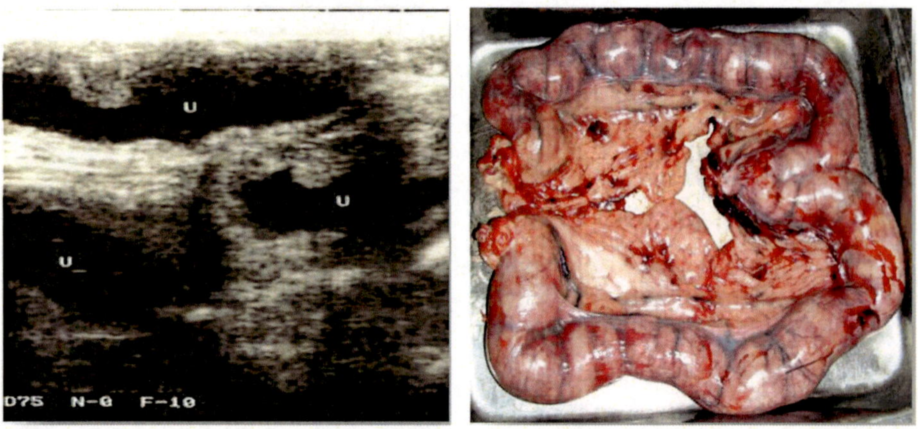

(A) **(B)**

Fig. 284: Trans abdominal sonogram of a Pomaranian bitch with purulent vaginal discharge showing anechoic fluid accumulation in uterine horns and thickened wall **(A)** suggesting pyometra. The bitch responded poorly to the routine parenteral antibiotic and intra-uterine antibiotic therapy. Hysterectomy revealed distended uterine horn with suppurating fluid **(B)** confirming sonographic diagnosis of pyometra.

Felines

Abscess

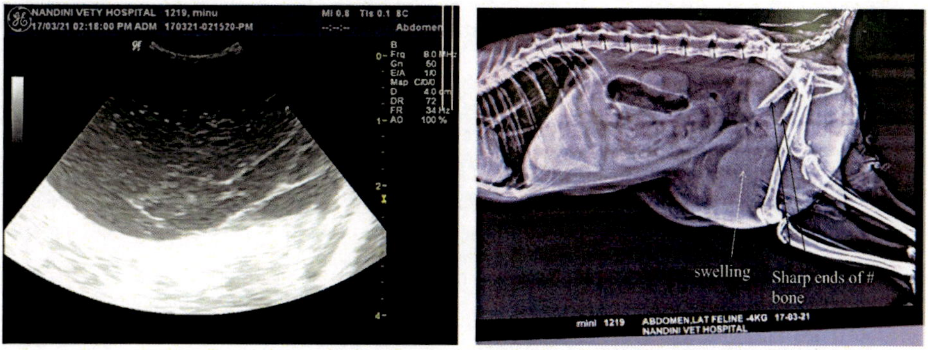

(A) **(B)**

Fig. 285: Trans abdominal sonogram of a female non-descript cat with marked soft odematous swelling in ventral caudal abdomen, pyrexia (104.5 °F) and anorexia showing mixed echogenic fluid with a thick wall in ventral caudal abdomen suggesting an abscess **(A)**. Radiograph of the cat **(B)** confirmed marked swelling with fluid. Abdominal pressure caused urination but no change in the swelling. Exploratory puncture yielded 150 ml of whitish foul smelling fluid akin to pus.

Gastroenteritis

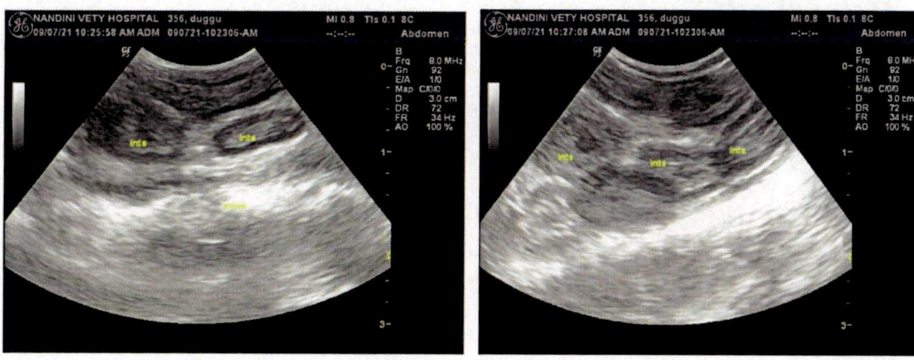

(A) **(B)**

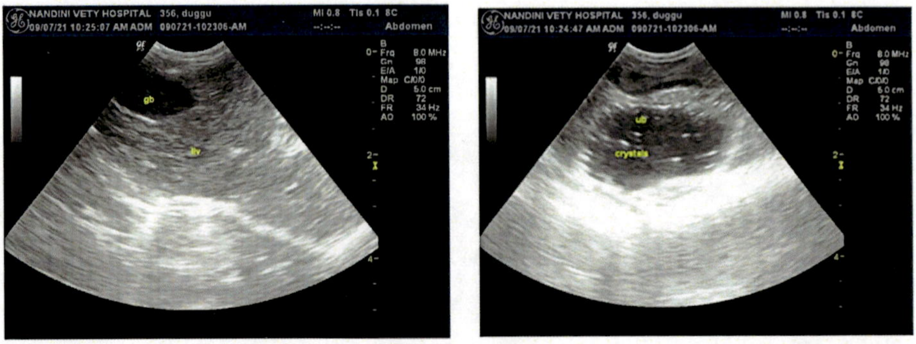

(C) (D)

Fig. 286: Trans abdominal sonograms of a three month old non-descript kitten (1.0kg weight) with hypothermia (temperature 93.5^{0}F), severe vomiting and diarrhoea showing intestinal loops distension, thickened intestinal wall with a loss of wall layering and conspicuous mucosal layer **(A and B)**; distended gall bladder **(C)** and echogenic particles in the urinry bladder **(D)** suggesting intestinal inflammation and crystalluria.

Hepato-biliary system

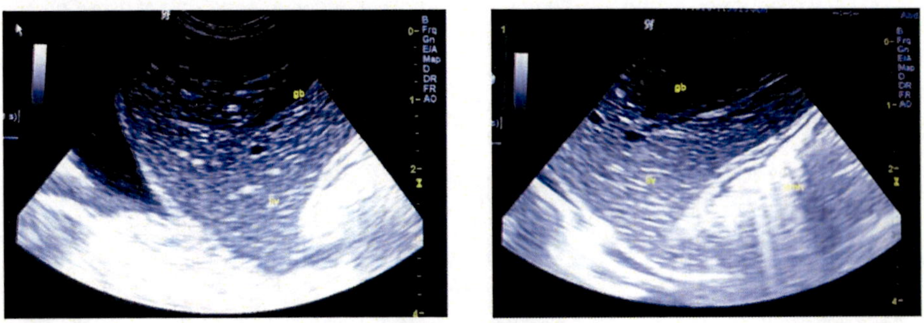

(A) (B)

Fig. 287: Trans abdominal sonogram of a six month old Persian cat showing hyperechoic liver with serrated margins **(A)** and distended gall bladder **(B)** suggesting liver cirrhosis/lipidosis. Lower values of glucose (56 mg/dl), total serum proteins (3.4 g/dl), albumin (1.4 g/dl), ALT (10 U/L), SAP (60 U/L) and BUN (13 mg/dl) lend further support to sonographic diagnosis as synthesis of liver enzymes is reduced owing to cirrhosis or fibrosis of the liver (Varshney, 2019, b).

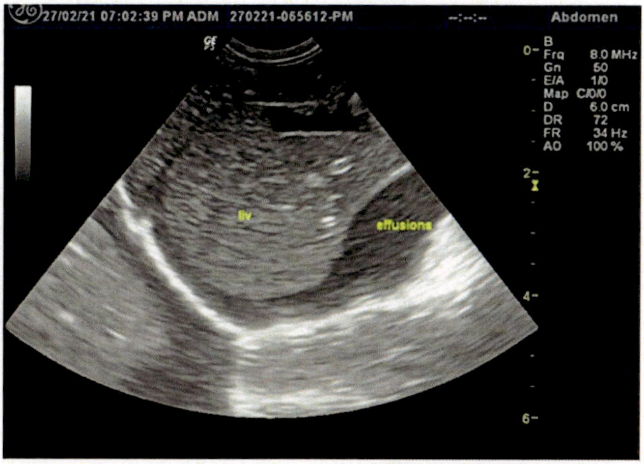

Fig. 288: Trans abdominal sonogram of a six year old female Bombay cat showing hyperechoic liver with serrated margins and accumulation of an excess anechoic fluid in the peritoneal cavity suggesting liver cirrhosis/lipidosis with ascites

Mammary Glands

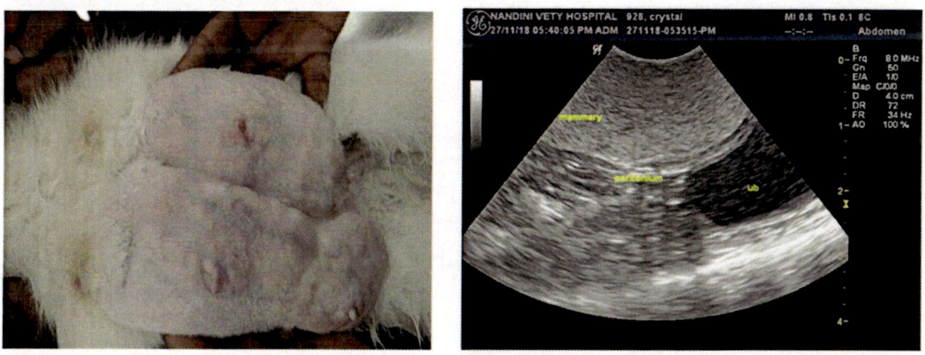

(A) **(B)**

Fig. 289: Trans abdominal sonogram of a cat with hard swelling of last pair of mammary gland **(A)** showing hyperechoic mammary tissues **(B)** suggesting feline mammary fibroepithelial hyperplasia. Increased serum progesterone (7.4 ng/ml) lend further support to sonographic diagnosis.

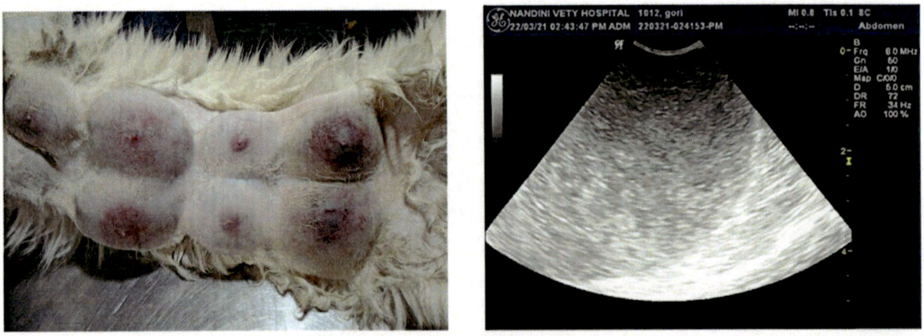

(A) **(B)**

Fig. 290: Trans abdominal sonogram of a 10-12 month old queen with swollen, firm bilateral enlarged mammary glands (four pairs) with erythematous skin **(A)** showing increased mammary echogenicity **(B)** as compared to normal or lactational mammary glands. Mass of granular and slightly hyperechoic texture with delimited margins suggested feline mammary fibroepithelial hyperplasia. Small irregular anechoic areas without acoustic enhancement are also visible in the sonogram. Increased serum progesterone level (28.15 ng/ml) and decreased serum estradiol (14.29 pg/ml)further supported the diagnosis of feline fibroepithelial hyperplasia. Treatment with cabergoline reduced the size of the mammary glands.

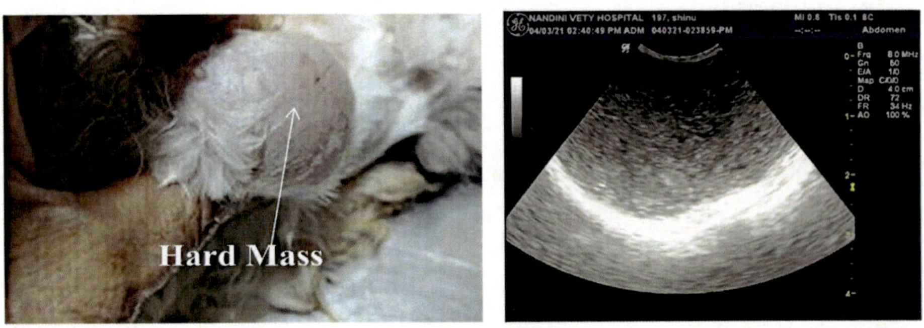

(A) **(B)**

Fig. 291: Transabdominal sonogram of an adult Persian cat with hard swelling in 2nd right thoracic mammary gland **(A)** showing heterogeneous echogenicity with irregular margins and thickened wall **(B)** suggesting mammary tumour.

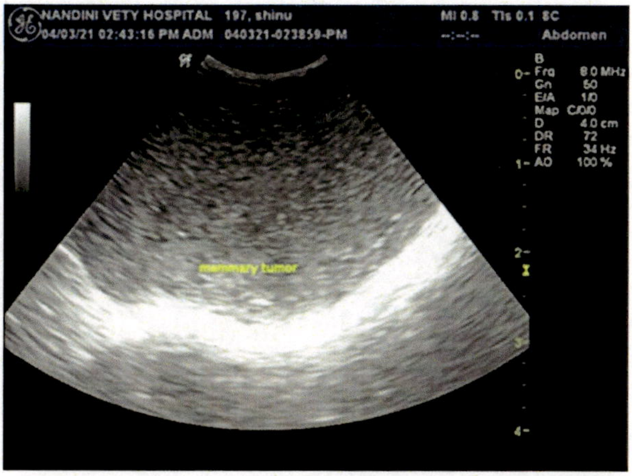

Fig. 292: Trans abdominal sonogram of a Persian female cat showing homogeneously mixed echoic structure of the last left mammary gland and thickened wall suggesting mammary tumour.

Subcutaneous Tissues

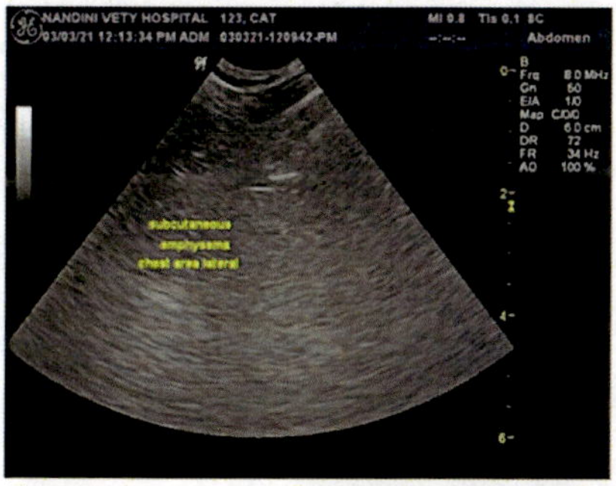

(A)

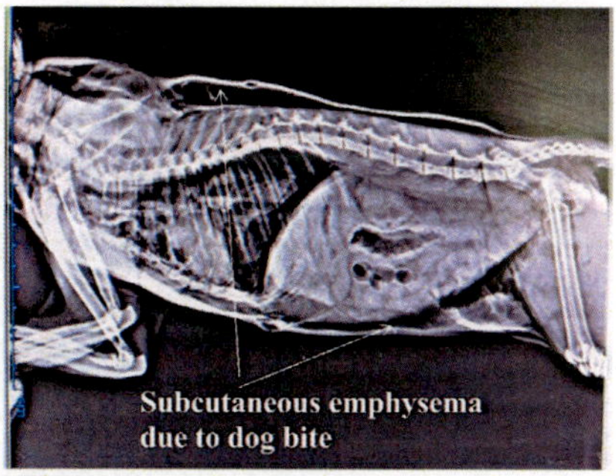

(B)

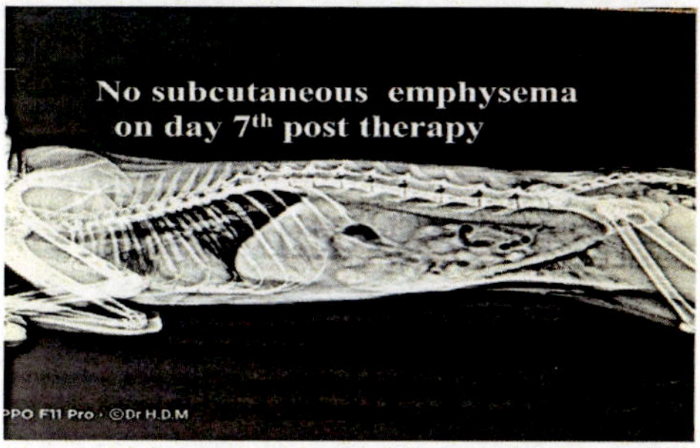

(C)

Fig. 293: Thoracic sonogram of an adult female Bombay cat with dog bite on dorsal chest showing hyperechoic punctiform collection of gas obscuring tissues in the far field and reverberation artifacts **(A)** suggesting subcutaneous emphysema. Radiograph of the same cat also revealed accumulation of gas (white arrows) subcutaneously **(B)** supporting sonographic findings. After seven days of treatment, x-ray revealed no accumulation of subcutaneous gas **(C)**.

Urinary system

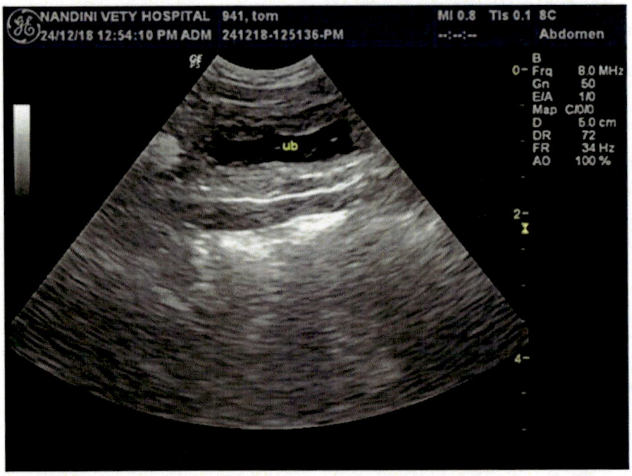

Fig. 294: Trans abdominal sonogram of a two year old tom cat with dysuria, hematuria and urinary incontinence showing thickened hyperechoic urinary bladder wall (> 3 mm) suggesting cystitis. Culturally negative urine with the presence of protein (+), occult blood (+) and erythrocytes (60-67 /H.P.F);within range values of serum creatinine (0.82 mg/dl), blood urea (28.73 mg/dl), ALT (37 I U/L), haemoglobin (12.4 g/dl),total erythrocytes (5.1 x10^6/mm^3), platelets (141,000/ mm^3), total leukocytes (6.6 x 10^3/mm^3), and packed cell volume (33 %), led to the diagnosis of idiopathic feline cystitis.

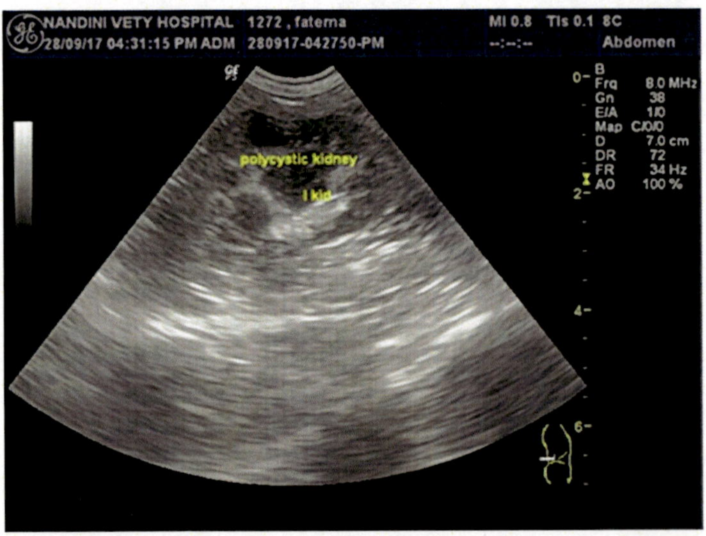

Fig. 295: Trans abdominal sonogram of a seven month old female Persian cat with pain in lumbar region and erratic blood mixed urine showing multiple hypoechoic cysts in left kidney (> 2 mm dia.). The cysts are anechoic/hypoechoic structures of smooth round/irregular margin and of variable sizes throughout cortex and medulla and loss of cortico- medullary junction demarcation (Varshney and Chaudhary, 2018).

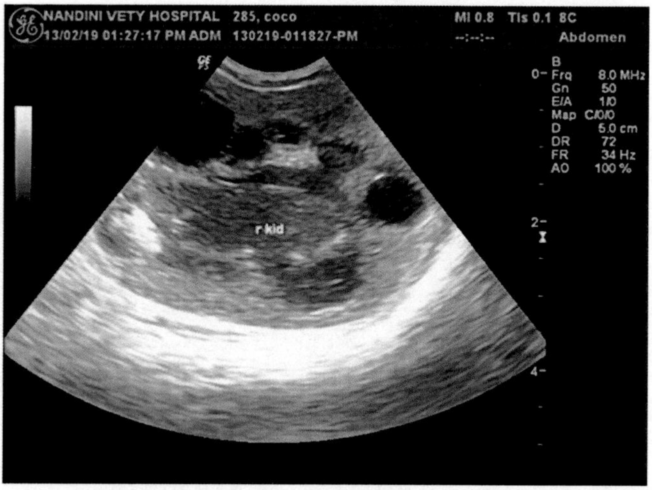

Fig. 296: Trans abdominal sonogram of a one year old male Persian cat with haematuria showing multiple smooth round /irregular margin anechoic structures of variable sizes throughout cortex and medulla and loss of cortico-medullary junction demarcation in right kidney suggesting polycystic kidney.

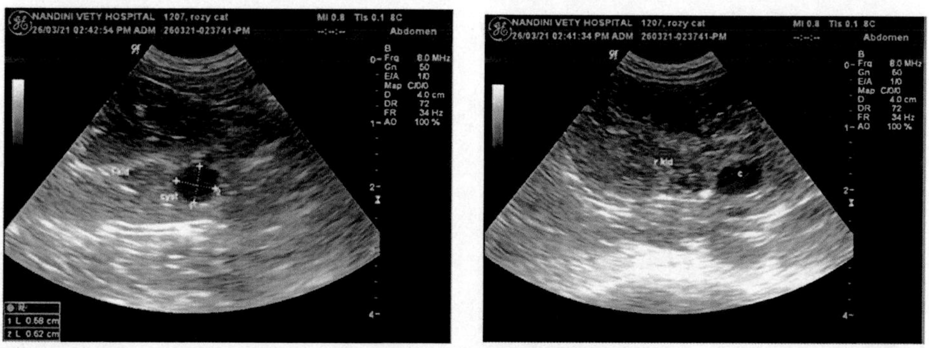

Left Kidney **Right Kidney**

Fig. 297: Trans abdominal sonogram of an eight month old female Persian cat with vomiting, weakness and constipation showing smooth round margin anechoic structures in both left and right kidneys suggesting cystic kidneys.

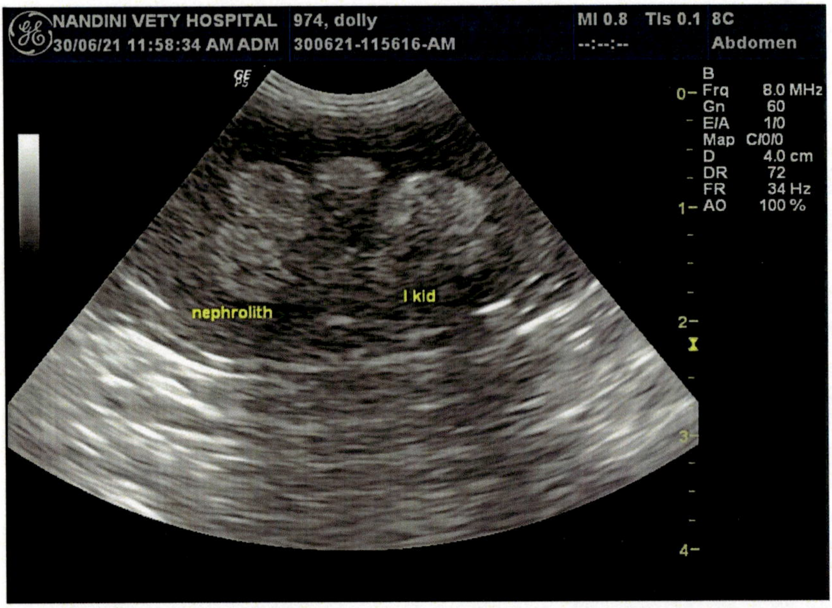

Fig. 298: Trans abdominal sonogram of a four and half year old female Persian Cat (Dolly) with anorexia for one month and occasional haematuria showing five brightly hyperechoic curvillinear foci with distal acoustic shadowing suggesting liths in the left kidney.

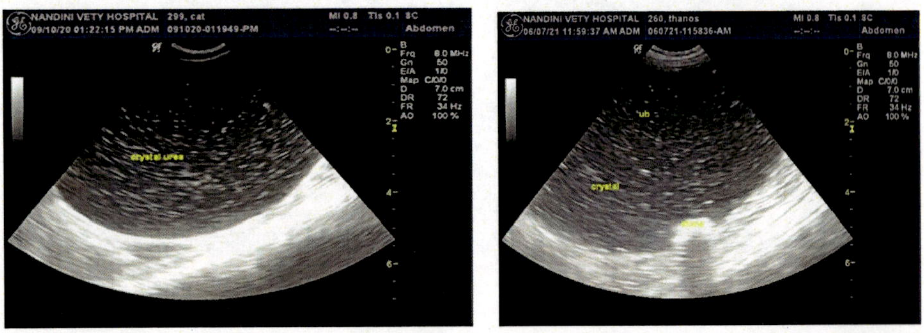

Fig. 299: Trans abdominal sonogram of a haematuric cat showing distended urinary bladder with hyperechoic crystals and a hyperechoic structure with acoustic shadowing suggesting crystalluria, cystolith and haematuria (Varshney,2019 a).

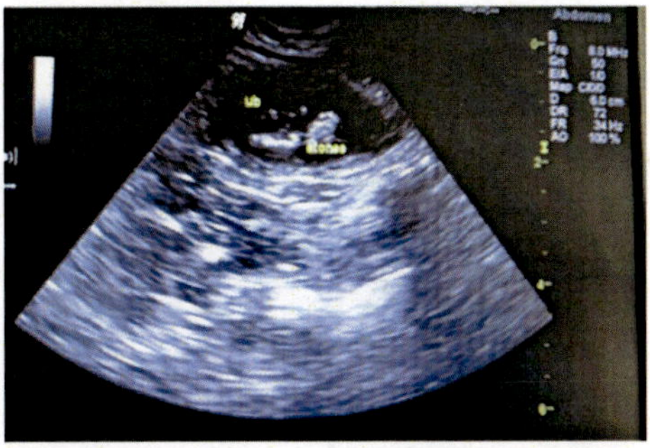

(A)

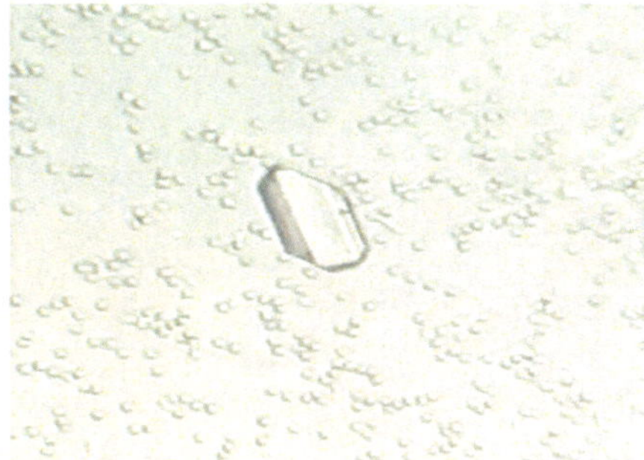

(B)

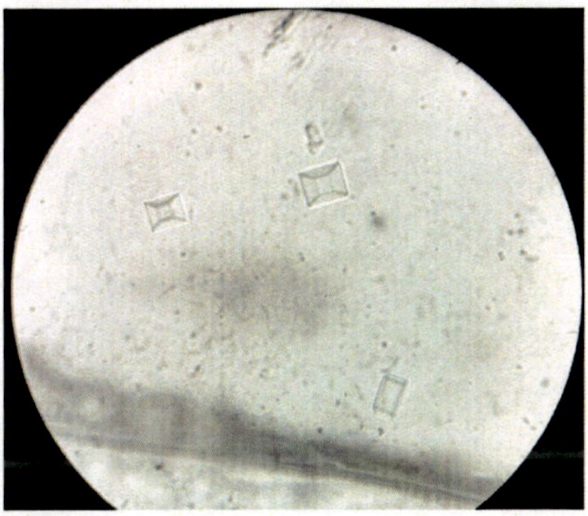

(C)

Fig. 300: Trans abdominal sonogram **(A)** of a haematuric cat showing hyperechoic irregular shaped urocystolith and thickened urinary bladder wall. Magnified view of the microscopic examination of the catheterized urine showed preponderance of the erythrocytes and crystals **(B, C)** resembling with that of struvite (Varshney, 2019 a).

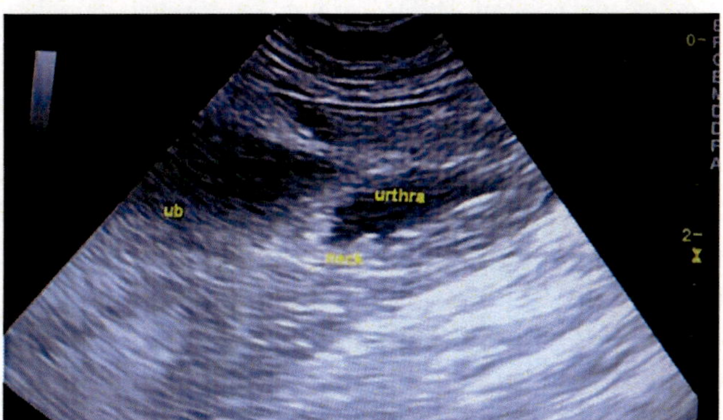

Fig. 301: Trans abdominal sonogram of a haematuric Persian cat showing an irregular shaped hypoechoic material without acoustic shadowing in the urethra suggesting blood and a few echogenic crystal in the urethra leading to no passage of urine (Varshney, 2019 a).

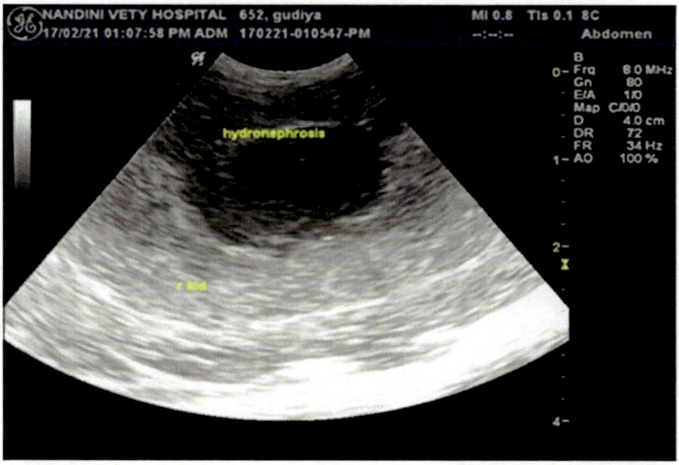

Fig. 302: Trans abdominal sonogram of a Persian female cat showing anechoic fluid in renal pelvis suggesting severe hydronephrosis.

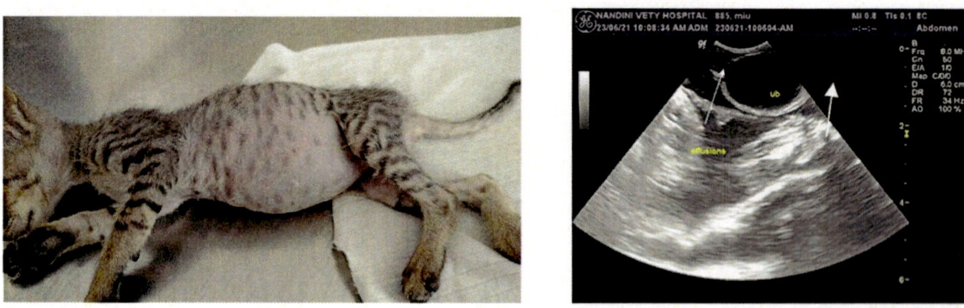

(A) **(B)**

Fig. 303: Trans abdominal sonogram of a nondescript kitten of 2.5 month with distended abdomen **(A)** showing break in the continuity of the bladder wall and anechoic fluid in the viscinity of the bladder **(B)** suggesting a leakage in the urinary bladder.

Uterus

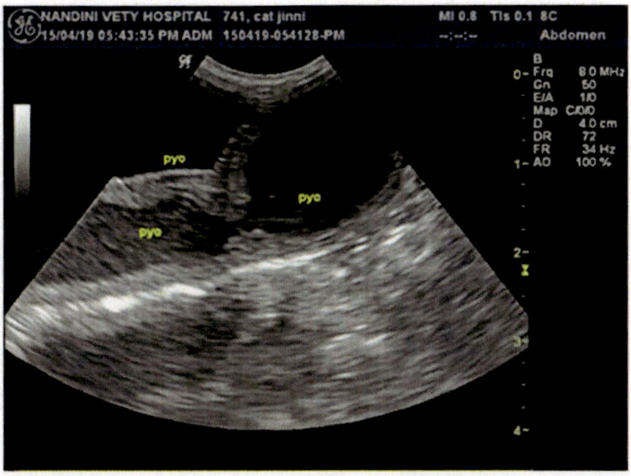

Fig. 304: Trans abdominal sonogram of a 10 year old female cat with an abdominal distension and purulent discharge from vagina for last 20 days showing an accumulation of anechoic/ hypoechoic fluid in uterine horns with thickened wall suggesting pyometra.

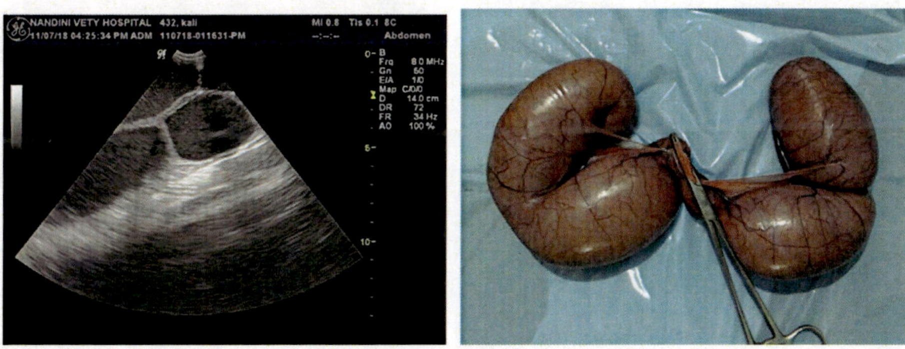

(A) **(B)**

Fig. 305: Trans abdominal sonogram of a five year old Persian queen (Kali) with vaginal discharge for 10 days showing anechoic fluid in the uterine horns with thickened uterine wall **(A)** suggestive of pyometra. Hysterectomy revealed grayish fluid filled uterine horns **(B)** confirming sonographic diagnosis of pyometra.

Indian Grey Mongoose

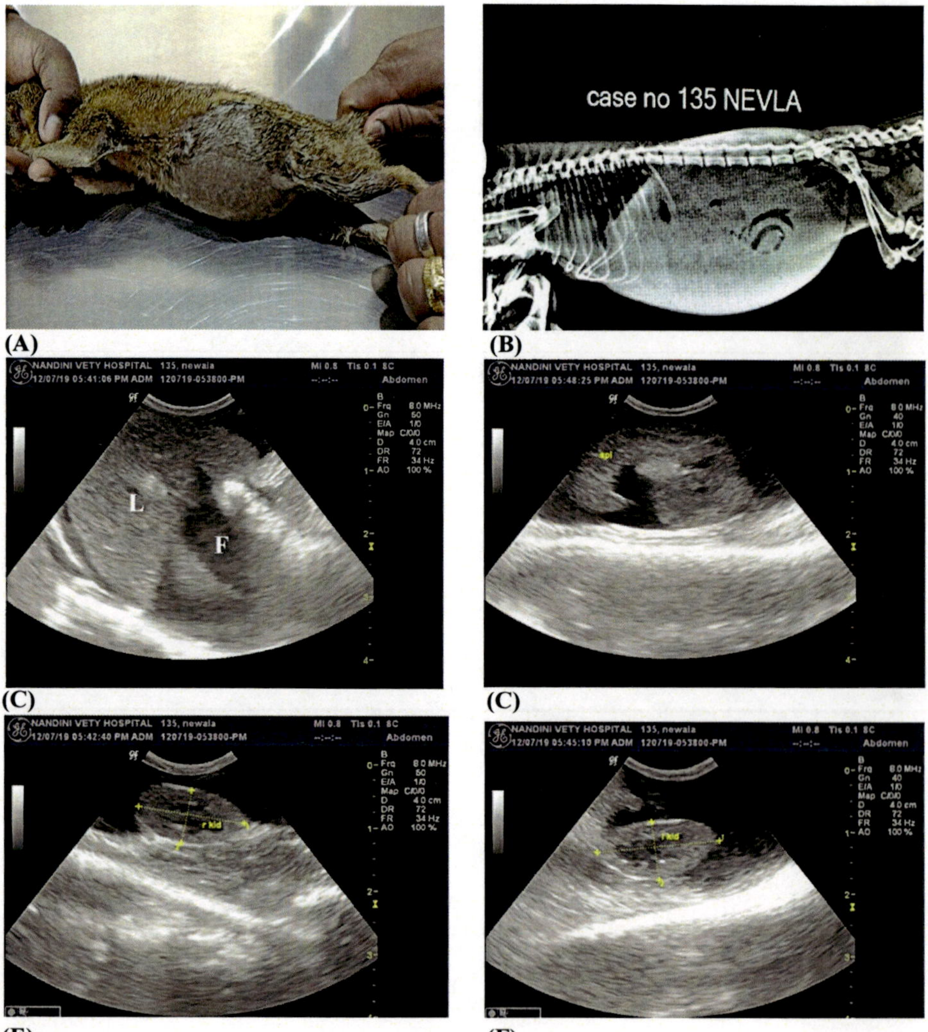

Fig. 306: Trans abdominal sonogram of an Indian gray mongoose **(A)** with radiographic ground glass appearance of abdomen **(B)** showing hyperechoic liver with serrated margins **(L)** and anechoic fluid marked as F **(C)**, hyperechoic spleen and fluid **(D)**, normal echotexture of right kidney(1.68 x 0.86 cm -E) and left kidney (1.94 x 0.95 cm-F) suggesting liver cirrhosis/fibrosis.

Rabbits

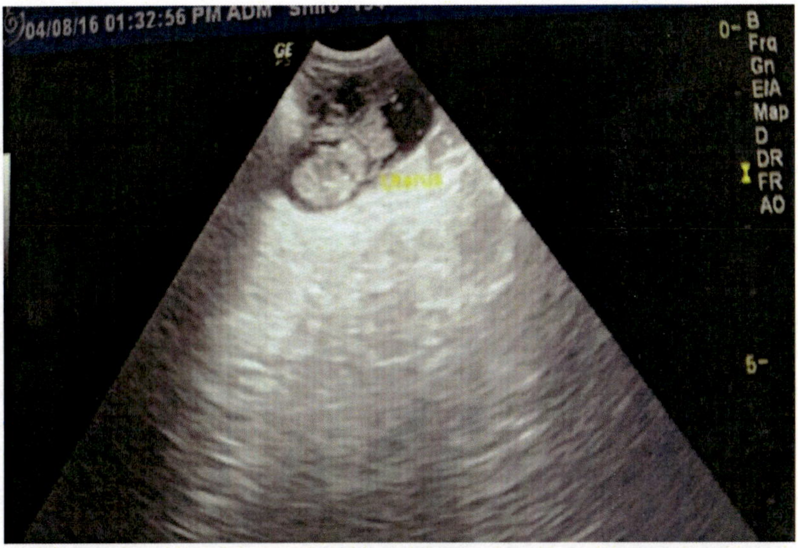

Fig. 307: Trans abdominal sonogram of a female rabbit (1.8 Kg) with uniformly red coloured urine for one month showing hyperechoic mass attached to uterine wall suggesting uterine tumour.

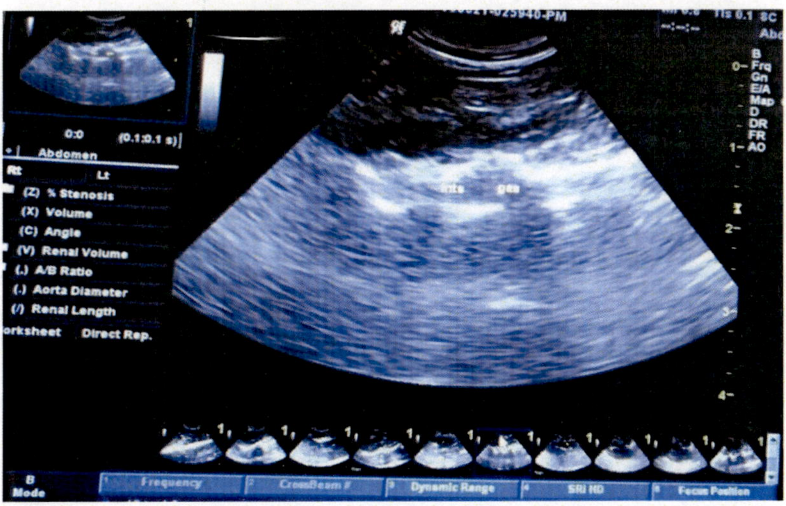

Fig. 308: Trans abdominal sonogram of a female rabbit (2.0 Kg) with mucoid faeces, abdominal pain, anorexia ,lethargy, hypothermia (97.2^{0}F) showing gaseous distension of the intestines. The history revealed that the rabbit was being treated with clindamycin by the owner himself. The clindamycin is contraindicated in rabbits as it is a common cause of cecal dysbiosis.

Chelonian

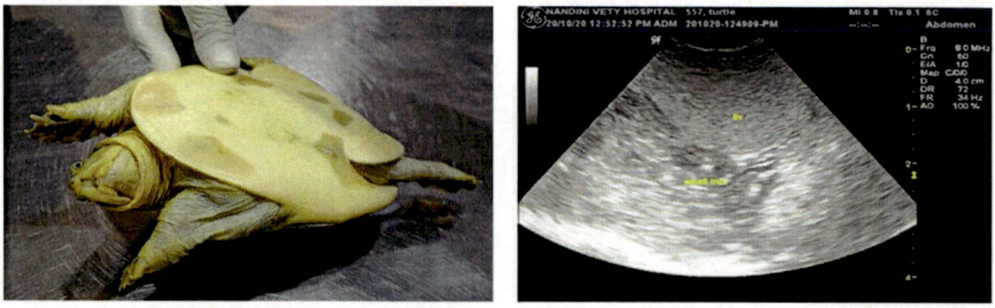

(A) (B)

Fig. 309: Soft shell turtle showing yellowish discoloration **(A).** Its sonogram **(B)** viewed through cervical windows showing hyperechoic granular texture of the liver with serrated margins suggesting liver cirrhosis/fibrosis/lipidosis.

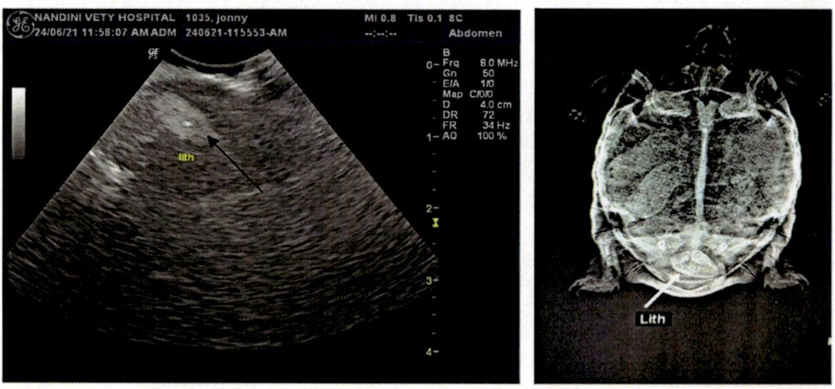

(A) (B)

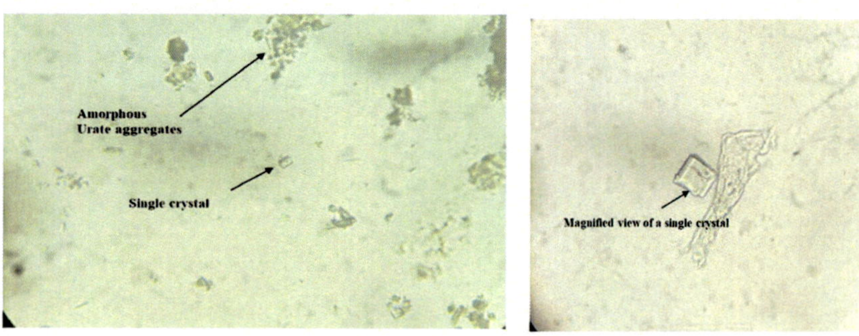

(C) (D)

Fig. 310: Sonogram (taken from right prefemoral acoustic window), radiograph and microscopic image of the cystolith of a three year old Star tortoise, weighing 600 g, with no passage of faeces and urine and swelling of cloaca. Clinical examination revealed hard palpable material. Sonogram **(A)** is showing irregular margined hyperechoic structure of 9.6 x 6.1 mm size with acoustic shadowing in the cloaca and hyperechoic particles in the urine suggestive of urolith. Radiographic examination **(B)** is also showing a radiopaque structure in the cloaca. The urolith was broken surgically. Microscopic examination of the lith showed amorphous urate aggregates **(C)**. Magnified view **(D)** of a single crystal is resembling with that of urate (uric acid) crystal. Based on the investigations , the tortoise was diagnosed with urate urolith.

Equines

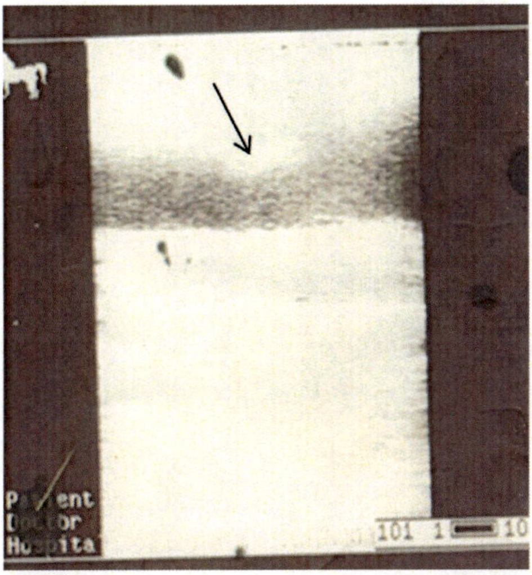

Fig. 311: A trans rectal sonogram of an eight year old mare with mild recurrent colic, posterior ataxia, hind limb incoordination, relative coolness of hind limbs(distal to tarsus), and per rectal detection of a firm area of aorta just cranial to aorto-iliac quadrification showing a pedunculated echogenic intraluminal mass originating from dorsal aortic wall just in front of aortic-iliac quadrification suggesting iliac thrombosis.Faecal examination showed preponderance of strongylid eggs. This iliac thrombosis was due to migrating larvae of *Strongylus vulgaris* (Hoque et al., 2002).

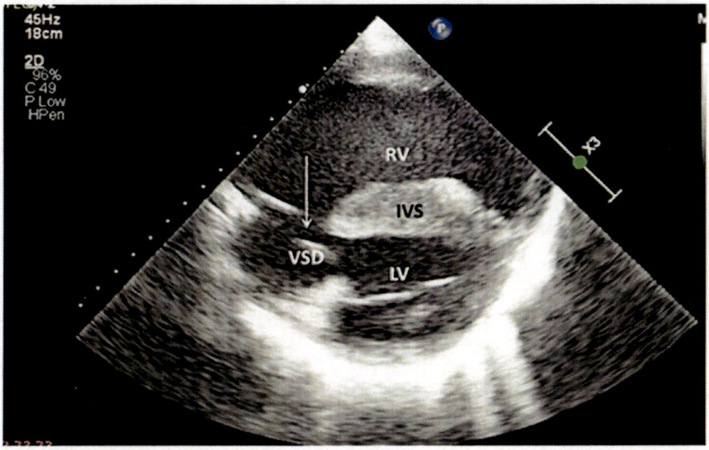

Fig. 312: 2-D echocardiogram of a one month old foal with shortness of breath, cyanosis, exercise intolerance showing ventricular septal defect (arrow) as echogenic region in ventricular septum.

Ruminants

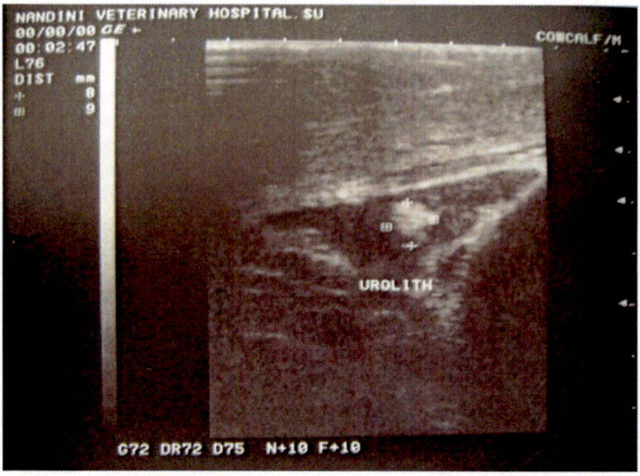

Fig. 313: Trans abdominal sonogram of a male cow calf with urinary incontinence showing a hyperechoic irregular shaped structure with shadowing in the urinary bladder suggesting cystolith.

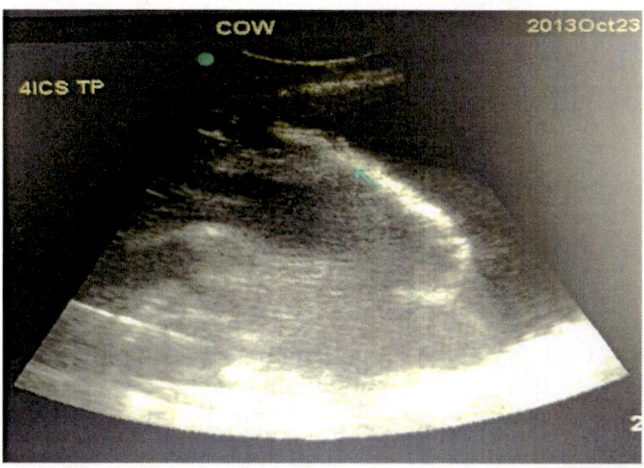

Fig. 314: Trans abdominal sonogram of an adult cow with brisket oedema showing hyperechoic curved metallic object (possibly wire) in the reticulum with thickened reticular wall suggesting traumatic reticulitis.

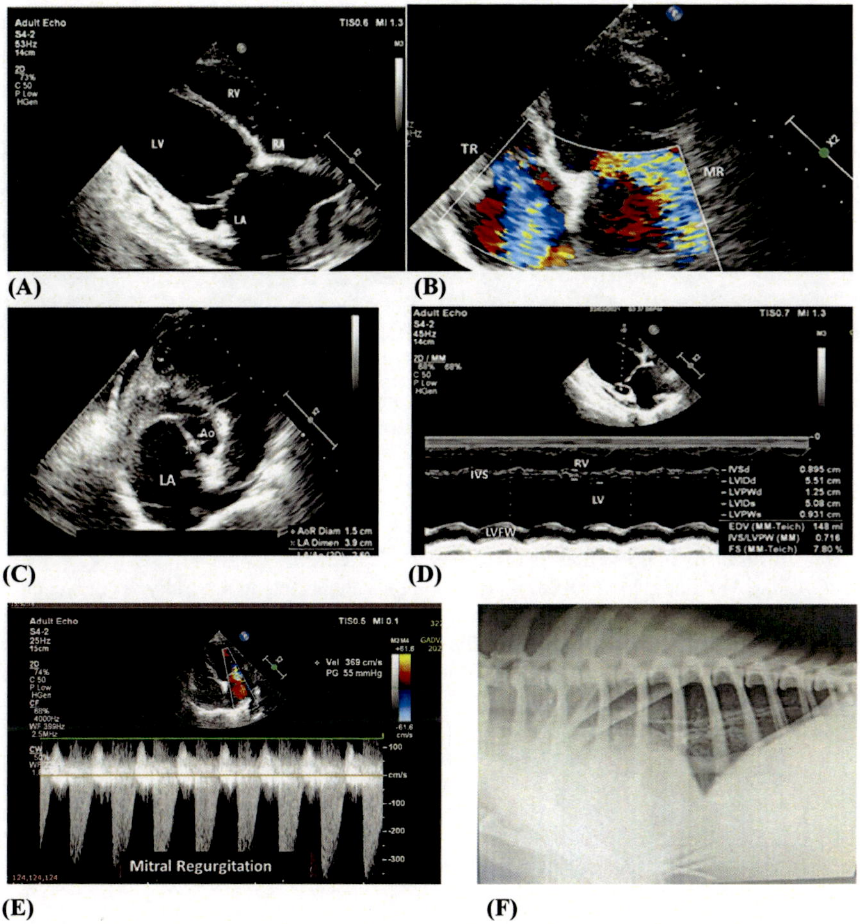

Fig. 315: Echocardiogram and X-ray of a one and half year old goat with the history of recent parturition, ascites, coughing and respiratory distress for last 10 days. Clinical examination revealed distended abdomen, pale mucus membrane, tachypnoea and tachycardia (HR 140 bpm). 2-D echocardiogram right parasternal long axis view **(A)** is showing enlargement of both atria and ventricles. RV = right ventricle, RA = right atrium, LV = left ventricle, LA =left atrium. Left apical 4 chamber view **(B)** is showing severe mitral and tricuspid regurgitation. Right parasternal short axis view at the level of aorta **(C)** is showing severe left atrial enlargement and an increased LA (left atrium):Ao (aorta) ratio (2.6). M- mode echocardiography **(D)** is indicating enlargement of left ventricle (LV), akinetic interventricular septum (IVS) and reduced movement of left ventricular free wall (LVFW) suggesting poor left ventricle function. The enlargement of left ventricle is associated with very low Ejection Fraction (EF 16.9%)) and Fractional Shortening(FS 7.8%). Continuous wave Doppler **(E)** is showing high mitral regurgitant (MR) velocity (3.69m/sec) suggestive of an increased pressure gradient (54.60 mm Hg) between the left atrium and left ventricle. Radiographic findings **(F)** are in tune with tracheal elevation and cardiac enlargement. Abdominal sonography showed free fluid in abdomen suggesting ascites. Based on these investigations, the goat was diagnosed with dilated cardiomyopathy and severe mitral and tricuspid insufficiency.

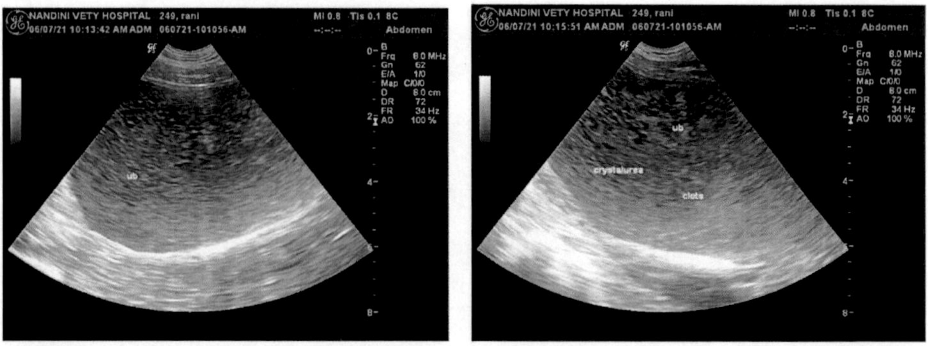

Fig. 316. Trans abdominal sonogram of an adult female goat (49 Kg) with micturation, dysuria, anorexia showing finely echogenic particles and aggregates of slightly echogenic material in urinary bladder suggesting crystalluria and haematuria.

References

Hoque, M., Varshney, J.P., Singh, G.R. and Maiti, S.K. (2002). Sonographic detection of aorto-iliac thrombosis in horse and its management. J. Rem.Vet .Corps.41:17-21.

Kumar, A. and Varshney, J.P. (2006). Studies on clinical variants in naturally occurring cases of canine ehrlichiosis. Intas Polivet 7: 94-101.

Saini, N., Uppal, S. K., Tandon, R., Randhawa, S.N.S. and Anand, A. (2017). A rare case of Ebstein Anomaly in a French Mastiff dog. J.Cardiol. Cardiovascular Therapy.7: 1-4.

Saini, N., Uppal, S. K., Tandon, R., Dhaliwal, P.S. and Anand, A. (2018). A rare case of bicuspid aortic valve in a German Shepherd Dog. Israel J. Vet. Med. 73:44-49.

Tiwari, Pooja, Varshney, J.P. and Hoque, M. (2001). Biliary obstruction in dogs: diagnosis and treatment. Indian J. Vet. Med. 21:115-116.

Varshney, J.P. (2019 a). Haematuria in cats due to struvitecrystalluria and its management. J. Canine Dev. Res. 15: 62-65.

Varshney, J.P. (2019 b). Liver cirrhosis ina Persian cat- A case report. J. Canine Dev.Res. 15: 66-69.

Varshney, J.P. and Chaudhary, P.S. (2018). Polycystic kidney disease in a PersianCat.The Blue Cross Book 38: 118-119.

Varshney, J.P., Hoque, M., Bandyopadhyaya, S. and Saghar, S.S.(2003). Fanconi's syndrome in Dobermann Dog- a case report. Indian J. Vet.med.23:127-128.

Varshney, J.P., Kumar, A. and Hoque, M. (2004). *Ehrlichia platys* and *B. canis* infection in a dog: A clinical report. J. Vet Parsitol. 18:35-37.